The Cure for Everything

The Cure for Everything

The Epic
Struggle for
PUBLIC
HEALTH

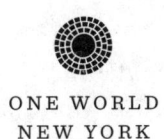

and a Radical
Vision for
HUMAN
THRIVING

Michelle A. Williams

with Linda Marsa

ONE WORLD
NEW YORK

One World
An imprint of Random House
A division of Penguin Random House LLC
1745 Broadway, New York, NY 10019
oneworldlit.com
penguinrandomhouse.com

Hardcover ISBN 978-0-593-59554-1
Ebook ISBN 978-0-593-59555-8

Printed in the United States of America on acid-free paper

1st Printing

First Edition

BOOK TEAM: Production editor: Mark Birkey • Managing editor: Rebecca Berlant • Production manager: Kevin Garcia • Copy editor: Stuart Calderwood • Proofreaders: Liz Carbonell, Kellyn Eaddy, Nicole Ramirez

Book design by Susan Turner

The authorized representative in the EU for product safety and compliance is Penguin Random House Ireland, Morrison Chambers, 32 Nassau Street, Dublin D02 YH68, Ireland. https://eu-contact.penguin.ie

In loving memory of my parents,
Angelita Verna Williams
Noel Alexander Williams

CONTENTS

The Tailor's Daughter, Near Misses, and the Tantalizing Promise of Public Health

"Of all the forms of inequality, injustice in health is the most shocking and the most inhuman."

—MARTIN LUTHER KING JR.

WHEN I WAS IN GRADUATE SCHOOL, I JUMPED AT THE chance to go on a field trip to the Dominican Republic, an opportunity to apply what I was studying in epide- miology to real problems. I was born in the Caribbean—my family emigrated to New York City when I was seven—and touching down in the DR felt like a homecoming. I soaked in everything—the heat, the bugs, the warmth of the direct sunlight, the bumpy rides on un- paved roads, and the verdant environment, so green and so lush. Even the smells, like the fresh fruits ripening on the vines, and the sights of familiar plants such as the breadfruit tree, reminded me of my roots and my early childhood in Jamaica.

The buildings in the small rural villages we toured were humble, mostly cinderblock or even more crudely constructed, with primitive cement walls, corrugated metal roofs, and dirt floors in dimly lit rooms. Most of the time, though, we sat out in plastic chairs on patios with thatched straw roofs that protected us from the blazing sun. But the structures were tidy and orderly, and they were shown off by our hosts with great pride.

We were there doing what is called "community-based participatory research," where the goal is to work with local residents to apply good science to better the life of the community. We struggled to talk with local leaders, however—the mostly male elders that did most of the speaking on behalf of the community—about the malnutrition that was stunting the growth of young children. Even though we saw it as a critical public health issue, they seemed indifferent. But in retrospect, I realize that they were probably more focused on jobs, housing, and other social determinants of health. Childhood nutrition was likely near the bottom of a lengthy list.

I also saw firsthand just how disruptive Nestlé's formula marketing campaigns were to young children. Local community health workers and our team leader, Gretchen Berggren, felt strongly about how Nestlé had marketed formula in the Caribbean (and in Black communities in the United States, too). To offset declining sales in the U.S. due to growing health concerns, the company strongly promoted formula feeding in poorer nations, and shrewdly linked using formula with social mobility, a tactic that targeted mothers and families who were aspiring to better their lot and climb the social ladder. To overcome built-in biases because of Nestlé's successful marketing campaign, we worked with local educators to teach mothers how much healthier breastfeeding was for newborns and infants than the formula they were consuming.

The people of the village were deeply engaged with us—they pushed back where they didn't agree or understand, which is exactly what you'd expect from an engaged community—but I could also see them putting what they were learning into practice. This was my first exposure to doing public health fieldwork as part of a team. Seeing the difference we could make in the life and health of a community— even during such a short trip—was transformative for me. Just a little bit of science could unlock a community's capacity to thrive. This, I realized, was what I wanted to do with my life.

A visit to Haiti the following year was an entirely different story. Even though it shares the island of Hispaniola with the Dominican Republic, the differences were stark. I had read the news reports about the nation's deep poverty, the political instability, and the horrific violence. But now I was seeing this harsh and unforgiving landscape up close, in real time. It was here that I first encountered starving children suffering from kwashiorkor, a type of malnutrition caused by a severe protein deficiency. The babies all had the bloated stomach; swollen ankles and feet; dry, brittle, and thinning hair; and skeletal limbs that we usually see only in regions of the world stricken by prolonged famines.

But I learned later that Haiti didn't just turn into this morass of chaos, extreme poverty, and violence overnight. What I was seeing had been more than two hundred years in the making, starting in 1804, when Haiti became the first independent Black-led Caribbean state, and threw out the French colonists, although they maintained a presence until 1809. France demanded reparations to the former slave owners and surrounded Haiti with gunboats until the government acquiesced. The United States intervened, too, and violently occupied the nation for nineteen years during the early twentieth century. It took the tiny island nation more than 122 years to pay off all of these debts, to the U.S. and France, which effectively siphoned off about 40 percent of the government's entire revenue to cover the penalties and debt service on loans until the late 1940s. This was the equivalent of $20 to $30 billion today. For generations, Haiti's revenues were poured into this double debt—to pay off the reparations and the loans they were forced to take on to pay it—instead of being used to build schools, hospitals, and basic infrastructure. Economists have compared Haiti's growth rate with its Latin American neighbors, and their models suggest the payments to France cost Haiti as much as $115 billion. To this day, Haiti remains trapped in a cycle of debt, poverty, and underdevelopment.

I'd gone with Dr. Gretchen Berggren as her student research assistant. She's dedicated her life to helping the children of Haiti by creating health-care projects that improve access to food and better diets to prevent the stunted growth so common among children in impoverished nations. She also developed strong community partnerships that eradicated tetanus in regions of Haiti where one in four children were victims of the potentially fatal bacterial infection. But I was also impressed by how she did what she did. She was a skillful problem-solver who would use every tool she could find, but she always did it in culturally appropriate ways. Dr. Berggren radiated a calming warmth and kindness that was a soothing balm to those around her, and she moved about gracefully even in the midst of the most heartbreaking, impoverished settings. Her example became my North Star as I navigated through the world.

On that trip to Haiti, we were given a tour of community-based clinics devoted to the nutritional needs of children, reproductive health clinics, and school-based public health. The people running the programs did their best, but the extreme poverty in their communities was overwhelming and a constant barrier to delivering quality care. In the Dominican Republic, we talked to mothers who were themselves healthy enough to breastfeed, which made it easier to make the case to them that their nutritious breast milk was much better than Nestlé's formula. But in Haiti, the mothers themselves were so malnourished that we couldn't honestly encourage them to breastfeed. It was hard to figure out where to even start. But we had to start somewhere. Dr. Berggren taught me that the mission of public health didn't change, even in the worst circumstances. Our job was to enhance the health and well-being of everyone, across lifespans and regardless of the external challenges. That didn't mean it was easy.

One incident that is etched in my memory happened as we headed home. Looking out of the car window on the way to the airport, I spied a group of kids playing. They were all naked or partially clad and rail-thin. Still, their spindly limbs were flying all over the place with a lightness that almost defied gravity. Their naturally brown skin was darkened to coal black by the filth of the field they were playing in, which was an enormous mound of waste. With a pang of recognition, I understood that these kids so easily could have been me, or my family, or my children. Dire poverty exists all over the world, but we have no control over where we are born. Being born in the wrong country or the wrong zip code is an accident of fate that shapes the lives of billions.

For years afterward, I was haunted by the fact that only chance had triggered the series of events that helped me evade the fate of these boys. It was chance that the ships that brought my African ancestors to North America ended up offloading them on Jamaican and not Haitian shores. While Jamaica is a poor country, too, it doesn't suffer from the soul-crushing poverty of Haiti that is born out of that country's specific historical traumas. It was only chance that there were enough opportunities for my parents in Jamaica—and eventually the United States—to gain a foothold on a better life.

My life has been defined by accidents and fateful near misses and lucky connections. I often wonder what would have happened to me if things had played out differently.

My parents were hardworking and made great sacrifices for their family. My dad was a master tailor who apprenticed at the U.S. military base in Guantanamo, Cuba, earning American dollars he sent home to give us a better life in Jamaica before we emigrated to New York. Once they arrived in the U.S., my parents routinely toiled at two and sometimes three jobs apiece. With their savings and with loans from our community's informal banking system, they bought a dry-cleaning business, which gave them some measure of independence. My mom worked sixteen hours a day, six days a week, while running a house and raising four kids, and we were all expected to pitch in.

They pushed hard for me to get the best education, and they wanted me to attend Bayside High School, one of the best public schools in New York City. In another accident of fate, in a city full of bad schools, I was able to get a seat at one of the best ones, instead of languishing in an underfunded institution where even the smartest kids didn't have the encouragement and mentorship that I did to help them realize their potential. My life would have taken a decidedly different course if I hadn't heeded the advice of those mentors.

The town of Bayside, which is a leafy neighborhood on Little Neck Bay in northern Queens, was once home to a swank colony of screen stars like Rudolph Valentino, W.C. Fields, and Groucho Marx. For me, going to school there meant taking long bus rides, an hour each way, from our less affluent neighborhood in Queens Village. There are days when the person I was then, a tall, shy teenager, bone-weary from volleyball practice and shivering in the cold at a dimly lit bus stop, doesn't seem all that far away. But if I hadn't gone to Bayside, I never would have met my social studies teacher, Mr. Greenspan. He became an early mentor, discussing the news events of the day with me like I was a peer and giving me books to read. One particularly memorable book was John Hope Franklin's landmark work *From Slavery to Freedom*. His influence changed the entire trajectory of my life.

I was awarded a volleyball scholarship to the University of Rhode Island, and even though I planned to major in biology, the coach there said I'd need to focus on athletics, not academics. I felt deflated because science was my passion, but the scholarship was tempting to an immigrant kid from a modest background. When I told Mr. Greenspan about my plans, though, he made no effort to conceal his disappointment.

"A state school?" he frowned. "You can do better. Much better."

He retrieved an application to Princeton from a drawer and threw it on the desk.

"This is where you belong."

Princeton.

The very thought took my breath away. It is one of the most patrician of the Ivy League universities, founded before our country was born and home to dozens of Nobel laureates. Still, Mr. Greenspan's encouragement was all I needed to see myself there, too, and I filled out the application that weekend.

I'm a tailor's daughter, and my father's words constantly echo in my head: Measure three times, then cut only once. I mull over things, but once I make a decision, I never look back.

When I got to Princeton, however, I came to a startling realization: I don't like the sight of blood. I was horrified that as a biology major I was going to be dissecting cats and mice. I scrambled to find a bloodless alternative and discovered the wonders of fruit flies, non-mammalian owners of big, beautiful chromosomes. Eric Wieschaus, a young fruit-fly geneticist, was in his first year as an assistant professor when I met him. I remember fumbling over my words when I asked to join his lab. His generosity was another one of those inflection points for me: Finding him allowed me to study biology and genetics in an unbloodied lab. Plus, he was brilliant. I was so gratified when he later shared a Nobel Prize in Medicine in 1995 for his research on the genetic control mechanism behind the development of embryos—all derived from his work with fruit flies.

But I found my true calling as a graduate student in public health at Tufts. Because much of the history of public health is rooted in sanitation projects, the university put their new public health program in the engineering department. Here again, it was just by chance—another potential near miss—that I met an epidemiologist, Annette Rossignol, who introduced me to the essential elements of fieldwork in public health, and a biostatistician, Clare Mahan, who taught me about the importance of impeccable data collection and statistical analysis. I discovered that I could marry my love for biology, my distaste for blood, and my growing desire to find solutions that impact people's lives.

What is public health? To me, public health is where health science is translated into policies and laws to support the optimal development of people everywhere: the work of protecting, promoting, and preserving humanity's capacity to thrive. Public health is based on a vision of social justice that sees health as a universal right and a public good. In medicine, physicians treat individual patients. In public health, we see our patients as whole populations. It is a big tent, with room for practically every social and biological science to come together. Public health is public wealth.

But what's most inspiring about public health is this: Its remarkable history shows us that *extraordinary progress for humanity is possible*. While we rightfully celebrate feats like mapping the genome, splicing human DNA, or finding better therapies for cancer or heart disease, these triumphs of medical science are dwarfed by the achievements of public health. Over the past century, public health has fueled our collective great escape from a world of unnecessary suffering and early death.

Through public health we've conquered smallpox and have almost vanquished polio. Life expectancy has nearly doubled in the past century, even in developing nations. HIV and AIDS are no longer a death sentence. Since 2000, child deaths have dropped by half worldwide. And tireless public and political advocacy campaigns, for everything from safer working conditions to seat-belt laws, food safety regulations to cigarette warning labels, have saved countless lives. Even the lowly toilet, when connected to the vast sewage systems constructed in the latter half of the nineteenth century that gave us clean water, has been credited with saving a billion lives and adding nearly two decades to life expectancy. Billions more lives have been saved through vaccinations, sanitation, and other public health initiatives—initiatives that, collectively, are largely responsible for the modern, technologically advanced world we live in today. These innovations are what enable us to travel widely and to live relatively disease-free in large, densely populated urban metropolises.

I've thought a lot about this history over the past few years in the aftermath of the worst global health crisis in a century. The horrors of the Covid-19 pandemic were a window into a world we thought we had escaped—we were marooned in our homes and faced with a fast-moving disease for which we had no treatments, vaccines, or easy solutions. This is what the world was once like, when we were unable to control outbreaks or cure infectious diseases, before antibiotics, and before childhood vaccines, when babies died in infancy or were sentenced to lives imprisoned in iron lungs because of polio.

I was dismayed by our botched response to the pandemic, an abject failure of public health. Our inability to contain the pandemic, especially in the United States, exposed deep fractures in our health system that were underscored by unthinkable losses: more than a million American lives, and at least six million globally, a number that includes more than 120,000 medical professionals, many of whom became infected because of drastic shortages of protective gear and inadequate safety precautions.

Hundreds of thousands of these people would be alive today if we had a better-functioning public health system, according to numerous mathematical models. At least one in every five hundred American families lost a parent or a caregiver, which means tens of thousands of children will grow up in families torn by grief. And the profound dislocations and psychological and economic aftershocks of our extended lockdowns will reverberate for years to come.

Why did our public health institutions fail us so profoundly?

The answer, of course, is complicated. The breakdowns around the pandemic are the result of decades of neglect that ironically had their origins in the groundbreaking scientific advances at the end of the nineteenth century. The discoveries by Louis Pasteur, Robert Koch, and many other pioneering researchers showed us that germs, and not bad air, were responsible for infectious diseases. Unfortunately, the unintended consequence of our increasing reliance on bacteriology was that we abandoned a different path to health: the eradication of social rot, which had once been the centerpiece of public health efforts, with an emphasis on costly sanitation projects, workplace reforms, and improving the infrastructure of filthy, air-deprived cities.

The reforms of the Progressive era of the early twentieth century, which saw the establishment of community clinics, outpatient pharmacies, and school-based nurses, led to the conservative backlash of the 1920s that branded public health measures as socialism, an ideological conflict that has dominated political debate for a century. Additionally, the rise of Big Pharma and for-profit medicine, especially after World War II, and the public health community's unwitting acquiescence to these seismic swings contributed directly to the failures of today. And it is only by understanding this history and unpacking how we got so disastrously far off track that we can begin to rebuild our public health system.

But we can also learn from the more recent past. What the pandemic *should* teach us is that the challenges and threats we face in the twenty-first century demand a public health response. Even though we spend far more on health care than any other nation, Americans' health, well-being, and overall life expectancy are much lower than those of other industrialized nations. This is because our deepest problems are not fixable by technology or simply taking a pill. Our real problems are ones that can only be truly treated by the preventive measures of public health: poverty, racism, gender biases, high rates of obesity, the lack of access to health care, the opioid addiction epidemic, and violence in all its forms—whether in the streets, in our schools, in our homes, or against women. Public health initiatives, unlike pills or technology, focus on the social side of medicine, and treat not just individual patients, but the whole ecosystem of communities and societies, ranging from preventing the emergence of more deadly zoonotic diseases like Covid-19, to confronting the systemic racism that is responsible for grave disparities in different racial groups' health and longevity, to coping with the catastrophic disruptions of climate change that will present the greatest risks to our health and well-being in this century.

With all of these headwinds, is it possible for future generations to live longer, healthier lives? Who will suffer and who will thrive? These are daunting questions, but the answers must be found in the collective decisions. Do we abandon public health or work to perfect it? Public health has enjoyed grand triumphs and endured abysmal failures, but despite the detours and mistakes throughout its history, it has enabled our steady progression toward relieving human suffering, increasing longevity, and allowing millions of people to realize their life's potential on a once-unimaginable scale.

This centuries-long great escape has fueled my optimism about our possibilities—and it is a vision of those possibilities, tempered by a clear-eyed exploration of our challenges, that is at the heart of this book. The stories you'll find in this book illuminate inflection points in this journey that show public health in action: in transformative social reforms, in scientific innovations, in government policies and the actions of compassionate communities, and in the efforts of brilliant and uncompromising public health heroes who have defied convention, often at great personal and professional sacrifice, to lead movements to make the world better. Each of these chapters shows how looking at our greatest problems through the lens of public health can clarify the challenges and their solutions, but also highlights what's really at stake: our lives.

But nothing in life goes in a straight line. Many of these interventions pushed society forward in aggregate, but at the expense of marginalized communities. Some solutions were steeped in the racism, classism, and misogyny that are so embedded in the way we do business that they're almost invisible.

I believe that public health really is our best hope. When it works, it helps us understand our world—how people live, where they work, where they learn, where they play, and what matters to their lives—and then it uses that information to help us collectively optimize human potential. What could be more vital for our present crises?

In short, public health is, to borrow a phrase, everything, everywhere, all at once. It starts with our homes and our immediate surroundings, but it also embraces the larger world: It safeguards us against the hazards of our built environment in ways large and small, explains how social inequities impact health, and applies the technological advances and discoveries that have extended our lifespans. Public health ensures that the water coming out of your pipe is free of lead. Public health looks at food insecurity and housing insecurity and connects the dots to show how those two insecurities contribute to a high burden of hypertension, diabetes, and other chronic diseases. Public health helps us see that chronic lung disease is preventable if we provide better, safer housing for low-income kids who are growing up in environments where dust mites and other environmental contaminants increase the risk for asthma. Public health makes sure that we have the right evidence available for making sure school lunches are nutritious and provided to those who need them, without stigma.

Public health makes sure that people wear seat belts and bicycle helmets. Public health does surveillance to detect threats, and to identify the factors that either increase or decrease risk. Public health ensures that we have the best science to help us create diagnostics and therapeutics, and then ensures that those diagnostics and therapeutics reach the populations that need them most.

Public health is understanding the factors that contribute to disparities in birth outcomes for African American, Hispanic, and white moms. And once we find out what those factors are, public health must be dedicated and devoted to minimizing those risks and bringing equity in health outcomes for all. Public health is working to reduce the burden of violence in our communities, including police and gun violence.

Public health looks at the systemic health-care disparities that have robbed the poor and disenfranchised of decades of life, resulting in huge longevity gaps between the healthy elites and the disadvantaged poor and communities of color, and seeks to build a more just and healthier future for all.

But all too often, we have not invested enough in the public health infrastructure and its workforce. Especially as we enter uncertain territory, it's worth remembering that clean air and water, vaccines, safe workplaces, unadulterated food and drugs, and all the other triumphs of public health, from the conquest of smallpox, polio, and other childhood diseases to safer streets, didn't just happen. These victories came after long uphill fights against the determined opposition of monied elites and their political minions. Even in the early nineteenth century, powerful business interests fought hard against imposing quarantines and shuttering the ports to prevent the spread of cholera, because they were bad for business.

Public health is an unseen pillar of our world and because we don't see it, we take it for granted—until we find ourselves engulfed in a catastrophe. This can literally happen in the blink of an eye, because of how epidemics quickly escalate from local outbreaks into larger—even global—conflagrations.

We saw that play out with Covid. The failures of the first Trump administration to safeguard Americans during the pandemic have been well chronicled, but it's worth repeating some of the more egregious errors. The pandemic's horrific first year came at the end of Donald Trump's first administration. Thousands were dying every day, frontline workers had no protective gear, tents needed to be set up in hospital parking lots to handle the overflow, and bodies were stored in refrigerated trucks because there was no room in the morgues.

This wasn't just a case of colossal bad luck for the Trump presidency. The administration actively discouraged masking and other preventive measures, minimized the outbreak, peddled dangerous nostrums, and vilified and silenced public health officials. This vilification—combined with some self-inflicted errors from public health officials made in the fog of the outbreak—caused an erosion of trust in public health that persists to this day. The White House even pushed the dangerous idea of herd immunity, which would have allowed the virus to rampage unchecked so that lockdowns could be lifted and presumably those who had been sickened would become immune to further infections. Trump's director of the National Institutes of Health, Jay Bhattacharya, formerly an economist at Stanford, was one of those championing this ill-advised policy. Public health has become a "tool for authoritarian power," he darkly warned at the time, "a political tool that's been used to enforce the biosecurity state."

The net result was catastrophic but predictable. In a damning analysis by *The Lancet* in February of 2021, researchers found that 40 percent of the nearly 500,000 Covid deaths in the U.S. during that first year of the pandemic were avoidable, which meant that as many as 180,000 Americans would be alive today if they had lived in any other industrialized nation. The *Lancet* researchers acknowledged that our disastrous response was partially the result of years of poor policy decisions, but they laid much of the blame on the response of the Trump administration. Unlike other nations' leaders, Trump minimized the threat, thwarted sensible actions as the infection spread, and often refused to cooperate internationally. The administration's failure to develop a coherent national strategy led to severe shortages of protective equipment and diagnostic tests; mask-wearing was politicized, and Trump even held indoor rallies where mask-wearing was discouraged and physical distancing was impossible. Little wonder that the U.S. had the grim distinction of leading the world in Covid deaths and confirmed cases.

Bear in mind that this devastation occurred when seasoned professionals like Anthony Fauci, head of the National Institute of Allergy and Infectious Diseases, and CDC director Robert Redfield, were at the helm. I shudder to think what will happen if we have another outbreak, whether it is Covid, bird flu, or another potentially deadly and highly contagious pathogen. Trump's unqualified officials in the top health spots have a few things in common: They have no experience managing large federal agencies or combating infectious disease, they have expressed varying degrees of skepticism about the efficacy of vaccines, and they still harbor deep resentments about how the government conducted the response to the pandemic, ranging from what they saw as unnecessary lockdowns to suppressing data on the purported origins of the epidemic. Deborah Birx, a veteran public health physician on Trump's White House Coronavirus Task Force, once called Covid contrarians a "fringe group without grounding in epidemics, public health, or on-the-ground common-sense experience." And today they are in charge of our nation's public health.

When I listen to some of Trump's health-care administrators talk, it reminds me of the broken clock that's right twice a day. They've picked up on some issues that the public health research community has been struggling with, such as how much fluoride we still need in our water now that we have it in our toothpaste. However, while skepticism is healthy and should be encouraged, it should also be based on what has been tested by science, not on fringe theories. The overall evidence is clear: Fluoride vastly improves dental health and prevents cavities.

On immunizations, I certainly sympathize with parents who are concerned about the multiple vaccines that are being given to their kids, when they haven't been given an adequate explanation or justification. The public health community—from directors of government agencies to pediatricians—probably need to better communicate the benefits of vaccines. And the fears of parents about vaccines are not unfounded. Vaccines absolutely do cause side effects in some number of recipients, especially when millions of people are getting them. This is true in the case of the yellow fever vaccine, which in rare instances can cause serious allergic reactions. In 1976, when 45 million Americans were inoculated with the swine flu shot, about 450 people developed a rare autoimmune disorder called Guillain-Barré syndrome, which can cause muscle weakness and paralysis (although there is still some controversy over whether the shot was responsible).

But in the big picture, vaccines are one of modern medicine's great miracles and have enabled us to live in densely populated urban areas, virtually eradicated deadly childhood diseases like diphtheria, polio, and measles, and have saved more than 150 million lives in the past fifty years alone, which translates to about six lives a minute. If you go to an old cemetery, you'll find dozens of graves for babies and children who died before the 1950s, but after that, there are hardly any. That's because the years afterward coincide with the start of widespread vaccine campaigns to inoculate children. "If you are unsure," one father posted, "the answer is, literally, written in stone."

Americans are still experiencing lingering feelings of grief, rage, and resentment because of all that we lost during the pandemic: loved ones, jobs, our children's educations. Those whose lives were derailed feel righteous anger. That legacy of bitterness has fueled mistrust in our institutions. But in our raw, vulnerable state, we cannot allow ourselves to fall prey to half-truths and outright falsehoods. They are distractions from the real root causes of why Americans are in such poor health.

The number-one killer in this country, especially of children, is not the fluoride in the water; it's guns, a subject you won't hear about much from the same politicians who vilify vaccines. Many of these vaccine critics—or the administration they work for—have normalized misogyny and sexual violence against women and have nothing to say about the lack of access to decent medical care, the role of poverty in health outcomes, or racial disparities in health outcomes. They're not talking about the truly wasteful health-care costs, such as the gross overspending on acute-care hospitalizations versus investments in primary care, health promotion, and disease prevention that genuinely save lives. And the bomb-throwers who are charged with dismantling institutions like the CDC have no understanding of the role the agency plays in preventing the spread of disease and why having "boots on the ground"—epidemiologists who investigate outbreaks—is imperative to track evidence in an apolitical way.

Right now, we're facing two crises. One is a problem of the status quo: We've made extraordinary gains in making life better for millions of Americans, but we've stalled out in significant areas. We've seen that with women's health, environmental justice, and other issues that affect less socially privileged, wealthy, or politically connected communities. The needle hasn't budged on deaths from gun violence or maternal mortality, to name a couple of seemingly intractable problems. These are the things that are hurting us, not vaccines or fluoride in the water. People are deeply and understandably frustrated by a profit-driven health-care system that makes it almost impossible to see their doctors and get the care they need to keep themselves healthy. What we haven't done—and what we need to do—is create equitable health care for everyone.

Unfortunately, when the power of the government is harnessed as a tool of corporate interests—a hallmark of the second Trump administration, in which billionaire oligarchs are in charge of key federal agencies—people become more vulnerable to disease and loss. We see this in Louisiana's "Cancer Alley." That's the nickname for the eighty-five-mile stretch of land between Baton Rouge and New Orleans where some two hundred petrochemical plants and refineries spew cancer-causing chemicals that blanket the air of surrounding communities, which are predominantly Black and poor and now have the nation's highest cancer rates. And it's the reason why Congress has failed to pass meaningful gun-control legislation, and why seventy-two countries, a number that includes every other developed nation in the world, ranging from Canada and the Czech Republic to Chile, Costa Rica, and India, have universal health insurance but we don't.

The other problem is that because we've stalled out in essential areas, people are desperate for solutions, which has fueled the creation of an entire social media ecosystem of conspiracy theorists and so-called health-care disruptors promoting bogus remedies. While these narratives proliferate, we have missed opportunities to tell stories that help people understand the extraordinary gains, both personal and societal, that they are enjoying because of public health.

I've dedicated my life to people who didn't have the lucky breaks I did, for whom the near misses meant the worst schools, the broken families, growing up in decrepit housing in neighborhoods racked by violence and sickened by bad air and dirty water. We are currently facing unprecedented challenges. There are many paths to meaningful action that will level the playing field. We need a twenty-first-century international public health movement. Unless this challenge finds its way to the top of the national and international agenda, this century could be a disaster movie without a happy ending. We can discuss this endlessly, but we must take action.

Or as my father would say: Make the cut.

The Cure for Everything

CHAPTER ONE

Every Life Matters

Public health was the driving force behind the formation of
our clean, modern cities. But the cumulative undertow of our original
sin has led to today's inequities.

M Y MOTHER DIDN'T KNOW HER EXACT BIRTHDAY.
The date on her passport was even different from the
one on her marriage certificate. This intimate piece of
personal information was not erased out of indifference or bureaucratic oversight but because of a failure of public health.

Let me explain.

My mother was born in 1935 in a rural village in Jamaica. In
those days, the custom was that the father would record the birth in
the town registry. But the frequency of infant deaths was staggeringly
high—more than one out of every ten babies didn't live long enough
to celebrate their first birthday. With such prohibitive mortality rates,
it became a grim routine practice to delay the registrar visit for the
first month or so after a child was born. The eventual registration
date became the birth date, sometimes even if it was six or seven

months later—a constant reminder of that undercurrent of painful uncertainty.

Jamaica was a crown colony then, part of Great Britain's globe-girdling empire, and wouldn't achieve independence until 1962, the year I was born. Still in the grip of its imperious colonial rulers, the island nation was plagued by severe economic hardship and civil unrest that frequently boiled over into violence at the height of the Great Depression. People were literally starving to death in the streets, and nursing mothers' breast milk was often so deficient in calories and vital nutrients that infants suffered gravely from malnutrition. Babies died from a wide range of ills, from starvation to simply being born prematurely because of a lack of prenatal care. But what killed them most often were infectious pathogens like pneumonia and diarrheal diseases that were transmitted in dirty water.

Children born in the United States that same year didn't face such daunting odds. Even at the height of the Great Depression in 1934, infant mortality rates in the U.S. stood at six deaths per hundred live births (6 percent). The difference was clean water. The introduction of two relatively inexpensive and easy fixes—chlorination and water filtration systems—in major American cities killed the microbes responsible for high rates of death from typhus, pneumonia, tuberculosis, and other infectious diseases throughout the latter half of the 1800s. Clean-water initiatives across the United States in the first forty years of the twentieth century slashed three-quarters of infant mortality and nearly two-thirds of child mortality, an astonishing achievement that is considered the most rapid health improvement in our nation's history.

Every life matters.

That's the first rule of public health, and it is the moral imperative of a humane, nurturing, and thriving society. Infant mortality rates are a prime indicator of how well a society is following that rule. Babies are the most vulnerable members of any society, totally dependent on others for their health and well-being. If these fragile new lives are nurtured and cared for in a supportive environment, the chances are that society is protecting all of its citizens.

In the 1930s, Jamaica was a place where life was cheap and not valued. The white British grandees who held power did little to alleviate that nation's grievous suffering, resulting in a terrible and largely preventable loss of life, and in wasted talent and potential. It should not have taken another seven decades to reduce infant mortality rates to the level already achieved in the United States under progressive reformers like President Franklin Roosevelt. But it did.

The creation of a society that values *every* life doesn't happen magically. It's a collective choice. At a critical juncture in U.S. history, nearly a hundred years before my mother's birth, we collectively chose to make an enormous investment in our future. In the first half of the nineteenth century, a coalition of politicians, progressive physicians, and social reformers, backed by the strong support of average citizens, embarked on a series of massive public health interventions that completely altered this country's trajectory. In the century following the Civil War, we saw a near-miraculous doubling of life expectancy, unlocking an entirely new set of tantalizing possibilities for the country. The civic measures that followed to improve public health, both large and small, are the very foundation upon which we've built our modern society.

The first fight of this opening era for public health was the battle to conquer deadly pathogens. Lethal contagions have plagued humanity since the dawn of civilization, but in the early 1800s, the rise of densely populated cities triggered an explosion of infectious diseases. The standard tools for stopping the spread of disease—isolation of the sick and quarantining the exposed—worked in sparsely populated rural areas but were woefully inadequate in cities. There, illnesses traveled with lightning speed along the fissures created by poverty. The haphazard, reactive approach to disease control had to change. We needed to get ourselves organized around prevention.

New York City was the epicenter of this seismic shift in the United

States. A dense urban metropolis, nineteenth-century New York was already an engine for economic growth and prosperity and a hothouse for the fledgling nation's science, art, and cultural pursuits. But deadly diseases engulfed New York with alarming frequency, from yellow fever, measles, and malaria, to cholera, typhus, and smallpox. These pathogens festered in filthy streets littered with garbage and human feces, and in the marshy swamplands on the southern tip of Manhattan. Newly arrived immigrants to New York in the early nineteenth century would encounter a fetid city core with garbage piled several feet high on the dusty streets.

New York's 1832 cholera outbreak would ultimately become a catalyst for transforming the city and laying the groundwork for eliminating infectious diseases that killed millions. Protecting public health became a public activity, a societal goal, and a critical cog in New York City's—as well as the nation's—meteoric rise.

Looking at the arc of how all of this evolved, and the forces that drove public health from its nascent stages in the early 1800s to where we are today, can show us what we need to do in the twenty-first century. Our lesson from this history is a mixed one: It is a story of death and malaise being met with collective determination and ambitious vision—but it is also a story of failure, a cautionary tale about what happens when anyone is excluded from that web of mutuality that protects us all.

Because the first and foremost lesson of public health is: Every life matters.

CHOLERA CHANGED EVERYTHING. THE DISEASE invaded almost every part of the United States in the nineteenth century, afflicting great cities like New York, Cincinnati, and Chicago, and claiming the lives of Iowa dirt farmers, New York longshoremen, Wisconsin miners, and Black field hands in the American South, as Charles Rosenberg noted in his book *The Cholera Years*. But there was a silver lining:

Cholera forced civic leaders to overcome centuries of complacency and indifference, midwifing the birth of our modern public health system and forging what would become an enduring social commitment to collective health.

Plagues are nothing new. They've ravaged humanity throughout history, causing seismic shifts in society and toppling empires. Roman soldiers brought back what is believed to have been smallpox after the war against Parthia, in what is now northern Iran, triggering a lethal pandemic that killed an estimated five million people and contributed to the collapse of the Roman Empire. Five hundred years after the birth of Christ, the Plague of Justinian, an early incarnation of the bubonic plague, claimed the lives of nearly 10 percent of the world's population. In the mid-fourteenth century, the Black Death, another variant of the bubonic plague, was the initial wave of what turned into a nearly five-hundred-year death march. In a scant eight years, from 1346 to 1353, it killed between 75 million and 200 million people, which comprised up to 60 percent of the populations of Europe, the Middle East, and Africa, according to some estimates, and led to the end of feudalism because of the scarcity of able-bodied laborers.

Diseases brought to the Western Hemisphere by explorers in the sixteenth century, including smallpox, led to the demise of the Inca and Aztec civilizations and claimed the lives of about 90 percent of the indigenous population. Native people on Caribbean islands like Jamaica were also hard-hit, and in 1518, the first smallpox outbreak in the so-called New World occurred in Hispaniola, which is now Haiti and the Dominican Republic.

In colonial America, there had been a patchwork of efforts to protect people from epidemics like the plague and smallpox. By the eighteenth century, isolation of the sick and quarantining the exposed were the standard tools for controlling diseases, a tactic designed for agrarian communities, but also used in the port cities that were most vulnerable to contagious maladies, like Boston, New York, Philadelphia, and Baltimore. It didn't work. In 1793 in Philadelphia, then the nation's capital, a yellow fever epidemic swept through the city, killing some five thousand residents, about 10 percent of the city's population.

But New York was the most vulnerable city of all. People from all over America and Europe flocked to Manhattan, which quickly became a teeming metropolis, and turned farmland, swamps, and uncultivated fields into shops, factories, homes, and the stately mansions along the East River where the city's wealthy dwelled in what is now the East Village. However, they brought with them the diseases that had beset Europe for millennia, like smallpox, typhus, measles, and scarlet fever. The overcrowded ships, which ferried immigrants from infected countries in Europe and sailors and traders who carried new strains of familiar diseases, were giant petri dishes for incubating and spreading lethal pathogens. Sickly passengers shared slop buckets and rancid water that spread the contagions.

Meanwhile, American metropolises were doubling in size seemingly overnight, as thousands of immigrants from other nations and migrants from rural areas flooded into cities seeking a better life. The sheer density in impoverished slums—whole families were crowded into damp and dismal cellar rooms with no ventilation or running water—created the ideal environment for the rampant spread of diseases. The tenement dwellers, who comprised half of a given city's population, were more susceptible to contagions because of their squalid living conditions.

Cities along the Atlantic seaboard in the United States were repeatedly devastated by deadly outbreaks of yellow fever and malaria. In the early part of the nineteenth century, more than half of all working-class children who lived in these crowded conditions died before their fifth birthdays because waves of diphtheria, scarlet fever, influenza, and measles killed thousands of them every year. Cities, in short, concentrated disease and misery in ways that were inconceivable in even the poorest rural regions. But when cholera arrived in North America in 1832, it set in motion a series of events that radically transformed society.

Cholera was the granddaddy of the epidemic diseases because the trade routes, which had become firmly established by the early 1800s, enabled it to spread worldwide, from Asia to North America's western frontiers. The disease had festered for centuries along the Ganges River in India, claiming millions of lives with dreaded swiftness, usually within forty-eight hours. Individuals could feel fine in the morning and be dead by nightfall. Some victims were stricken so quickly that they died in the street. And it was an agonizing death. The pathogen causes sharp muscle cramps, fever, and uncontrollable diarrhea and profuse vomiting, leading to severe dehydration. In the end stages of the disease, victims become parched, screaming for water to quench their unslakable thirst, their bodies racked by excruciatingly painful spasms.

But an outbreak that began in 1817 at a traditional annual religious festival in Calcutta was the origin of arguably the world's first truly global pandemic. When the three-month festival ended, pilgrims carried cholera home with them to other parts of India. Hundreds of thousands of Indians died, according to some estimates, and at least 10,000 imperial troops in the occupying "presidency armies" of the East India Company, which ruled India, also perished.

Over the next fifteen years, the contagion sailed from port to port, transmitted by travelers or in contaminated kegs of water or the excrement of victims. There were cholera outbreaks along trade routes in China and Japan, and in Iran and Russia before it spread through Europe, landing in England in October of 1831. Cholera ultimately claimed more than 31,000 lives in England alone.

With growing dread, civic leaders and residents in the United States, in cities up and down the Atlantic coast, read reports about how cholera raged uncontrollably throughout Europe. Health officials and apprehensive New Yorkers knew their crowded, filthy city was ripe for an epidemic. However, they didn't know exactly how the disease spread.

In those days, medical professionals pinned the blame for cholera on "noxious air," and generally believed infectious diseases were primarily caused by "miasma," an atmospheric malaise emitted from rotting organic matter. "People are literally dying in consequence of inhaling the unhealthy miasma of filthy streets," said Dr. John Griscom, a leader in the early public health movement who served as the city inspector of New York City in the 1840s. We know now, however, that cholera is spread by drinking water or food that has been contaminated by the feces of an infected person.

In New York, at the time, heaps of garbage, animal manure, and human waste littered the streets, sometimes piled three feet high, and flowed freely into drinking-water sources at a time when sanitation was nonexistent. The tainted water was so foul that residents would drink beer or wine instead or mask the taste of the water with tea. Local government was dominated by the graft-ridden Tammany Hall. Corrupt city officials stole the funds appropriated to clean the streets and relied instead on roaming herds of thousands of wild pigs to eat the trash. Local residents looked after the pigs, which they would later slaughter for food, and city streets were transformed into giant feeding troughs. The Board of Health and the civic leaders responsible for enforcing sanitary regulations were ineffectual at best.

On Friday, June 15, 1832, a steamboat arriving from Albany carried unwelcome news: Cholera had broken out in Quebec and Montréal. North America's last great barrier to the epidemic—the Atlantic Ocean—had been breached.

By Sunday, New York Mayor Walter Bowne banned all ships from docking in the New York harbor. Towns along the Erie Canal instituted stringent quarantine regulations that they hoped would create enough of a barrier to halt the influx of immigrants from Canada. But these restrictions were too little, too late. Cholera had already hitchhiked on immigrant ships that docked in Quebec and then piggybacked on infected passengers who traveled from ports in Canada down the St. Lawrence and Hudson rivers into the United States. Desperate émigrés, many of whom had braved treacherous transAtlantic voyages on rickety, overcrowded ships in stormy seas, easily circumvented these restraints. Passengers frantic to reach New York jumped off the canal boats and continued on foot, even in the face of armed militias. Immigrants on ships headed to New York, some of which reported cholera deaths on their passage from England, disembarked in nearby ports like Perth Amboy in New Jersey before boarding ferries to New York.

In late June of 1832, cholera emerged in Manhattan. On a Monday evening, June 26, a recent émigré from Ireland named Fitzgerald came home from work complaining of severe stomach cramps. The pain worsened during the night, so he called a doctor the next morning. When the physician arrived, Fitzgerald was starting to recover but his two kids were seriously ill, doubled over with agonizing stomach cramps. They died the next day, and his wife succumbed on Friday. Within the next few days, doctors saw a handful of other patients with the same symptoms: severe intestinal cramps, diarrhea, and vomiting. Most of them died. These physicians all came to the same conclusion: It was cholera.

Yet there was official silence on these cholera cases. Despite impassioned pleas by prominent physicians to warn the public, the Board of Health and Mayor Bowne insisted that these cases were nothing out of the ordinary, presumably because of fears that the news would trigger a massive business shutdown and disrupt economic stability. Still, rumors about the contagion spread. Panic quickly engulfed the city. Once-crowded streets were now deserted, and more than 100,000 residents fled in an exodus from New York reminiscent of what we saw in the early stages of the Covid pandemic.

But the poorest residents, the immigrant Irish Catholics and African Americans, were sitting ducks with nowhere to go in the teeming Five Points neighborhood, the impoverished slum where the outbreak began. They were forced to drink the only available water, from contaminated wells, and lived in overcrowded tenements, which hastened the spread of the disease. The most wretched dwellings were unfinished basements, sludge pits with walls that dripped slime, sewage, and moisture after every rain. It was impossible for people who lived in these places to maintain even the most basic sanitary practices or cleanliness.

But they garnered little sympathy from their more affluent and established neighbors, who filtered their understanding of disease through the rigid moral prism of Christian rectitude. Cholera and every other sort of pestilence were seen as the scourge of the sinful, a punishment for their moral depravity, and epidemics were largely blamed on the poor and on recent immigrants who were mostly Irish Catholics. If they became ill, it was their own fault. As long as their suffering didn't threaten the more affluent, one historian observed, the attitude was: "Who cares?"

However, these indifferent New Yorkers unknowingly violated the first rule of public health—every life matters—and they soon paid the price. Within weeks, the entire city was under siege by the disease. Civic leaders set up five emergency hospitals in schools and other buildings. Swamped undertakers could not keep up with demand, and bodies piled up on the streets. On July 20, at the epidemic's peak, more than one hundred new cases of cholera were reported. By August, the number of cases began to dwindle, and the outbreak largely ran its course and ended in September. But within those two months, the disease killed more than 3,500 of the city's approximately 250,000 residents, a death toll comparable to more than 110,000 in today's New York City of eight million. Most of the victims were poor immigrants.

THE ARRIVAL OF CHOLERA DOVETAILED with another crisis: Supplies of clean, fresh water had become increasingly limited as the city grew. The island of Manhattan is surrounded by brackish rivers that are unsuitable for fresh water. Residents were forced to rely on cisterns, wells, and natural springs. But these water sources were soon unable to handle New York City's growing population. By the late 1820s, civic leaders struggled to find a source of potable water, fruitlessly scouting rivers and ponds outside the city that could supply New York's residents. Without water, New York would simply dry up.

The twin crises of water and epidemic provided the impetus for a bold plan: the construction of the Croton Aqueduct system, which would ferry clean water from the Croton River more than forty miles away—a monumental engineering feat for its time. The plan had been previously rejected because of its multimillion-dollar price tag and the logistical challenges of creating a water delivery system that stretched from Westchester to Manhattan. But in an election held in April of 1835, voters approved the project by a three-to-one margin, in a result that would forever change the city.

The aqueduct opened to public use on October 14, 1842. The aqueduct was built on an incline and carried water by gravity for forty-one miles. Traveling at a little less than two miles per hour, it took twenty-two hours to complete the journey from the Croton River to the Harlem River and over the High Bridge at 173rd Street, before emptying into two reservoirs in Manhattan between 79th and 86th streets, at Sixth and Seventh avenues, and to fortified holding tanks in what is now Midtown Manhattan. The $13 million price tag translates to more than $480 million today, which was an enormous infrastructure investment for a city of about 325,000 residents.

But clean water was not enough.

Panic gripped the city once again in November of 1848, when a ship from Europe docked at Staten Island with a handful of its French and German passengers suffering from cholera. Seven died and were buried at sea, while others were rushed to local hospitals. Gradually, the disease spread through Staten Island and made the jump to Manhattan in May of 1849. The city's population had more than doubled since the previous outbreak, and residents now numbered more than 500,000. This time cholera killed some 5,000 New Yorkers. During these years, mortality rates skyrocketed to almost double what they were at the beginning of the century. And cholera wasn't the only killer. As late as 1850, the average age of death for a New Yorker was less than forty years old, due to shockingly high child mortality rates.

Only three out of five children lived past their fifth birthdays, the others felled by dysentery, infant diarrhea, and successive waves of the highly contagious diseases of childhood, especially scarlet fever, diphtheria, pneumonia, and measles, which were responsible for the deaths of hundreds of children every year.

By that time, a coalition of progressive physician reformers, humanitarians, publicly minded civil servants, and democratically accountable politicians were pushing for even more profound and ambitious public health projects to clean up cities and rid them of disease. Driven as much by social and economic concerns as by medical ones, these broad-based campaigns, which enjoyed the support of the communities, were the genesis of the modern public health movement. The connection between bad living conditions, urban density, and the incubation and spread of disease had become blindingly obvious, as it was that the poor, living in dire circumstances, were the most vulnerable.

The efforts of this group of early public health crusaders were inspired by the nineteenth century's "Great Sanitary Awakening," the reform movement that took hold in western Europe, greatly influenced by Edwin Chadwick, a London lawyer and secretary of the Poor Law Commission in 1838, who was convinced that the environment played a crucial role in the development of diseases. To prove his point, he directed the commission to do an analysis of the life and health of the London working class, and later of the entire country. The results of this analysis revealed the wide disparity in longevity between economic classes. The landed gentry lived, on average, to age thirty-eight; tradesmen died at twenty-two on average, while laborers could expect to live only seventeen years. To remedy this situation, Chadwick proposed building drainage networks to remove sewage and waste, cleaning up the water and the garbage-filled streets, establishing national and local boards of health, and appointing district medical officers.

Chadwick was a prophet ahead of his time, unfortunately. It wasn't until the 1860s that the British Parliament agreed to fund an immense sewer network in the wake of what became known as The Great Stink in 1858; sewage and industrial waste dumped into the Thames River had backed up, releasing an overwhelming stench that enveloped London throughout the hot summer months of July and August. Here again, public health initiatives were ignored or delayed until a crisis forced action.

However, in France, sanitary projects had been underway for a decade. In 1848, Louis-Napoleon Bonaparte, nephew of Napoleon I, became the first elected president of the French Second Republic. He won a resounding victory because he guaranteed Parisians that he would clean up the city. This would not be the first time—or the last—that public health was on the ballot. After twelve years in exile in London, Bonaparte was shocked by how dingy and dirty the over-crowded and disease-riddled Paris was. The city had grown to more than a million residents in his absence and was beset by a cholera outbreak that claimed the lives of 19,000 Parisians.

Bonaparte had promised to end poverty and improve the lives of working-class people in Paris, many of whom were living in the same horrid conditions as their counterparts in New York; in some cases, twenty people were crammed into one room with no light, windows, or toilets, and shared a common courtyard that was used as a make-shift outdoor latrine. Bonaparte embarked on a grand public-works program that turned Paris into a vast construction site for nearly two decades at a staggering cost of 2.5 billion francs (which translates to 75 billion euros or approximately $78 billion in today's money). French authorities tore down some 12,000 buildings, built wide bou-levards and parks (including the Bois de Boulogne, which had been inspired by London's Hyde Park), constructed an elaborate sewage system, and installed gas lamps along the widened cobbled streets, which were soon filled with café terraces.

These massive public health infrastructure investments were driven by a coalition of progressive civil servants like Chadwick, who were armed with the scientific data to clearly demonstrate the ben-efits of their proposals, socially minded politicians like Bonaparte who recognized their importance, and the widespread public support that made it all happen. The combination of fresh social and medical science, popular advocacy, and democratically directed civic action is what formed the Sanitary Movement.

Here in the United States, similar movements took hold. The combination of new data, advocacy, and desperate need led several states to establish sanitary commissions. While the notion of urban clean-up campaigns doesn't sound particularly sexy to our modern ears, they were vital to the creation of the sophisticated metropolises of today. The Sanitary Movement led to wide-ranging urban reforms, including citywide sanitation surveys, tenement improvements, initiatives to keep accurate counts of deaths and illnesses to better track what was happening in the community, and investigations to shed light on the conditions that were responsible for mortality. Major infrastructure projects brought clean water to growing cities, and garbage was regularly collected from the streets. Even the pigs were relieved of their duties: In 1849, New York City police rounded up more than 20,000 wild hogs from the streets of Manhattan and banished them north of the city.

But civic leaders grappled with how to continue building upon these reforms. By the 1840s, New York City had become a critical hub of world trade, and wealthy shipping tycoons regularly visited London and admired the city's well-manicured public grounds. Momentum had been building among the city's elite to build a grand park that would match the resplendent green spaces of Europe. They wondered why New York didn't have lush tree-lined landscapes to rival those that blanketed London. At the same time, sanitary reformers believed that open spaces provided invaluable relief from the congestion of the growing city and cleansed the air of disease.

In 1849, a group of wealthy and influential New Yorkers hatched the idea of a landscaped public park like Hyde Park. These civic leaders envisioned a vast urban oasis that would improve the city's health with its open spaces, calming natural scenery, and cleaner air, and provide a needed antidote to the smoke, dust, and debris of the rapidly industrializing and expanding metropolis. It would become, in the words of the pioneering landscape architect Frederick Law Olmsted, "the lungs of the city" that would "uplift" and have "a manifestly civilizing effect" on the city's downtrodden and offer a place of "healthful recreation for the inhabitants of the city of all classes" that would create a needed break from the hustle and bustle of nineteenth-century urban life.

After years of debates and legal jockeying over the location, size, and cost of the park, the state legislature enacted a law that set aside more than seven hundred acres in the middle of Manhattan, between Fifth and Eighth avenues, from 59th to 106th streets (and later expanded northward to 110th Street).

In 1857, the new Central Park Commission held a design contest. Calvert Vaux, the brilliant London-born architect who had helped lay out the grounds between the White House and the Capitol, joined forces with Olmsted. Though he lacked architectural training, Olmsted was a visionary who was convinced that Vaux's naturalistic designs could be a blueprint for transforming unremarkable terrains into Edenic environments in the hearts of bustling cities. A lengthy tour of England's majestic green spaces had convinced Olmsted of their salutary value, and he viewed these publicly built pleasure grounds as a tool of social democracy where the rich and poor met on common ground.

Olmsted was an unlikely champion of the less fortunate. Born in 1822, he was the scion of a wealthy Connecticut merchant family whose ancestors arrived in the United States in the early 1600s. A public intellectual, he was a brainy dilettante and didn't find his true calling until later in life, when he was able to integrate his love for pastoral environments with his desire to help humanity. He was greatly influenced by the growing social-medicine movement and traveled widely throughout Europe. In 1850, he had visited England's public gardens and subsequently wrote the book *Walks and Talks of an American Farmer in England*. Inspired by the grand parks he saw there, he became convinced that natural scenery, fresh air, and the outdoors could be restorative not just for physical health but for mental health, too. This, coupled with his desire to uplift the poor, who were most affected by the city's health crises, informed his visions for a majestic urban oasis.

Central Park gave Olmsted the chance to put his ideas into practice.

The Vaux-Olmsted proposal, which was selected over thirty-two other entries, reflected Olmsted's conviction that these open green spaces should provide an egalitarian sanctuary where everyone could breathe clean air. Their plan combined long stretches of open, rolling meadows and formal gardens in the English tradition, and incorporated the latest thinking on the importance of good sanitation—with drainage systems for the land, well-circulating waterways, and state-of-the-art sanitary facilities. Construction began in 1858. More than five million cubic yards of stone, earth, and topsoil were moved, and crews built thirty-six bridges and arches, constructed eleven overpasses, and planted more than 500,000 trees, shrubs, and vines. The first section of the park opened in 1858, and the park was finally completed in 1876 at a cost of more than $14 million ($360 million today).

But initially, Olmsted and Vaux's vision of a "people's park" was far from reality. Olmsted and the Central Park Board discouraged the working classes from enjoying the grounds and limited sports and active recreation activities. Swimming or fishing in the ponds, playing musical instruments, setting off fireworks, holding parades, posting bills, and displaying flags were strictly taboo. Deputized "park keepers" enforced rules that forbade swearing, throwing stones, picking flowers, or annoying the birds. The wealthy could tour the park in stately carriages without disturbing the carefully cultivated natural landscapes and comprised about three-quarters of park visitors in the 1860s. They were welcomed because "they know how to behave themselves," Olmsted noted, while men who dared to play ball were called "rude fellows." So much for "uplifting" the poor.

But New Yorkers would be, well, New Yorkers, even 160 years

ago, and collectively, they wouldn't stand for this nonsense. Throughout the 1860s, the working classes and immigrants fought against the restrictions and spearheaded drives to allow music, boating, and beer sales, especially on Sunday, which was normally the only day when they weren't working. It would take another century before we would fully appreciate the mental and physical health benefits of leisure-time physical activity. Today, the park welcomes more than 42 million visitors each year, and over the decades, it has evolved into the egalitarian and salutary urban oasis that Olmsted envisioned.

SOMETIMES, HOWEVER, PUBLIC HEALTH COMES from sources other than the vaunted enterprises of the wealthy and powerful. Public health can show up in something as simple as people coming together to create a community where they can center their lives on health, safety, and well-being. Seneca Village was a prime example of this. Home to New York's largest African American community in the mid-nineteenth century, Seneca Village was a sanctuary, an affordable and peaceful refuge for people escaping slavery and from the city's unrelenting dangers and violence; a place to interact in a sustainable way with nature, in a remote location that protected its residents from the disease outbreaks and unhealthy conditions of the teeming tenements in lower Manhattan, where most New Yorkers lived. In Seneca Village, African Americans created a safe oasis, a grassroots, poor people's public health movement—and a brilliant example of how the collective action of communities to build healthful spaces from the ground up was just as essential to improving people's lives as the costly top-down projects generated by the Sanitary Movement.

Seneca Village was spread out over 750 acres of land between 83rd and 89th streets along the western edge of what is now Central Park and was one of several residential settlements scattered throughout the sparsely populated uptown. The community was surrounded by farms and pristine countryside dotted with hills, trees, streams, and rocky outcroppings. A nearby spring, called Tanner's Spring, was thought to be the water source for the community. They endured harsh winters and it wasn't an easy life. Even ferrying buckets of water from nearby streams could become a treacherous undertaking in icy conditions. But settlers were infused with a pioneering spirit, and it became a real, organized village with streets and churches and schools, a good place to raise a family and a lot healthier than crowded downtown.

But Seneca Village was demolished to make way for Central Park.

More than 1,600 working-class people were living in the area that became Central Park. All were evicted under eminent domain. The Central Park commissioners rationalized their land grab by maintaining that the area was occupied by marginal vagrants in ramshackle dwellings who, according to one observer, "lived off the refuse of the city, which they daily conveyed in small carts, chiefly drawn by dogs." Newspaper stories called Seneca Village residents "wretched and debased squatters," and dismissed their flourishing community as a "shantytown" and a "n****r village."

Nothing could have been further from the truth. Black New Yorkers had owned their own land in the village for decades and put down deep roots. In September of 1825, Andrew Williams, then a thirty-year-old bootblack, bought three lots of land in what is now the Upper West Side of Manhattan for $120, equivalent to about $3,600 today. A week later, the African Methodist Episcopal Zion Church purchased six lots in the same tract with the intent of using the land for a cemetery. One of the church's trustees, Epiphany Davis, a store clerk, acquired twelve lots for $578 ($17,000 today). Among the other Seneca Village landowners were Albro Lyons Sr. and his wife, Mary Joseph Lyons, who had inherited the property from one of Mary's relatives. The couple were educated and affluent pillars of Manhattan's African American elite and dedicated abolitionists. They also ran a boardinghouse for Black sailors near the East River docks that doubled as an Underground Railroad station. It sheltered hundreds of escapees fleeing bondage. Seneca Village may have even been a railroad stop.

Within a few years, nearly a dozen houses had been built on the land, and many of them were two stories tall. Families grew, children attended the neighborhood school that was opened later, residents planted gardens and grew their own food, raised livestock, fished in the nearby Hudson River, and worked as laborers or in service jobs. Seneca Village became a rustic middle-class hamlet of mostly free Blacks.

Only a few decades before, colonial New York was an epicenter of the slave trade, with more Africans held in shackles than in any other city in the country aside from Charleston, South Carolina. Nearly half of all households had enslaved servants. The city's economy was built largely around the slave trade—first by the Dutch and then by English merchants. They supplied the ships that trafficked in human beings kidnapped from the Africa coast, bought and sold slaves in the taverns of their own city, and profited from the trade of the commodities that enslaved people produced: sugar, tobacco, coffee, chocolate, and cotton. Enslaved people performed almost all of the heavy labor in constructing New York's infrastructure—the roads, the docks, the hospitals, the prisons, the churches—and they even built the wall on Wall Street.

Enslaved New Yorkers weren't freed until 1827, making New York one of the last Northern states to abolish slavery. Life was treacherous even for emancipated African Americans in the city. Slave-catchers were a constant threat. They routinely patrolled the streets, abducting both free Black people and fugitive slaves. Despite the Black population's enormous contributions to the city's growing prosperity, they were largely excluded from sharing in that wealth, and laws were enshrined to restrict African Americans economically and politically. They were relegated to the most menial, low-paying jobs, and forced to live in the most squalid conditions. While the poor and newly arrived immigrants were also stuck in terrible living situations, it was far worse for Black people, who had scant opportunities to better their lot or enter the higher-paying skilled trades and become carpenters, cabinet makers, bakers, or silversmiths. And even if they somehow did become master craftsmen, it rarely improved their circumstances, because most whites refused to work next to them.

They were also targets of racial violence that escalated when enslaved people were freed, which resulted in the torching of African American churches and other institutions. In October of 1834, this swelling tide of resentment and hatred spilled over into the streets, in a race riot that lasted nearly a week. Thousands of angry white rioters ransacked the Five Points district and destroyed the homes and churches of white abolitionists. The rebellion was finally quelled by the local militia. Through all this tumult, Seneca Village remained a beacon of safety, and the distance even insulated them from the deadly 1832 cholera outbreak that killed thousands of New Yorkers.

By the early 1830s, Andrew Williams, who had made his living repairing worn boots at an establishment in lower Manhattan, had painstakingly built a roomy two-story house of his own. Ambitious and industrious, Williams moved in with his wife, Elizabeth, who worked as a domestic, and their two children, Eliza and Jeremiah, in what they thought would be a home for their family for generations.

By 1855, the area was an integrated enclave that was home to about 225 people, two-thirds of whom were Black. The rest were mainly Irish immigrants who had fled their native land during the great potato famine when widespread crop blight led to more than a million deaths from starvation. And Seneca Village was no longer considered a remote hinterland. The built-up city had reached the streets in the '40s, with its population at over half a million; one of the Croton Aqueduct reservoirs had been built just south of the settlement; and 86th Street had been constructed in the 1830s as a major crosstown thoroughfare.

Archaeological evidence indicates that some residents were prosperous enough to afford luxuries like fine china, porcelain, candlesticks, shoes, and toothbrushes. The Irish and the African Americans lived together in relative harmony, they sat together in the integrated All Angels' Church, which was founded as a missionary parish, they married one another, and they were buried side by side in cemeteries.

Most residents were employed, their children attended the local school, and half of them owned their own homes, according to census records.

Property owners throughout the proposed Central Park site fought hard to preserve their way of life and spent two years petitioning the court and appealing decisions in a vain attempt to save their homes. But by 1856, the mayor issued final notices to inhabitants to clear out. Andrew Williams left reluctantly. After thirty years, he felt his land was worth at least $4,000 and he wasn't satisfied with the paltry $2,335 that he was given. But he refused to be daunted by this setback. Within sixty days, he bought a parcel of land in Astoria, Queens, in an area settled by Quakers that was friendly to African Americans, and he began to rebuild. But the Williams family, like so many others before and since, were robbed of the generational wealth that they had rightfully accumulated when Seneca Village became a casualty of New York City's grand visions.

THE STORY OF THE SANITARY Movement and of the creation of Central Park—and of visionaries like Olmsted—reminds us that we can improve our world, our communities, and our neighborhoods. We have the power to identify how we're being harmed and to initiate projects that help us thrive—through clean water and air, with verdant places to play and breathe—to connect our humanity with nature.

We have great power to transform our world.

Frederick Law Olmsted's advocacy of the salutary effect of green spaces has found new currency today. Growing evidence indicates that the way we've arranged our "built environment"—where we work, live, play, and shop—is profoundly toxic, and one of the chief culprits behind disability and death in the twenty-first century. Zip codes are more important than genetic codes as a predictor of health and longevity, numerous studies show, and up to 60 percent of our health is determined solely by where we live. Access to parks and pools and spending time in nature are linked to reduced anxiety, depression, stress, and even mortality. It's probably no surprise that Central Park and other urban havens became sanctuaries during the Covid pandemic's lengthy lockdowns. Green spaces make for happier, healthier cities, and proper ventilation and better sanitary practices can stop the spread of infectious diseases.

However, we must match these ambitious endeavors with the moral clarity that ensures that no one is left behind, displaced, or harmed. We need Central Park. But we also need the Seneca Villages, the places where public health advances came from the grassroots and unlikely innovators. But the fate of Seneca Village is also a cautionary tale of how marginalized communities get left behind by well-meaning government initiatives that cause collateral damage. Today, predominantly white neighborhoods on average have 44 percent more park space per resident compared to communities populated mostly by people of color, according to a 2021 report by the Trust for Public Land. Because of residential segregation, which is largely the result of redlining—an exclusionary banking practice that prevented Black Americans from qualifying for mortgages—and racial covenants, many communities of color have been relegated to the bleakest environments, with decaying infrastructure, polluted air, dirty water, and the most concrete, the most asphalt, and the least vegetation.

This is the unfinished business of public health: that the great escape afforded by strategic infrastructure investments in public health did not reach all of us. To this day, some Americans remain trapped in conditions that inspired the Sanitary Movement of the nineteenth century. More than two million people in the United States don't have indoor plumbing, and even more live with inadequate systems for pumping out human waste, according to the EPA. Witness what's happening in parts of the rural South, like Lowndes County, Alabama, which lacks basic sanitation and where seasonal downpours flush raw sewage into backyards or even underneath the floorboards of homes. Or the ongoing water crises in Flint, Michigan; Jackson, Mississippi; or even suburban New Jersey, where failures to make sustained investments or maintain vitally important infrastructures leads to modern-day public health emergencies. This is especially true throughout South Asia and Africa. Large populations with huge untapped human potential are held back from thriving because of the lack of basic sanitation, which fuels the prevalence of diseases that were eradicated in the West a century ago. Progress—the great escape—isn't universally experienced, nor are these escapes permanent. It takes only one natural disaster, or a traveler from abroad carrying asymptomatic cholera, or even Covid, to spark an outbreak here and reverse our good fortune; witness how quickly thousands of Americans seeking shelter from Hurricane Katrina were thrown back into the same horrific conditions that sparked the Sanitary Movement 150 years earlier. And this impermanence is one of the humbling features of public health work.

We must never forget: Every life matters.

CHAPTER TWO

War Changes Everything

The Civil War ushered in a new era in public health.

O UR SOCIETY IS STRONGER WHEN WE TAKE CARE OF EVERY-one. This isn't simply a moral imperative—it's enlightened self-interest. We've seen this play out time and again: Inequality creates a sick and vulnerable society, and divisions by race, sex, and class weaken our capacity to thrive. Equality and inclusiveness builds strength because it enables more segments of society to flourish and contribute to the greater good. And that lesson was played out in the very clear illustration of how the Civil War was fought and won: We must stick together, and we must care for the lesser among us.

The South was a feudal state, which made it fundamentally weak on a number of levels. The slaved-based economy was unstable because it was built and reliant upon the cruel exploitation of anyone, and not just the enslaved, who weren't members of the planter aristocracy or their willing minions, a tiny sliver of the population who controlled most of the wealth but refused to contribute to civic well-being. In stark contrast, the North, while admittedly a racist, sexist, and class-conscious society, embraced progress and inclusiveness and invested in civic goods. There was still some room for women to organize their charitable impulses and contribute their expertise, for a handful of Black surgeons to heal the sick, and for social reformers to make the public safe, all of which immeasurably aided in the resounding victory of the Union Army and resulted in the saving of lives.

BUT THE LESSONS LEARNED FROM the Civil War were not fully embraced. The North mirrored the South's callousness and carelessness when it came to camps for the formerly enslaved. These lessons were largely forgotten as well during the later failures of Reconstruction, when one out of every four of the newly emancipated perished from disease or neglect. Even in the post-war years, during the second wave of the Industrial Revolution, thousands of immigrants were seen as expendable and forced to work in hazardous conditions that often led to their early deaths.

And this is a lesson, too: Strength is not inherent to any society; it is built and cultivated—such as the creation of Head Start, for example, so no child would be left behind even if they were poor, or of Medicare, which lifted millions of the elderly out of poverty—and it can be abandoned and lost, too.

A Union victory was hardly assured in the pivotal summer of 1861. In July, when the first full-scale battle of the Civil War was fought at Bull Run on the outskirts of Manassas, Virginia, it led to an unexpected Confederate rout. The Union Army was relatively small and disorganized, and ill-equipped to deal with the aftermath of the bloodbath on the battlefield. Men paralyzed by gunshot wounds or choking on their own blood and vomit lay dying on burnt fields, surrounded by the mangled bodies of their fallen comrades. The horrified soldiers who survived quickly fled, leaving few behind to rescue, much less treat, the hundreds of injured soldiers, or to bury the dead.

The critically wounded soldiers remained stranded on the battlefield for days, the first two of which were spent in drenching rains, while the rest streamed into the nation's capital, becoming a sick, hungry, unruly mob that slept in Washington's muddy, filthy, and overcrowded streets, a breeding ground for infectious diseases, like dysentery, typhoid, and cholera.

Our common perception of Civil War medicine is of physicians surrounded by the amputated limbs of wounded soldiers. The real work, however, wasn't in fixing bodies broken by battle, but in fighting disease: The chaotic conditions of the war triggered the worst outbreak of epidemic diseases ever seen in the United States, a medical Armageddon that claimed hundreds of thousands of lives. Millions of soldiers, many of whom were rural recruits who had never been exposed to contagious diseases, were packed into crowded training camps that were denser and larger than most American cities. Hundreds of thousands of newly emancipated former slaves and families were uprooted in the crossfire and fled to refugee camps behind Union lines as the armies advanced into the South. Exposure to the elements, starvation, and the cramped, unsanitary conditions in those camps made them vulnerable to diseases like measles and smallpox, for which they had no natural immunity. Latrines were often just a few feet away from sleeping, cooking, and eating areas, and human waste seeped into drinking-water sources, generating huge outbreaks of dysentery, typhoid fever, and deadly chronic diarrhea.

At the dawn of the war, the divided nation's fragmented medical establishment and patchwork public health system was ill-equipped to deal with this impending crisis. America's health infrastructure was minimal. Almost all health care in those years happened in the home; only those who didn't have families to take care of them were consigned to hospitals, which were mostly threadbare facilities that were little better than almshouses. Even the United States Army medical staff was minuscule: a surgeon general, thirty surgeons, and eighty-three assistant surgeons. Of that number, twenty-four left to fight for the South and three were dismissed for "disloyalty," which meant the

Union's medical corps had only eighty-seven men at the war's outset. And hardly any of the doctors who were later recruited had military experience. Many were humble country doctors toiling in small private practices or in the few charitable hospitals that treated the destitute. They were ill-prepared for wartime medicine, a job that required routinely treating dozens of patients a day and containing mass outbreaks of pneumonia and dysentery. They had only a handful of useful medications in their kit: quinine for malaria, the anesthetic chloroform, and morphine—and others that were not useful at all, like mercury, which was used to treat diarrhea and was toxic.

Out of sheer necessity, the Civil War became a watershed in the evolution of public health. In four short years, the crucible of war radically transformed the practice of nineteenth-century medicine. The policies and techniques that the military institutionalized became standard practice after the war, ushering in an entirely new era in medicine. The entire nation, in both the North and the South, was put on a war footing, giving the government and military vast powers, and a rapid centralization of the state through the army. When the Union Army occupied New Orleans in 1862, for instance, they took over management of the city. The region had been plagued by epidemics of yellow fever for decades, but the military immediately took steps to control these outbreaks. Incoming boats were quarantined to stop the spread of disease, and sweeping sanitary reforms were strictly enforced in a way that the government or even individual reformers had been unable to do before the war. "And this happened over and over again across the country," said Jonathan S. Jones, a Civil War historian at the Virginia Military Institute. Unfortunately, Black soldiers and the newly emancipated people were relegated to inferior care, if they received care at all.

On April 25, less than two weeks after the bombardment of Fort Sumter set the war in motion, Dr. Elizabeth Blackwell, who was the first woman to earn a medical degree in the U.S., realized that there needed to be an organized way of systematically collecting and distributing lifesaving supplies, such as bandages, blankets, food, clothing, and medical supplies, to soldiers. The fiery British-born physician organized a meeting of nearly sixty women, mainly volunteers who wanted to help with the war effort, at the New York Infirmary for Indigent Women and Children, a hospital she founded with her physician sister, Emily, in 1857 in what is now New York City's East Village.

Support for Blackwell's initiative mushroomed almost overnight. A few short days later, Blackwell, along with the Reverend Dr. Henry Bellows, a Unitarian clergyman involved in public health, presided over an overflow assembly of some four thousand women at Cooper Institute to form the Women's Central Association of Relief for the Sick and Wounded of the Army (WCAR). Throughout the war, WCAR played an instrumental role in relief efforts, dispatching tons of food, medical supplies, blankets, and clothing to the front lines; raising tens of millions in today's dollars to support Union troops; and, of even more enduring importance, spearheading the training of female nurses. Largely because of WCAR's efforts, the Civil War marked a turning point in the profession of nursing: Over the course of the conflict, more than 3,000 women served as paid nurses (although some estimates put that figure as high as 15,000), which began the transformation of nursing to a female-dominated field.

Across the nation, hundreds of relief societies had cropped up in the anguished months following secession to help frontline troops. As the war raged on, women throughout the Northern states met in homes and churches to answer the call for supplies for the wounded, including rolled bandages, blankets, sewed or knitted clothing, and money to provide financial support for soldiers' families.

The leaders of the relief effort, which was comprised of women of all ages who wanted to do their part for the war effort, recognized that all these diverse programs across the country needed to be coordinated. They proposed the creation of a national sanitary commission that would be modeled on the one formed by the British government during the fighting in Crimea.

Because federal officials turned a deaf ear to the women's pleas, they enlisted male colleagues to argue their case. In May of 1861, Dr. Henry Bellows led a delegation of male physicians who lobbied Congress for the creation of an association that would coordinate and streamline these volunteer activities. In June of 1861, a reluctant President Lincoln, who felt an independent group was unnecessary—like a "fifth wheel to the coach," he reportedly said—bowed to their pressure and signed an executive order for the establishment of the U.S. Sanitary Commission, with a mandate to organize national relief efforts during the war.

Frederick Law Olmsted had earned a national reputation in his nearly three years serving first as the designer and later as superintendent of the construction of Central Park, which was one of the largest public-works projects in the antebellum United States. Because of his proven administrative skills and extensive experience running a large, civilian-based operation, he was viewed as a competent manager, which is precisely what was needed in these troubled times, and he became secretary general of the commission. Bellows would serve as president.

On a sweltering day in July of 1861, Olmsted arrived in Washington, D.C., to take the reins of the newly formed Sanitary Commission. He was dismayed by the chaos, "inefficiency and misery" he witnessed in the city's muddy streets, he noted in a letter to his wife in New York. "Many regiments are but a mob . . . a disintegrated herd of sick monomaniacs . . . pale, grimy with bloodshot eyes, unshaven, unkempt, sullen, fierce, feverish, weak, and ravenous." Worse, he found that the army's moribund Medical Bureau had done virtually nothing to prepare for war: Medicine and trained medical staff were in short supply, officers and soldiers disregarded the military's sanitary regulations, and the army's leadership was dismissive of the new research coming out of Europe in the wake of the Crimean War about the necessity of sanitary measures to reduce cases of the diseases that had devastated combatants in that conflict.

Olmsted, who was then thirty-nine and walked with a limp after a recent carriage accident had left him permanently disabled, thought the war wouldn't last much longer and the Southern rebellion would be put down quickly. He rolled up his sleeves, resolving to "overcome in some details the prevailing inefficiency and misery," and got to work to improve sanitation in Union Army military camps. It turned out to be a monumental undertaking, and Olmsted found himself frequently at odds with government bureaucrats, and, in the words of Sanitary Commission treasurer George Templeton Strong, the "lethargic, paralytic, ossified" Medical Bureau.

Within days of the Union defeat at Bull Run, Olmsted dispatched seven Sanitary Commission inspectors to thirty of the regiments to inventory conditions. Their frontline interviews produced an inflammatory report indicting the military and civil government for poorly distributed rations, weak military organization, and incompetent officers. The report showed how the ill-prepared soldiers' exhaustion and lack of food was partly responsible for the Confederate rout. They also made recommendations on selecting proper camp locations, installing drainage systems, disposing of waste, ventilating tents, and preparing food, all strategies aimed at reducing disease. Not surprisingly, the report wasn't well received by government officials, who viewed Olmsted as a meddlesome annoyance, but it set the stage for his tireless work to improve the lives of Union troops.

In April of 1862, Olmsted and a team that consisted of four surgeons, twenty male nurses, and six medical students, steamed down the Potomac along the Virginia peninsula leading a small flotilla, including a beat-up ocean liner that they turned into a floating hospital. With his penchant for efficiency and order, Olmsted divided the ship into two wards so that soldiers stricken with contagious diseases could be quarantined. Meals were served and medications were distributed at specific times, while triage stations were established on land to categorize casualties before they were transferred to the ship. The medical crew accompanied General George McClellan's army, a force of more than 120,000 men that was about to launch a major offensive to capture the Confederate capital of Richmond. The two-month siege, known as the Peninsula Campaign, turned into a war of attrition with high body counts—more than fifty thousand soldiers from the North and South were killed or wounded. In the swampy, mosquito-infested coastal lands, malaria was rife but the Union Army lacked enough quinine to prevent the disease's spread.

Olmsted frequently found himself on the front lines, organizing the transfer of hundreds of wounded and sick Union soldiers from land to the hospital ship. He and his team worked tirelessly throughout the long months of the campaign to prevent the men on the battlefields from bleeding to death or starving. Sanitary Commission volunteers staffed food stations, offering hot soup, fresh bread, and pots of coffee to famished troops returning from the front, many of whom hadn't eaten in days, and supplied the army with cots, beds, food, and medicine. But the military operation ultimately led to a humiliating Union defeat. By the end of the campaign, Olmsted estimated they had treated more than eight thousand sick and wounded soldiers. With no end to the war in sight, the misery and bloodshed of that spring prompted Olmsted to famously declare that the war had created "a veritable republic of suffering."

In the spring of 1862, however, Olmsted finally found a kindred spirit and staunch ally when Congress appointed a new surgeon general, William Hammond. Tall, brilliant, and imposing, Hammond, who later founded the field of neurology in the United States, was a progressive thirty-three-year-old dynamo who had studied at New York University and was on the faculty of the University of Maryland School of Medicine. As surgeon general, Hammond was deeply influenced by the work of Florence Nightingale, the British founder of modern nursing who pioneered the sanitary methods that saved countless lives, and the approaches that she urged the British medical department to adopt during the Crimean War. He instituted a series of reforms that overhauled the Army Medical Corps, improving efficiency and greatly reducing battlefield deaths for years afterward. As the war intensified, the Northern army "realized it needed to beef up its medical apparatus," said Jonathan S. Jones. "And they started to bring in new younger doctors, in their twenties and their thirties, who were not mired in the old ways of doing things."

Hammond raised entry requirements for physicians in the Army Medical Corps, weeding out dead wood and promoting people based on competence, not rank or social connections. Modernized medical care led to a dramatic decrease in mortality, but advances in clinical medicine alone were inadequate. It took attending to other social determinants, like nourishing food, clean water, and proper disposal of human waste and garbage, to prevent deaths.

So Hammond expanded the number of field hospitals, housed them in a series of tents, and introduced pavilion-style infirmaries that were airy and well-ventilated, an innovation first devised by Nightingale to prevent the spread of disease. He required hospitals to maintain more complete records, centralized the dispensing of medications, and dispatched regular inspectors to check for cleanliness and ventilation. Working in tandem with Olmsted and other members of the sanitary commission, he created a new ambulance wagon corps to quickly transport the wounded from the front lines and transfer them to trains or hospital ships. Supply lines became more efficient and more quickly delivered food, medicines, and supplies to the troops.

In 1862, Hammond commissioned the construction of a new army hospital on fifteen acres of wooded countryside in what was then a rural area on the outskirts of Philadelphia. It was intentionally located outside the cramped and crowded city, based on the idea that breathing the pure country air would help soldiers recover. Dr. Isaac Hayes was put in charge. A graduate of the University of Pennsylvania medical school, Hayes had achieved some renown as a ship's surgeon. He sailed on one of the many expeditions to find the lost Arctic explorer Sir John Franklin, and later worked on other Arctic expeditions. The organizational skills that enabled him to map out the logistics of a multiyear trek into the frigid Arctic served him well. He laid out plans for a massive facility from scratch, and the buildings were constructed within forty days.

Satterlee Hospital became the second-largest hospital in the country. It was like a small city, with thirty-three wards that contained a total of 4,500 beds in canvas tents and wood-frame structures. The facility, which cost more than $200,000 ($6 million in today's money), was cutting-edge for its time, and its trappings and amenities laid the foundation for our modern hospitals. Each ward was outfitted with the latest equipment: iron stoves for heating, rooftop exhausts to enhance ventilation, piped-in hot water for bathtubs and basins, and water closets (rudimentary toilets) that were connected to a twelve-foot trough that emptied waste directly into a sewer.

The hospital contained three industrial-sized kitchens staffed with enough cooks and equipment to turn out meals for thousands, and a laundry that ensured the patients' clothes and linens were kept clean. At its peak, it also housed a barbershop, a clothing store, a dispensary, a library, a post office, a reading room, a printing office, and even an observatory where a local band performed for sick and wounded soldiers. Hayes was aided by a team of more than forty doctors, an additional forty medical "cadets" or medical students, and more than a dozen pharmacists who devised systems for delivering medicines to the wards. Hayes recruited nearly a hundred Roman Catholic nuns as the core of his nursing staff.

More than 50,000 patients would be treated at Satterlee throughout the war, and only 1,100 of them died, an extraordinary achievement considering the relatively primitive state of Civil War medicine and sanitary conditions in that time before the era of germ theory. One of Hayes's most important innovations was sharply restricting the number of amputations. As a Quaker, Hayes believed in the sanctity of the human body and the importance of keeping it intact. It's quite likely that performing fewer amputations reduced the number of patients who suffered from shock and life-threatening infections, and thereby saved lives. The hospital's overall success in limiting mortality in the middle of a catastrophic public health crisis proved that their strategies worked. By the end of the war, there were 400 Union Army hospitals modeled on Satterlee, with about 400,000 beds.

Medical teams treated more than two million patients, who were transported to the hospitals by train or ship. Mortality rates hovered around 8 percent.

In the summer of 1863, the Union and Confederate armies marshaled their forces in the vicinity of Gettysburg. Olmsted and his team anticipated there would be extensive casualties in the coming battle and began transporting food and medical supplies to rural Pennsylvania. As a result, the Union hospitals were ready when the fighting started in what became the war's bloodiest battle and decisive turning point. "Our regular wagon force was on the ground during the battle," Olmsted wrote to his wife, "and the wagons visited all the field hospitals as fast as they were established and hours before they received supplies from other quarters."

After the Battle of Antietam, which featured the bloodiest single day of the war—a day when nearly 23,000 Americans from the North and South were killed, were wounded, or went missing—Sanitary Commission agents arrived within three days and delivered to hospitals "ten thousand shirts and drawers, five hundred bottles of stimulants [alcohol], two thousand sponges, several tons of soup, and other nice articles of nutriment," according to Olmsted. Not surprisingly, one soldier thankfully wrote in a letter to his family, "What could we do here without the Sanitary Commission. Many of our medicines, our stimulants, blankets, bedding for the field hospital come from the S.C. I would rather have Mr. Olmsted's fame than that of any general in this war since its beginning."

The Union Army benefited from applying basic public health measures that had helped contain epidemics in cities—providing clean water, adequate food, and shelter from the elements, and building latrines far from campsites—and that followed the sanitary principles championed by Florence Nightingale. But the Confederacy was truly another country entirely. There was little in the way of a civilian public health infrastructure in the American South to use as a foundational starting point. While Northern cities were industrializing and laying the groundwork for what became our modern public health system, the South prided itself on being a mostly rural land.

There were well-trained Southern doctors who attempted to raise the standards of medical care, but the overwhelmed Confederates lacked the infrastructure and resources necessary to adequately care for the thousands of soldiers wounded in battle or sickened by malnutrition, exposure, and disease. A case can be made that it wasn't only industrial superiority that gave the North its advantage, but also the reformist elements in the Union. That inclusiveness and fairness and equality, however imperfect, harnessed the power of free African Americans, who were among the most dedicated soldiers, and the beneficence of women's relief organizations that aided Union troops, while the U.S. Sanitary Commission pushed hard for needed changes in the military's medical system, which saved countless lives.

In the South, slavery and a sclerotic feudalistic economy undermined even token relief efforts. Municipal governments in the South were controlled by this wealthy planter class, who refused to pay to clean up the region's few cities. (Sanitary reforms weren't implemented until the early twentieth century in most states of the former Confederacy.) And if Black people lived in constant peril in places like New York's Seneca Village, where they were easy prey for slave catchers even if they were free people, in the South, they were chattel with no more rights than livestock. The only time they were provided even token care was when their health threatened a slaveholder's finances. Their continued exploitation in the face of deadly disease outbreaks was justified by the prevailing idea that although they were inherently inferior, they were better built to withstand the onslaught of epidemics.

Frederick Law Olmsted witnessed this firsthand. In December of 1852, years before the Civil War started, the then thirty-year-old journalist embarked on a journey through the antebellum South as an undercover correspondent for a newspaper that would later become *The New York Times*. He traveled for more than fourteen months on horseback and by steamboat and stagecoach through the heart of the

Deep South, and later to New Orleans and Texas. Shaken by what he saw, he denounced the South as a "stronghold of evil" and believed that Black Americans were "entitled to the inalienable rights of man." He could barely conceal his revulsion as he recounted one appalling incident after another of overseers brutally whipping slaves in the fields, often just to make an example of them to others held in bondage. "Under the slave system of labor, discipline must always be maintained by physical power," he wrote. "The steady input of violence into the Southern economy was equally a device for time-saving and profit-maximization as well as a powerful, self-perpetuating mechanism of dehumanization of the enslaved."

Olmsted was struck at every turn by the backwardness of the slave system, the waste of talent, time, and natural resources, and the profound poverty, not just among those who were enslaved but of the poor whites who weren't much better off than the serfs of Czarist Russia.

The monopoly of King Cotton was harmful, in Olmsted's view, because the one-crop economy was reliant on imports, and it throttled economic engines because it prevented the diversification key to the growth of a modern industrial society. The stranglehold that plantation owners had on politics meant they had little motivation to improve conditions of the less fortunate, and the stagnant economy offered few opportunities for poor whites to better their circumstances and there was virtually no middle class. "The citizens of the cotton states, as a whole, are poor," he noted in another dispatch on June 11, 1853. "They work little, and that little, badly; they earn little, they sell little; they buy little, and they have little—very little—of the common comforts and consolations of civilized life."

But it was the uncontrolled pestilence and the offhand dismissal of the welfare of the enslaved inhabitants that troubled him most. Malaria was a constant threat. When he was traveling in South Carolina, he was warned repeatedly by locals about the disease. Virtually all plantation owners, their overseers, and their families abandoned their plantations as summer approached and quarantined themselves far from the malaria-riddled wetlands. Only the enslaved were left behind to fend for themselves in the swamps and rice fields.

This was particularly true of yellow fever. The viral disease was endemic in the Deep South, especially in New Orleans, which had the subtropical climate and dense population that made it a model breeding ground for the lethal pathogen. An acute hemorrhagic fever that we now know is spread by mosquitoes, yellow fever causes severe symptoms, including jaundice, chills, nausea, headaches, fever, convulsions, and delirium. In its final stages, victims would bleed through their eyes, noses, and ears, and vomit blackened, coagulated blood, before lapsing into a coma.

New Orleans was battered for decades by waves of epidemics. In the sixty years before the Civil War, the city suffered more than twenty-two yellow fever outbreaks during the hot, humid summers, which claimed the lives of more than 150,000 people. Locals lived in constant terror of the insidious malady that wiped out as much as 10 percent of the city's population during outbreaks, killing about half of those who became infected. The filthy streets and the swamplands surrounding the city provided the ideal conditions for incubating disease and contaminating the water supply. Diseases were also spread by the thousands of sailors and steamboat workers who streamed through New Orleans, along with the steady waves of immigrants who flooded into the port city from Ireland, Germany, and France. Aside from New York, New Orleans, gateway to the Mississippi Valley and the booming cotton industry, was the number-one destination for Europeans in antebellum America.

The summer of 1853 was particularly deadly. More than 12,000 people died in New Orleans alone, accounting for nearly one out of every fifteen residents, and the surrounding rural regions were hard hit, too. People were dying at such an alarming rate, faster than graves could be dug, that it gave rise to the popular saying that soon people would have to dig their own graves. But enslaved Black people, many of whom had been forcibly transported to New Orleans to be sold in the nation's largest slave market, fared the worst. Solomon Northup, the author of *Twelve Years a Slave,* was among them. He contracted smallpox when he was in the New Orleans slave mart, according to Kathryn Olivarius, a historian at Stanford University and author of *Necropolis: Disease, Power, and Capitalism in the Cotton Kingdom.* "When he was sold upriver," she said, "he survived yellow fever and very nearly died."

Ironically, yellow fever created a strange social hierarchy in New Orleans between those who survived a bout of the disease and were therefore presumably immune to the virus (or "acclimated," in the local parlance), and the "unacclimated." Those who couldn't prove they were immune had difficulties finding a job, a place to live, or even making social connections because people feared they would die. "If you're unacclimated, you basically languish in professional and social purgatory," said Olivarius. "Without this immunity credential, you can't ever climb the ladder and you're always stuck on the ground floor. It became quite literally part of your identity, the way that you described yourself and your position in society."

Longtime residents were thought to be immune because they were presumed to have survived a mild bout of the illness in childhood. But newcomers to the city were scapegoated. The Whig politicians in power in New Orleans had no incentive to use tax dollars on sanitation and quarantine. Their rationale was that most of the people who were dying from yellow fever were immigrants and out-of-towners—and they usually voted for Democrats. High mortality was profitable to the powerful because workers lived a precarious existence—making them grateful for any kind of wage—and were vulnerable to the whims of New Orleans's arcane social order and at constant risk of being felled by disease. Rather than asking the powerful moneyed classes to pay for the safety-net infrastructure projects that were being constructed in Northern cities, civic leaders thought the best solution to combat yellow fever was to let the workers become sickened and acclimated—or die. According to Olivarius,

Every elite person in New Orleans—every merchant, every enslaver, every banker, every politician—claimed to be immune. Their attitude was that "we got acclimated and we survived so you have to do this for yourself." This reinforces this immune hierarchy and is a major disincentive for the political elites to spend any kind of tax money on drainage, sanitation or quarantine because they believed that nothing could stop yellow fever.

In the perverse logic of the slave system, enslaved people were believed to have "inherited immunity" to yellow fever because the disease began in Africa and spread to America through the European slave trade. This, the theory went, is what enabled them to pick cotton and cut sugar cane under the sweltering subtropical sun in swamplands without getting infected. The labor-intensive "cotton economy would entirely collapse without the labor of immune Black people," said Olivarius. "If Black people are naturally resistant to yellow fever, Black slavery is natural, even humanitarian, because it protects white people from spaces and labor that would kill them."

But in private, the slaveholders knew the truth. "Acclimated" enslaved people sold at a premium, 25 to 50 percent more than enslaved people who were "unacclimated," and the slave markets shut down in August, September, and October, presumably to protect the health of their valuable property. "They'll loudly publicly proclaim this line that all Black people are naturally immune but when their actual financial lives are on the line, they of course only purchased acclimated slaves," said Olivarius.

There was this whole sub industry of getting people "safely" through the acclimation process. In all of the slave marts, in the auction houses on Esplanade Street in New Orleans, medical doctors were on retainer so they could be called upon if someone got sick before they were sold. The death of an enslaved person wasn't a human tragedy, but a problem for their bottom line. And a lot of prominent doctors in New Orleans moonlighted and made extra money doing this slave auction health care. Yellow fever was an engine of wealth creation for every medical professional.

The deaths in New Orleans from yellow fever were the result of callous indifference bordering on criminal negligence. In 1862, Benjamin Butler, the Union Army general in charge of the occupied city, imposed strict quarantines and instituted a rigid program of garbage disposal and sewage drainage. "The war was actually the healthiest period in New Orleans history to date and there weren't any reported deaths from yellow fever, even though hundreds of thousands of people and soldiers were coming in and out of the port each year," said Olivarius. "There might have been a few cases of yellow fever, but they were quickly suppressed, and the Union army cleaned up the city." Here again it was shown that when the basic tenets of public health are rigorously applied, lives are saved.

The South's failure to work for the greater good, and instead to preserve a corrupt and barbaric system and institutionalize neglect and inequality for most of its citizens—a practice that served only the interests of a wealthy, white, aristocratic class—was the mark of an inherently weak society. This is precisely what made it virtually defenseless against a stronger, more robust and inclusive society like the North, and even the most elite Southerners became vulnerable to disease and the catastrophic losses of war. This lesson applies not just to the South but to all societies around the world that fail to invest in their people.

Even today, the lack of infrastructure investments has translated to unsanitary conditions in parts of the rural South, like Alabama, that are reminiscent of backward regions of developing countries. And even in northern locations like Baltimore, Maryland, or Flint, Michigan, or Portland, Oregon, or New Jersey, the lack of access to clean water in the twenty-first century—the twenty-first century!—has been caused by a complacency in the federal and state governments that has led to a public health crisis that should never have happened.

THE INSTITUTIONAL INDIFFERENCE OF CIVIC leaders in the states of the former Confederacy persists to this day—a legacy of the monstrous system of bondage in which human lives were expendable—and continues to undermine not only the health of Black Americans but of all residents. In many ways, and for large swaths of people living in red states, not much has changed. States that were part of the Confederacy rank near the bottom or dead last in virtually every metric of health and well-being. In some cases, they have worse outcomes than those of developing countries that lack the advanced medical infrastructure that we have in the United States.

The reasons are attributed to the usual factors: These states have more people who are overweight, who smoke, drink alcohol, or abuse drugs, and who are less likely to have health insurance or even a regular family doctor. But dig a little deeper and the real reason becomes clear: Their poor health is the result of centuries of institutional neglect, the seeds of which were planted when those first slave ships arrived in the Western Hemisphere. While there are regions where progress has been made, parts of the Deep South remain trapped in an economy that hasn't progressed much beyond the nineteenth-century slave system and is often governed by a political class bankrolled by and beholden to monied interests. It remains reliant on exploiting workers, both white and Black, perpetuating union-busting and Jim Crow discrimination to keep wages down, and gutting child-labor laws and safety protections for the largely immigrant workforce toiling in slaughterhouses and meat-packing plants.

We saw this with the refusal of red states—like Mississippi, Alabama, South Carolina, Tennessee, and South Carolina, many of which have the nation's worst health outcomes—to take the Medicaid expansion funds as part of the Affordable Care Act. This translated into the loss of tens of millions of dollars in federal health-care subsidies that left more than two million Americans without health insurance and led to the shuttering of dozens of rural hospitals. This scenario was repeated again at the end of the Covid pandemic. When we emerged from the pandemic, red states like Arkansas and Texas moved swiftly to drop thousands of families and children from health insurance coverage under Medicaid when the Biden White House lifted insurance coverage mandates that had protected the poor during the Covid outbreak. In Arkansas alone, 11,000 newborns lost health insurance virtually overnight.

During the Civil War, however, while the North may have had distinct advantages in their military might and in their approach to public health that aided in their ultimate victory, the Union forces—as well as policymakers and politicians—neglected to understand the underlying lesson—the importance of inclusivity for all segments of society—when it came to the newly emancipated. The formerly enslaved were never integrated into the public health system during or even after the war, and were either abandoned or exploited for their labor and as cannon fodder.

That opportunity to rectify our country's callous mistreatment of emancipated African Americans was lost when Reconstruction was abandoned in the early 1870s. But this backtracking is not unique to the South or to the post–Civil War years. The vast disparities in health have been a persistent and pervasive problem over time and across the country. Going forward, similar opportunities were lost when efforts to pass universal health insurance during FDR's administration were stymied by the American Medical Association, and LBJ's vision of the Great Society was abandoned. We saw this repeated when the Obama administration passed the Affordable Care Act, which Republican lawmakers did their best to repeal, chip away at, or undermine in its full implementation. The fundamental right to health care has been consistently denied to a large swath of the American population. The fragmentation of our health system is what led to the massive vulnerability and loss of life when the pandemic, a true health emergency, struck. The overarching result is that we not only have poorer health outcomes than any other industrialized nation, via such metrics as maternal and infant mortality, but also the highest death rates during the pandemic among developed countries. When we don't learn these lessons, inertia, racism, and sexism weaken our society in these pervasive and pernicious ways.

We'd like to think that the Civil War was a moral crusade on the part of the North to end the barbaric institution of slavery, but the reality is that while slavery was the casus belli for the South, the North fought, initially at least, to preserve the Union—although the collapse of slavery was the ultimate outcome. Even though Lincoln has been lionized throughout history as the Great Emancipator, the Emancipation Proclamation in 1863 wasn't entirely inspired by benevolent impulses. In the harsh realpolitik of war, historians say, it was largely a savvy political maneuver calculated to beef up the Union Army's manpower by enlisting Black soldiers while at the same time cutting the South off at the knees by drastically depleting the workforce that their labor-intensive economy relied upon.

But after emancipation, when freed slaves came pouring into the Union Army refugee camps, no provisions were made to supply them with adequate food, clothing, and shelter. "[I]n the effort to dismantle the institution of slavery, very few considered how ex-slaves would survive the war and emancipation," notes Jim Downs in *Sick from Freedom: African-American Illness and Suffering During the Civil War and Reconstruction*.

> An abstract idea about freedom became a flesh-and-blood reality in which epidemic outbreaks, poverty, and the suffering threatened former bondspeople as they abandoned slavery and made their way toward freedom . . . sickness compounded by the inability to secure clothing, shelter, and food left many freed people dead and caused inordinate suffering among those who survived.

Historical accounts reveal in wrenching detail the horrors that the formerly enslaved faced when they escaped bondage. Their treacherous passage to safety—evading Confederate guerillas, vengeful plantation owners and their brutal slave patrols, with no food or water, and carrying nothing but the ragged, threadbare clothes on their backs—was grueling and dangerous. Many perished on the perilous journey. While the Union Army didn't subject them to the constant threat of violence, cruelty, and torture as did their brutal slave masters, they were met, at best, with apathy and negligence.

If they somehow made it to the overcrowded and unsanitary Union camps, the newly emancipated often encountered open hostility from soldiers and the military brass, who blamed them for the war and were reluctant to offer any aid because they felt their sickness and vulnerability to disease were a result of their inherent inferiority. The formerly enslaved were left to their own devices and reduced to begging for scraps of uneaten food, worn-out clothes, and unused tents to shelter their families. "The fear of dependency ran like a cancer throughout the rhetoric of Union officials in the Civil War South," notes Jim Downs in *Sick from Freedom,* echoing the sentiments that still have currency today. "Both federal leaders in Washington and local military officers in camps feared that any gesture of help or support would encourage former bondspeople to become dependent on federal aid and assistance."

The story of James Miller and his family is especially poignant and, unfortunately, typical of the horrors that formerly enslaved people endured when they sought sanctuary. In November of 1864, the weather in rural Kentucky was unrelentingly harsh. Camp Nelson, a Union stronghold spread over four thousand acres about twenty miles south of Lexington, was battered by bone-chilling winds, frigid temperatures, and drenching rainstorms. The camp housed roughly eight thousand soldiers and about five hundred newly emancipated slaves. It even had a training ground for Black recruits. Joseph Miller and his wife and four children, who had escaped from chattel slavery, were permitted to stay in the camp and provided with food and shelter as long as the elder Miller joined the Union Army. However, the military, as often happened, failed to keep their side of the bargain.

On November 22, a windy and rainy morning when temperatures dropped below freezing, Union Brigadier General Speed S. Pry ordered the evacuation of all the freed people from the safety of the camp. Union soldiers on horseback invaded the makeshift village of tents and huts that Black soldiers had built for their families and forced them out. Some were still asleep and barely had time to gather their clothing and meager personal belongings before soldiers began tearing up their tents. The weather that morning was "the coldest of the season," one Union official later said. "The wind was blowing quite sharp, and the women and children were thinly clad and mostly without shoes."

Joseph Miller begged the guards to allow his family to stay because his seven-year-old son was sick. "I told the man in charge of the guard that it would be the death of my boy," Miller reportedly said. He told them he was a soldier in the Union Army and his family had no place to go. But the guard responded that if the family didn't "get up on the wagon, he would shoot every last one of them." Heartsick, Miller watched as his family was transported to an unknown destination.

After completing his duties that day, Miller left the camp to search for them. He walked over six miles before he discovered "an old boarding house belonging to the colored people," he recalled. In one corner of a frigid room, he found his family "shivering with cold and famished with hunger." His son had frozen to death earlier in the day while being transported to the boarding house. Miller was grief-stricken, but under orders to return to the Union camp that night. The next day, he walked back to the boarding house. With no place to bury his son, he carried the child six miles back to the Union camp and buried him in an unmarked grave that he dug himself. Within three weeks, Miller's wife, Isabella, and his son Joseph Jr. had perished. Ten days later, his daughter Maria died. By the day after the New Year, Miller's last remaining family member, his son Calvin, was dead, too. A few days later, on January 6, 1865, Joseph Miller passed away. The cause of his death is unknown. But considering the circumstances, he could have been infected by disease, weakened by malnutrition, or frozen to death from exposure to the elements. "Or perhaps," Downs speculated, "he died from a broken heart."

The Miller family were among the hundreds of freed slaves who perished from starvation and exposure at Camp Nelson in the waning days of the war. The wrenching "displacement, deprivation, and ultimately death" that befell the Miller family typified the suffering of the roughly 500,000 freed slaves who sought refuge in Union camps during the Civil War; estimates of mortality in slave refugee camps range from 25 to 50 percent, where victims perished from malnutrition, exposure, or the diseases that ravaged the camps. "The medical crises"—and the public health failures—"that freed slaves endured," noted Downs, "suggest that sickness and death may not have been the unavoidable consequences of war, but the very price of freedom."

The cruel treatment of newly freed people wasn't confined to military and refugee camps, where scarce resources were stretched thin. In 1862, an outbreak of smallpox occurred among formerly enslaved people who had gathered in a vacant lot in the nation's capital after fleeing farms, homes, and plantations in Maryland and Virginia. Yet the federal government failed to acknowledge the outbreak, and Lincoln, even as he was drafting the Emancipation Proclamation, ignored it because it was largely seen as a "Black epidemic." Appalled, the Medical Society of the District of Columbia roundly denounced the government's inaction. "It is generally admitted that small-pox is one of the diseases due to domiciliary circumstances, and is at all times a preventable disease," the doctors contended. "It has been stated over and over again by eminent authorities, that there need not be a single case of small-pox in any city; if the authorities will but take the proper steps to check it."

Despite the availability of a vaccine, nothing was done to treat or stop the spread of the highly contagious virus, which is easily transmitted by human contact. In the absence of quarantines, the disease spread through the South when former slaves searched for work. Smallpox continued to be a scourge in Black communities throughout the nineteenth and early twentieth centuries, a plague so fierce that sympathetic white physicians worried it would lead to the extinction of the Black race. The disease claimed at least 60,000 lives during the Civil War and Reconstruction.

Reports of the desperate circumstances of the formerly enslaved filtered back to sympathetic people in the North. In February of 1862, abolitionists met at the Cooper Institute and formed the National Freedman's Relief Association, which went on to create similar committees in Massachusetts, New York, and Pennsylvania to provide resources for newly freed people. Harriet Jacobs, who was enslaved during her childhood and escaped to the North where she became a prominent abolitionist, feminist, and writer, left her home in Philadelphia and boarded a train to Washington, D.C., to visit newly freed slaves, and to write about their circumstances for Northern reformers like William Lloyd Garrison, the famed abolitionist.

The city had been overwhelmed by enslaved people escaping from bondage and seeking asylum, and many of them were homeless, destitute, and gravely ill. Wartime Washington was chaotic. Main thoroughfares were rutted and potholed from all the war traffic, side streets were filled with pigs, goats, cattle, and chickens, and gutters for drainage were clogged with weeds, which meant rains constantly flooded the muddy roadways. In an account for Garrison's publication, *The Liberator,* Jacobs wrote that she had visited Duff Green's Row, a government camp for the newly emancipated. Their conditions were deplorable, and people were suffering grievously.

"I found men, women and children all huddled together without any distinction or regard to age or sex," she observed. "Some of them were in the most pitiable condition. Many were sick with measles, diphtheria, and scarlet and typhoid fever. Some had a few filthy rags to lie on; others had nothing but the bare floor for a couch." Yet there was no one to offer comfort or aid to the sick and dying. "Each day brings its fresh additions of the hungry, naked and sick," she wrote in

September of 1862. "In the early part of June, there were, some days, as many as ten deaths reported at this place in twenty-four hours." Jacobs did her best to soothe the agonies of the dying, and offered them clothing, blankets, and words of comfort: "Those tearful eyes often looked up to me with the language: 'Is this freedom?'"

A year later, in 1863, as Ulysses Grant's army advanced through the Mississippi Valley, thousands of previously enslaved Blacks were freed. The Black Americans liberated by Union forces were considered seized property and referred to as contraband. The military began setting up what became known as contraband camps throughout the occupied South to house these wartime refugees. Camp Barker, which was in a rural area in the northwest of Washington, D.C., was one of the larger of these encampments, and homed about 40,000 people.

In 1863, the military created an infirmary, which they initially called the Contraband Hospital but later changed to Freedmen's Hospital. Built on a parcel of swampland in northwest D.C., the camp had unhealthy living conditions and its hospital lacked basic supplies and water. The damp environment and overcrowded conditions were a breeding ground for infectious illnesses, including respiratory infections, which raged unchecked. The sickest patients were treated in one-story barracks and tents that were converted into wards and included an isolation area for patients with smallpox. Hospital activities were moved to several sites before the facility was transferred permanently to the buildings that had once housed Campbell Hospital, a large pavilion-style facility with a capacity of six hundred beds, a supply of fresh water, and a waste-disposal system.

In January of 1863, not long after the Emancipation Proclamation, a surgeon in Toronto, Canada, who had been closely watching developments in the United States, wrote to President Lincoln, imploring him to consider hiring him to work with "some of the colored regiments . . . [so I can] be in a position where I can be of use to my race." His name was Alexander T. Augusta, and he'd been born a free man in Norfolk, Virginia, in 1825, but was forced to relocate to Canada to pursue his medical education because of racial discrimination. He received his medical degree from Trinity College of the University of Toronto in 1856—the first African American to graduate from a medical school in what was then called British North America—and he had a successful practice in the Canadian city until the Civil War broke out in 1861.

Unlike many "country doctors" who trained through apprenticeships at makeshift operations that were little more than diploma mills, Augusta obtained a medical degree from an established university and was recognized as a fully trained physician. But it wasn't easy. Initially, he had applied to the University of Pennsylvania but was rejected because of his race, although William Gibson, the chair of the school's department of surgery, recognized his gifts and tutored him privately for three years. Augusta applied to medical school again, this time in Chicago, but was turned away once more. Sadly, this pattern—and the consequences of discriminatory practices in medical education—persists to this day and is likely to worsen, given the recent Supreme Court decision to roll back affirmative action. We will talk more about this in a later chapter.

The 1850s were a period of escalating political instability in the United States, and the passage of the Fugitive Slave Act in 1850 imperiled even free Black Americans living in the North. This prompted Augusta, along with many others, to emigrate to Toronto. After graduation, he had a successful private practice, headed up the Toronto City Hospital, a twenty-five-bed charitable facility, and operated a pharmacy. Augusta was a prominent figure in Toronto, and advocated abolitionism and anti-racist activities. He served as president of the Association for the Education of Coloured People in Canada, to improve educational opportunities for Black children, and he mentored promising students. But he never forgot his American roots, and he offered to provide Lincoln and the Secretary of War, Edwin M. Stanton, with letters attesting to his character and competence from his colleagues in Toronto.

Trained surgeons were at a premium, so he was invited back to the United States. Once he returned, however, he faced unrelenting racism and countless indignities. When he arrived for his medical examination, the medical board president was enraged that no one had told him the candidate was Black and rejected him out of hand. The racist white doctor was overruled, and Augusta became the Union Army's first Black surgeon and officer. In May of 1863, Augusta took over as the first Black executive officer in charge of the Freedmen's Hospital.

But he discovered that a Black man wearing a major's uniform aroused deep-seated hostility. The thirty-eight-year-old physician found himself attacked by a gang of ruffians when he boarded a train in Baltimore that was headed for Philadelphia. They tore the epaulets from Augusta's uniform, and a police officer refused to intervene. Augusta managed to get help from a federal provost marshal and, at his insistence, his attackers were found and later convicted of assault. However, the provost marshal's office was surrounded by a mob that demanded that they "lynch the scoundrel" and "hang the Negro." Augusta was only able to reach Philadelphia when he was escorted by several plainclothes police officers with revolvers drawn.

Unfortunately, this sort of treatment wasn't unusual in a city like Baltimore, which bordered the South. Augusta noted in a letter to the Washington newspaper *National Republican,* "where it is considered a virtue to mob colored people." But the worst racism he faced was from white doctors, who couldn't abide a Black doctor who held a higher rank, and constantly complained to the secretary of war. The army stopped commissioning Black physicians; instead they were hired as contract doctors without military rank or standing. Augusta knew he needed to be surrounded by surgeons he could trust, and he recruited several of his colleagues from his days in Toronto, including Anderson Abbott, who was his protégé in Toronto and later succeeded him as the head of the Freedmen's Hospital, along with John Rapier Jr., William Powell Jr., William Ellis, Charles Purvis, and Alpheus Tucker. This cadre of surgeons formed the nucleus of the medical corps that would serve Black Americans during and after the war, at the Freedmen's Hospital and nearby contraband camps. Augusta was later transferred to South Carolina and then Georgia, where he worked at Lincoln Hospital in Savannah with Harriet Jacobs and her daughter Louisa. "The hospital was the city poor-house," Harriet Jacobs observed. "The doctor is faithful in the discharge of his duties, but has very little to work with. . . . We have to depend on our friends to assist us in relieving the wants of these poor creatures."

While at Lincoln, Augusta was promoted to the rank of lieutenant colonel by brevet in recognition of his wartime service. He returned to Washington in 1867 to work again at Freedmen's Hospital, which is the oldest institution in the world primarily dedicated to providing patient care and professional training for Black Americans. In September of 1868, it became the teaching hospital for the Howard University Medical School. Augusta was a founding member of the school's medical department, where he taught anatomy, and he was the first Black to be on the faculty of a medical school in the United States. In a photo taken in 1869 of the inaugural medical faculty, Augusta sits in a chair, his back ramrod straight and his hands resting on his thighs. He is surrounded by his seven white colleagues, and is staring intently into the camera as if to say: "I belong here."

When he died in December of 1890, Augusta was buried with full military honors at Arlington National Cemetery.

More than 750,000 soldiers lost their lives in the Civil War, the greatest toll of any war in American history. Roughly two-thirds of them died from diseases, which was a staggeringly high number. But these mortality rates were far lower than the mortality rates from infections in Crimea, in which eight out of ten men there died from disease, and not on the battlefield. The death toll was far greater for the Confederacy—one in four Confederate soldiers died or were incapacitated versus one in ten for the Union Army—because the Union had better medical care, food, shelter, and sanitation systems. And in the camps and hospitals where stringent sanitary guidelines were enforced, deaths from diseases dropped dramatically. The unstinting efforts of public health officials to improve troops' living conditions on the battlefield and the investments in basic public health measures helped the Union win the war and spared thousands of soldiers from needless suffering and death.

The lessons learned from the war added greater urgency to the Sanitary Movement, which had been stalled throughout the antebellum United States. After the war, the doctors, nurses, and medical volunteers who worked in the hospitals and camps returned to their homes with a renewed sense of purpose and pushed for sanitary reforms. They had seen firsthand that proper sanitation, clean water, the use of disinfectants, and enforced isolation and quarantines saved lives and gave them real power in preventing the spread of disease long before the discovery of germs. In 1866 and 1867, New York and Chicago instituted the nation's first municipal boards of health, and by the 1870s, most major cities had established public health departments.

Deaths from cholera and yellow fever dropped dramatically. Many of the strategies and policies that had been instituted on the battlefields and in the camps became standard practice. When there was a cholera outbreak in New York in 1866, strictly enforced quarantines and the use of disinfectants and basic sanitary techniques stopped the spread of disease; it was the first time that the use of scientific techniques contained an epidemic, according to Charles Rosenberg in *The Cholera Years*. Community hygiene, the mandatory use of smallpox vaccinations, and even filling out paperwork to keep count of illnesses and deaths—the vital record-keeping that tracks the health of a community—became routine. "This created the impulse from 1865 throughout the 1870s for state-sponsored sanitary reforms," said Jonathan S. Jones. "It was a big turning point in American medicine."

But these reforms were not shared equally with Black soldiers and the newly freed Black Americans. More than 180,000 African Americans served as soldiers in the Union Army; about 40,000 of them perished, but only about 10,000 died in combat. Most Black soldiers died from disease. It wasn't until the Korean War, when the U.S. Army became fully integrated (almost a century later!), that Black soldiers received the same care that was afforded to white soldiers.

After the war, thousands of newly emancipated people languished in refugee camps with few resources and were heavily reliant upon the charitable impulses of former abolitionists. About a quarter of the approximately four million freed slaves either died or were stricken by illness in the years between 1862 and 1870, according to research by Jim Downs. The formerly enslaved endured conditions so horrific that they were "dying by the scores," wrote one military official in Tennessee in 1865. "Sometimes 30 per day die and are carried out by wagonloads without coffins, and thrown promiscuously, like brutes, into a trench."

In February of 1865, slavery was outlawed when Lincoln signed the Thirteenth Amendment into law. A month later—before General Robert E. Lee surrendered to Ulysses S. Grant at Appomattox Courthouse on April 9, 1865, which effectively ended the war—the Freedmen's Bureau, formally known as the Bureau of Refugees, Freedmen, and Abandoned Lands, was established by Congress. Its mission was to relieve the immense suffering of millions of formerly enslaved people and poor whites throughout the South and help them become self-sufficient by providing food, housing, and medical aid, setting up schools, and offering them legal assistance.

It was a massive undertaking. In the fall of 1865, there were only eighty doctors and twelve hospitals to serve the medical needs of more than four million newly emancipated people. Within three years, the Bureau had expanded to more than nine hundred officials in posts from Washington to Texas, and millions of people were under their jurisdiction. By 1869, over half a million patients had been treated by Bureau physicians and surgeons, and sixty hospitals and asylums were in operation. However, the bureau was formally disbanded in 1872, and derailed from many of its lofty goals by a lack of money, racism, and the revanchist politics of the post-Reconstruction era that saw a resurgence in power of the embittered former plantation owners.

"No sooner had Northern armies touched Southern soil than this old question, newly guised, sprang from the earth,—What shall be done with slaves?" W.E.B. Du Bois asked in an eloquent and insightful essay that appeared three decades later, in the March 1901 issue of *The Atlantic Monthly*, about the circumstances surrounding the creation of the Freedmen's Bureau. The pioneering social scientist characterized the formation of the bureau as "one of the most singular and interesting of the attempts made by a great nation to grapple with vast problems of race and social condition."

In the aftermath of a disastrous war that left the Confederate states in ruins, Du Bois illuminated all the reasons why the well-intentioned enterprise was reviled in much of the South.

In a time of perfect calm, amid willing neighbors and streaming wealth, the social uplifting of four million slaves to an assured and self-sustaining place in the body politic and economic would have been a herculean task; but when to the inherent difficulties of so delicate and nice a social operation were added the spite and hate of conflict, the hell of war; when suspicion and cruelty were rife, and gaunt Hunger wept beside Bereavement—in such a case, the work of any instrument of social regeneration was in large part foredoomed to failure.

CHAPTER THREE

Public Health's Most Celebrated Act of Civil Disobedience

*Once germs were discovered as the culprits behind infectious diseases,
we conquered the ills that had once felled empires. But public health
initiatives that dealt with societal inequities were derailed.*

SCIENTIFIC KNOWLEDGE IS A PUBLIC GOOD BECAUSE IT IS AN essential foundation of a thriving society. The most beautiful scientific solutions are driven by data, compassion, care, justice, and simplicity. It is a public good that comes from the creativity and persistence of people who want to understand how nature could be harnessed in ways that help all of us to thrive. Science manifests in many ways, ranging from devising vaccines and therapeutics for infectious diseases to trying to understand how racism and discrimination get under our skin to promote premature aging, or weathering. When we talk about the breadth of the scientific endeavor and tie all scientific discoveries together, they bring about a myriad of solutions that can prevent or treat disease and promote public policy changes that enable all of us to live better, longer, and safer lives.

We saw this with the enactment of Medicare in 1965, a landmark change in public policy that gave the elderly access to decent medical care. This enabled millions of Americans to live healthy and fulfilling lives in dignity without being hobbled by chronic ills that are preventable or manageable. The introduction of vaccines during the Covid pandemic is another instance in which public health policy and scientific discovery came together to save lives. Overwhelmed ER doctors on the front lines saw the results right away. Fewer people were showing up in emergency departments, and the patients who did come in weren't as gravely ill. Deaths plummeted and the economy was resuscitated.

Arguably, the modern era of public health based on a firm foundation of science began with the research of a shy British physician. His name was John Snow, and his story has been told countless times. His rigorous research and meticulously gathered data identified the environmental factors that were the root causes of the cholera outbreaks that plagued London in the mid-nineteenth century—a perfect example of how science saves lives. John Snow created an entirely new paradigm and provided the template for all of the public health scientists who followed.

In the ensuing decades, scientists like Robert Koch and Louis Pasteur proved that tiny microbes were the culprits responsible for the diseases that killed millions, a discovery that launched a golden age in public health. Clean-water initiatives and vaccine campaigns conquered scourges like cholera, typhus, and diphtheria. Infant mortality rates dropped, and life expectancy increased by nearly thirteen years, from age forty-seven in 1900 to sixty by 1930. Public health embraced programs in the community, helping pregnant mothers, babies, and the poor. But public health soon became a victim of its own success. Community-based programs soon took a back seat to the academic microbe hunters, who came to dominate the field. Anything else that had a long-term impact on public health—toxic environments, lack of access to health care—was dismissed or ignored. And perhaps it is no surprise that the Black community and other marginalized groups suffered the most from this seismic shift.

But like so many other nineteenth-century inflection points in public health, it all started with cholera. In August of 1854, six hundred people perished in just ten days as cholera swept through Soho in London's West End. Medical professionals believed that infectious illnesses were primarily caused by "miasma" or "noxious air" emitted from rotting organic matter. But Snow, an obstetrician who pioneered the use of anesthesia, was skeptical that cholera was spread by foul air. Based on his research and observations of how the disease affected victims, he gradually became a disciple of the then-controversial germ theory, namely that microscopic agents were responsible for the epidemics that ravaged crowded cities.

Cholera directly attacked the lower intestines, causing agonizing abdominal pains, and the constant vomiting and severe diarrhea that led to the grave dehydration that killed victims. If cholera was genuinely transmitted by breathing in foul vapors that entered the body, Snow reasoned, it would have, at least initially, made its presence known as a general fever and in the lungs—which it did not. He became convinced that cholera was a water-borne illness spread by as-yet-unidentified pathogens, transmitted in fecal matter on the hands or soiled sheets of victims or by drinking or eating foods prepared with tainted water.

In those days, residents of London didn't have running water. They got their water from local wells or the various water companies that tapped into the highly polluted Thames River. Water was pumped into reservoirs adjoining the river, and sand filtration systems were used to remove impurities. The clean water was then bottled and delivered to pubs, other businesses, and homes.

During an earlier cholera outbreak, in 1848, which killed 53,000 people in England and Wales, Snow systematically traced the pathway of the disease, using data from vital records, surveys, and chemical testing, and discovered that the common thread among its victims was that they had ingested contaminated water. From the registrar general, he got the names and addresses of all the people who had died of cholera, and he visited each home to find out where they got their water. His research was exhaustive—and in the process, he established some of the methods still used today by epidemiologists.

One of his case studies was of residents of Thomas Street, in a poor section of London, where there were two courts close together consisting of a small number of houses or cottages. People in Surrey Buildings started getting sick when wastewater was dumped into the street and seeped into a channel that polluted their well. In contrast, their neighbors at Truscott's Court had a different water source and weren't hit much by disease. The same pattern held true when Snow looked at the spread of cholera among the more affluent residents of Albion Terrace, who were mostly tradespeople and professionals living in detached row houses. When one resident became ill and the wastewater contaminated the water supply, more than half the residents were stricken with cholera, and half of those died. However, people in only one row of houses were sickened, because they tapped into the same polluted spring. Yet people in "all the surrounding houses were quite free from it," Snow noted in his August 1849 report, *On the Mode of Communication of Cholera*.

Here again, the common element was the water; air pollution couldn't explain the disease's transmission, because all residents living in the area were breathing the same air. But local authorities were firmly in the miasma camp, and disregarded Snow's suggestion that cholera epidemics—which had resisted attempts at containment through quarantine and isolation—could be stopped by simple sanitary measures and cleaning up tainted waters.

When another cholera outbreak hit London in 1854, Snow built upon his previous research and compared the death rates of people getting their water from the Southwark or Vauxhall Companies, which still tapped into a dirty section of the Thames, to that of the Lambeth Company, which had shifted its water source in 1852 to a much cleaner spot upriver, beyond where sewage was dumped. Snow, an ardent student of the then-nascent field of data analysis, realized immediately that this was a natural experiment, a simple form of the randomized trial that is still a fundamental tool of epidemiology. "No fewer than three hundred thousand people of both sexes, of every age and occupation, and of every rank and station, from gentlefolks down to the very poor," he noted, "were divided into two groups without their choice, and, in most cases, without their knowledge."

Combing through the data collected by the city's Registrar General revealed stark differences. During the first four weeks of the epidemic, mortality rates were 107 of every 100,000 inhabitants who used either the Southwark or Vauxhall water, while only 8 out of every 100,000 customers of Lambeth died. "In other words," noted Snow, "the disease was between thirteen and fourteen times as fatal to the population having the impure water [Southwark and Vauxhall] as to that having the improved supply [Lambeth]."

Still, civic leaders remained unimpressed. Out of sheer frustration, Snow embarked on the gumshoe-detective sleuthing mission that would change medical history. That fateful August, when cholera went on its deadly rampage through Soho, striking more than three hundred people in forty-eight hours and killing hundreds within days, Snow collected the names of all the cholera fatalities and plotted them on a map of the area. He discovered most of them clustered around a water-well pump on Broad Street.

Then he talked to people in the area who didn't fall ill. A workhouse for inmates that had only a handful of deaths had its own well, while workers at the local brewery preferred to drink beer. Armed with his map as evidence, he appealed to local authorities to have the pump handle removed, to prevent people from using the contaminated well. (Later research revealed that washing the soiled diapers of an infant who died of the disease had contaminated the water by the pump.) They refused. Frustrated, Snow removed the handle himself, and cases of cholera, which had already begun to diminish, plummeted.

Even though John Snow's removal of the Broad Street pump

handle is heralded as the event marking the birth of epidemiology, his real achievement was earlier, when he compared the disparities in fatalities between residents ingesting water from the different water companies. Epidemiology, which is a fundamental science of public health, does a number of things. It looks at the frequency, distribution, and determinants of disease in human populations rather than individuals, which allows scientists to detect signals that may not be obvious by just examining one or two patients. The lessons learned are then used to fuel positive changes in health and wellness on a scale far greater than that of clinical medicine. In this particular instance, Snow compared two distinct but evenly matched groups to tease out the different variables, which enabled him to identify the source of the cholera infections. He realized that what the people who were sickened had in common was drinking the same contaminated water. Beyond that, Snow's discovery is widely viewed as one of the first validations of the modern germ theory of disease. So, in one act, the scientific and methodological bases for public health were affirmed.

This is a well-studied piece of history, but it still moves me like a great work of art. John Snow's defiant act of civil disobedience deeply resonated with me early in my career. It was an act of profound beauty, and I greatly admired this quiet contrarian, a vegetarian who never married and died of a stroke at the age of forty-five. There was an elegance about his work because it was simple, clear, concise, and reproducible, derived from clear methodology and application of the science. He was driven from that purest of emotions, the desire to do good and eliminate unnecessary suffering, and his work unlocked the potential for humanity to move closer to a more just and thriving society.

While his work wasn't flashy or sexy, sometimes there is nothing sexy about implementing scientific knowledge. Sometimes, it is simply laborious grunt work, with years going by without any payoffs or breakthroughs. But Snow persisted. Based on his observations, he sensed there was something in the water, but it was something we couldn't see. And it required a humility, a tenacity, and a belief in statistics—in the science—to motivate his actions. He couldn't convince civic leaders of what he knew to be true, but he created the foundation upon which the entire discipline of epidemiology—the basic science of public health—was built.

It was scientific knowledge that prompted his act of defiance, but knowledge by itself doesn't save lives. It's the social and political will to use the science to make changes happen that saves lives. All of the microbiology in the world would not have saved that next family from contracting cholera. What saved them is that science led to action. Public policy for the greater good.

John Snow's work lives on in big and small ways across the globe. His groundbreaking research inspired fundamental changes in water and waste management that made possible the thriving cities of today.

Snow was a bookish mathematical whiz fascinated by numbers. His willingness to spend hours combing through handwritten columns of figures, and his uncanny ability to see patterns in seemingly unrelated statistics and track down the source of disease outbreaks was made possible by his mastery of the then-relatively new field of data collection. Statistics and data gathering became indispensable tools for helping epidemiologists pinpoint the source of outbreaks and gauge their magnitude and severity, to better deploy methods of containment.

Even though Snow is celebrated as the father of epidemiology, the use of statistics to compare the health of different populations had its roots at least two centuries earlier. John Graunt, an affluent businessman in seventeenth-century London, tracked births and causes of deaths using the city's Bills of Mortality, which is the first known instance of recordkeeping of health-related population data. What Graunt immediately noticed was that deaths from causes other than the plague occurred at a regular and predictable rate year after year. But the plague behaved quite differently: Some years thousands succumbed, while at other times the death toll would be negligible.

Graunt concluded from these observations that the plague had a different origin from the other ills that routinely killed Londoners, such as consumption (tuberculosis), syphilis, jaundice, and scurvy, and that it was probably not spread by fetid gases in the air; otherwise, it would strike with the same regularity as these ailments. Graunt and Snow were not alone—their and others' discoveries laid the foundation for what would become the fast-growing scientific discipline of epidemiology during the Victorian era. This was a period of great intellectual ferment that saw the publication of Darwin's groundbreaking *On the Origin of Species* in 1859, which was based on similar techniques for making comparisons of different groups.

John Snow's contemporary Florence Nightingale was also an early advocate of using statistics to prevent, control, or limit the ravages of diseases. Although she is widely celebrated for her bravery as a nurse, leading corps of women onto battlefields of the Crimean War to care for wounded soldiers, and as a trailblazer in pushing for the sanitary reforms that transformed medicine, these achievements eclipsed her profound contributions as a pioneering epidemiologist and statistician. In 1858, in recognition of her research, she was the first woman elected to the Royal Statistical Society.

Nightingale was born in 1820 to a wealthy family that encouraged her academic pursuits, and she had a classical education. As a child, she was captivated by numbers, and her father hired a mathematics tutor when she was twenty. Although a woman of her stature was expected to marry a man who came from the same social class, Nightingale believed that nursing was her calling—an ambition that dismayed her parents because the profession was then viewed as menial labor. Over their strenuous objections, she enrolled as a nursing student at a German hospital in 1850. She exhibited her exceptional talents early, and within a year after her graduation, she was promoted to superintendent of nursing at a British hospital, where her efforts to improve sanitary conditions significantly lowered death rates during a cholera epidemic.

But her greatest challenge, and one that would define her life and revolutionize medical practice, came when she was recruited to lead a corps of nurses to tend to ill and injured soldiers in the Crimean War.

On November 4, 1854, when she and her fellow nurses arrived at Barracks Hospital in Scutari, Turkey, they were horrified by what they saw. The hospital itself was sitting on a large cesspool, which contaminated the water and spread its nauseating smell throughout the halls. The walls and ceilings were filthy. There were no beds, blankets, furniture, or cooking utensils, and there was a severe shortage of the most basic supplies, such as bandages, soap, towels, and even sinks to wash dirty linens. Rats, fleas, and other vermin ran rampant. There were six dead dogs under one window, and a dead horse soaked in an aqueduct for weeks.

Emaciated, weak, and dying patients lay in their own urine and feces on makeshift stretchers throughout the building. Soldiers suffered from frostbite and gangrene, and were stricken with dysentery, cholera, and typhus, living in what Nightingale called "utterly chaotic, unsanitary and inhumane conditions." Worse yet, medical records were woefully inadequate: There was no systematic reporting of soldiers' ailments or causes of death, which meant the medical staff was flying blind when it came to allocating resources and managing diseases. And the deaths of hundreds of men who were buried in unmarked graves weren't even reported, leaving bereft families with no news of the fate of their loved ones.

The dictum "If you can't measure it, you can't manage it" is one of the guiding principles of data collection today. Nightingale intuitively understood this and knew the importance of keeping scrupulous records of the number of soldiers killed, injured, or diseased. She also kept track of such factors as cleanliness—whether patients were regularly bathed, if there were fresh linens and clean facilities—and the placement of latrines and ventilation. Careful documentation with statistics, she believed, could demonstrate whether a specific intervention was effective.

Over that long, harsh winter, she and her team embarked on a prodigious effort to improve sanitary conditions at the hospital, which housed more than 2,300 soldiers. She somehow found hundreds of scrub brushes and recruited the least-ill men to scour the hospital from floor to ceiling. They established regular protocols for bathing patients, who had only been washed every six weeks because of staffing shortages, and set up laundries to clean bed and body linens and kitchens to serve the starving men nutritious meals. In the evenings, Nightingale would wander the hospital halls, checking on patients by lamplight.

When she returned to England in August of 1856 after the war ended, she worked with William Farr, the renowned statistician who headed the vital-statistics office at the General Register Office, to analyze the data she had collected in hopes of convincing the government of the need for sanitary reforms. They came to some startling conclusions. Seven times as many soldiers died from preventable diseases while they languished in squalid camps than from battlefield injuries. Also, the sanitary reforms that Nightingale and her team had instituted at Barracks Hospital had reduced mortality by more than 30 percent. Less than a decade later, Frederick Law Olmsted would employ Nightingale's sanitary strategies during the Civil War, which helped tilt the balance in favor of the Union Army.

In the U.S., as the Industrial Revolution took hold in the mid-nineteenth century, the systematic use of standardized health statistics—births, deaths, and causes of mortality—became widespread, and prompted the creation of city and state public health agencies that helped reduce the spread of disease, especially after the Civil War. During New York City's 1866 cholera outbreak, the recently formed public health board collected data that enabled officials to track the spread of disease and target strategies—including inspections, immediate case reporting, complaint investigations, evacuations, and disinfection of possessions and homes—where they would work best at keeping cholera in check.

Even before John Snow, there had been hints that microscopic organisms were responsible for disease, but the medical establishment refused to acknowledge this possibility. Even something as obvious today as handwashing to prevent illnesses was met with steep resistance in 1847, when a young Hungarian obstetrician, working at the

Vienna General Hospital, suggested that doctors' failure to perform this simple act was responsible for killing one out of every ten women who had just given birth. In the mid-nineteenth century, doctors routinely began their day performing bare-handed autopsies on women who had died the day before of childbed fever, a lethal infection that caused raging fevers, painful abscesses in the abdomen and chest, and deadly sepsis. Afterward, they would help deliver babies in the hospital's maternity wards.

But the young doctor, Ignaz Semmelweis, noticed that only about 4 percent of women died when their babies were delivered by midwives, and yet the maternal death rate was more than double when deliveries were performed by doctors in the best hospitals in Europe and America. Semmelweis correctly surmised that there was some type of "morbid poison," invisible particles that the doctors carried from the autopsy suite and transmitted to women about to give birth in the delivery rooms.

As a consequence, he made handwashing mandatory among the medical students and junior doctors in his department at the Vienna General Hospital, ordering them to use a chlorinated lime solution to thoroughly remove the smell of decay that lingered after performing the autopsies. Mortality rates on his obstetric service plummeted, from 7.8 percent to less than 2 percent. Yet his success at saving lives was contrary to accepted medical wisdom, and his colleagues were incensed by the implication that they were somehow responsible for their patients' deaths. They ignored his warnings. Another twenty years would pass before handwashing became accepted. In 1867, British surgeon Joseph Lister, who was looking for ways to prevent surgical infections and gangrene, also suggested that handwashing and scrubbing surgical instruments could stop the spread of disease. By the 1870s, surgeons regularly scrubbed up before surgery. This simple, unsexy hygiene practice saves countless lives. Later reinforced by advances in bacteriology, simple handwashing remains an important pillar of public health.

But it was Louis Pasteur's research that conclusively proved germs were the culprits behind many diseases. In the mid-1850s, the French scientist was dean of the science faculty at the University of Lille, in northern France near the border with Belgium, when he was hired by a local distillery to find out why their beer was turning rancid. Peering through a microscope, he saw tiny organisms that he believed were making the beer sour. He called them germs, because they seemed to be germinating or growing, and he discovered that these microbes could be killed by heating the liquid, in one of the first demonstrations of pasteurization. Pasteur began a series of studies on broader aspects of fermentation and soon discovered that living organisms caused alcohol fermentation, and that specific microbes triggered the production of lactic acid, which was responsible for the souring of milk. By 1865, he proved the link between germs and disease.

In the late 1870s, the German scientist Robert Koch, who is considered the founder of bacteriology, applied Pasteur's research to human diseases. He proved that the bacillus anthracis was, in fact, the cause of anthrax, and he later identified the mycobacterium tuberculosis and the vibrio cholerae. Within the next several years, American and European scientists discovered the bacteria responsible for many infectious diseases, including leprosy, diphtheria, typhoid, yellow fever, and the bubonic plague. New methods of controlling or even preventing the spread of disease, such as pasteurization, vaccinations, and better water purification techniques, were widely adopted.

The results were nothing short of miraculous. These breakthroughs were a watershed in the history of medicine, enabling the conquest of many of the diseases that plagued humanity throughout history. Almost overnight, life expectancy increased, jumping nearly a decade from thirty-nine years in 1870 to forty-eight years at the turn of the century. Cities, no longer at the mercy of periodic outbreaks of yellow fever, cholera, and other infectious ills, thrived and prospered. The practice of medicine, which had previously been a hit-or-miss proposition in a profession overrun with quacks peddling worthless nostrums, was utterly transformed. Now doctors just had to find the infectious pathogen, kill it, and cure the disease.

During the Spanish–American War in 1898, to cite one notable example, more soldiers died from yellow fever and malaria, which plagued Cuba for generations, than in combat. But in 1901, U.S. Army physician Walter Reed, who was part of the American occupying force on the steamy tropical island nation, began an extensive mosquito-eradication campaign; research by Cuban doctor Carlos Juan Finlay suggested that the insects were the carriers that spread the yellow fever virus. Within a year, yellow fever had been vanquished, and cases of malaria had plummeted, too.

Humanity, at long last, was gaining the upper hand against the scourges that had bedeviled civilization for centuries. Clean water eliminated the diarrheal infections that killed children, antitoxins were devised for diphtheria, and infant mortality rates tumbled. For the first time, parents had some assurances that all of their offspring would survive into adulthood. "Before 1880, we knew nothing; after 1890 we knew it all; it was a glorious ten years," William Thomas Sedgwick, bacteriologist and former president of the American Public Health Association, said.

In the wake of these achievements, massive engineering projects were launched to clean up contaminated drinking water, which was the source of water-borne infections like cholera and typhoid fever. In 1874, for example, Milwaukee, Wisconsin, a midsize midwestern city of 100,000 people, spent $1.9 million—which translates to $52 million in today's money—to build a waterworks that pumped 16 million gallons per day from Lake Michigan. However, the results of costly clean-water campaigns were dramatic. In 1893, Chicago stopped using water from the shores of Lake Michigan and built a four-mile water-intake crib out in the deeper, unpolluted part of the lake. Over the next two decades, the city invested in water sanitation and chlorination projects that experts estimated reduced overall mortality by 56 percent by 1925.

In the late nineteenth and early twentieth centuries, local health agencies broadened their services and began offering clinics and medical-education workshops in their communities. In New York and

Baltimore, public health nurses did home visits, and these and other cities set up health clinics in schools to deal with tuberculosis and infant mortality. The United States had more than 500 tuberculosis clinics and 538 baby clinics by 1915, which were largely operated by city health departments.

But it was at this juncture that medical science retreated from the costly infrastructure initiatives and the community-based programs that have been the foundation of public health efforts throughout the late nineteenth and early twentieth centuries. The energetic, social, sanitary, moral, and religious reforms that had previously driven the science of public health were replaced by more individualistic clinical-medicine measures that were viewed as a more effective way to achieve the same goals. This is where interventions shifted from being community-based to an emphasis on individual patients.

With the acceptance of germ theory in the 1890s, state public health boards opened laboratories to identify the exact causes of each disease—the pathogens that were the culprits—and the best methods of preventing them. In cities like New York, public health laboratories produced vaccines and antitoxins to control smallpox, diphtheria, and other infectious diseases. Public health champions like Charles V. Chapin, who served as the superintendent of health for Providence, Rhode Island, for nearly fifty years, called for a new direction that would revolutionize the practice of public health and convert it to a more biomedical science and laboratory-based profession. Echoing the sentiments of others, Chapin believed that public health should focus on finding germs and controlling diseases; time and money spent on cleaning cities and upgrading the harsh environments that made people sick was wasted. Civic infrastructure investments were scaled back.

The irony is that both approaches were steeped in science. But the physical sciences, the engineering sciences, as well as the social and behavioral sciences that drove public health initiatives and helped communities thrive, took a back seat to individualized medicine. For the world to benefit, however, all these sciences needed to be brought together—the biomedical sciences combined with the diverse scientific disciplines that come together under the umbrella of public health—in service of humanity and the planet.

The ascendence of bacteriology also marked the beginning of the drive to make public health more of a professional discipline. In 1873, the newly founded American Public Health Association had its first annual meeting in Cincinnati. Previously, public health had been the province of an unorthodox coalition of political appointees and voluntary social reformers. Public health officers were normally physicians, but their ranks were also filled by nurses, engineers, mathematicians, chemists, and even lawyers. Public health is a big tent where all disciplines come together to serve one common goal: to protect, promote, and preserve the health of populations.

But there wasn't an agreed-upon standardized set of required skills. To remedy this, the first professional public health training program in America, the Harvard–MIT School of Health Officers, was founded in 1913 and offered classes in sanitary engineering, preventive medicine, and allied subjects. Three years later, Johns Hopkins University launched its School of Hygiene and Public Health, and other universities soon followed that example. The rise of academic medicine meant that public health education would center on the laboratory.

Public health became the province of experts as it became more based on scientific research. "Prevention and control of disease were no longer tasks of common sense and social compassion, but of knowledge and expertise," Barbara Rosenkrantz noted in *Public Health and the State: Changing Views in Massachusetts.* "Health reforms were guided by engineers, chemists, biologists, and physicians."

Medicine and public health's drive toward becoming science-oriented and creating higher professional standards resulted in major victories in the conquest of diseases. But there was a serious downside to this change. Perhaps not surprisingly, the acceptance of germ theory disproportionately benefited whites. Between 1890 and 1900 in New England, there was a 30 percent reduction in death rates from typhoid fever for white Americans living in cities. For Black Americans living in cities, rates dropped only 2 percent. During the same period, death rates for Black Americans actually increased, from 67.2 to 72.7 per 100,000 people, while it dropped for whites.

The consequences of this shift away from the environmental and behavioral causes of ill health—all the factors that had a long-term impact on health—were ignored. The more systemic, structural determinants of health—dilapidated housing, lack of clean water, and adequate sanitation—received diminishing interest and investments, and the costly infrastructure projects that benefitted populations were largely abandoned—which effectively left the most vulnerable even further behind. Bacteriology became dominant, rather than a subfield of public health, which was now focused on laboratories where bacteria were incubated, rather than on the big-picture public health perspective.

Unfortunately, all of the factors that undercut public health measures—a strictly bacteriological approach that ignored the social factors responsible for disease, the institutionalized neglect of Black Americans and impoverished communities, the dismissal of the firsthand experiences of public health physicians, and the vilification of scientists who challenged what had quickly become the prevailing dogma, namely that germs caused all diseases—coalesced in the hunt to find the origin of pellagra.

Pellagra had reached epidemic proportions among the poor sharecroppers, tenant farmers, and cotton mill workers in the South in the early years of the twentieth century. However, the single-minded focus on finding an infectious agent sidetracked the search for the real cause for decades, resulting in untold suffering and thousands of needless deaths. This regrettable episode is only one example of how concentrating exclusively on germs with the same institutional blindness that once characterized the insistence on foul air as the source of illnesses, and neglecting to investigate other factors that play crucial roles in sickness, led to grave public health failures.

Pellagra is characterized by the four D's: dermatitis, diarrhea, dementia, and death. In the early stages, sufferers develop a thick, scaly, pigmented rash on skin exposed to sunlight, a swollen mouth, and a bright-red tongue, and experience such symptoms as severe abdominal pains, vomiting, and diarrhea. Left untreated, pellagra can affect the nervous system, causing dementia, memory loss, and hallucinations, and eventually can lead to death. Pellagra was rare in the United States but had been common among European peasants in agricultural regions where it was first identified in 1735.

In 1907, however, the incidence began to skyrocket in the U.S., and, initially at least, seemed to mostly afflict impoverished communities in the South. Then the disease was diagnosed in patients in mental hospitals, and as pellagra rapidly claimed more victims, there were outbreaks among inmates in prisons, children in orphanages, and even in the general population in the rural South. By 1912, 30,000 people had been diagnosed, and 40 percent of them had died of the disease. All told, it is estimated that the epidemic of pellagra caused more than three million cases and 100,000 deaths until it was brought under control in 1940.

In his 1911 annual report, Walter Wyman, the nation's surgeon general, warned that pellagra could become a "national calamity." National conferences were convened, pellagra commissions were formed, and a hospital in Atlanta dedicated to the care of pellagra patients opened in October of 1911. A privately funded field study in cotton-mill districts in Spartanburg, South Carolina, was conducted in 1913. Based on extensive house-to-house surveys, the commission concluded that there was no relation between diet and the disease, and that pellagra "is in all probability a specific infectious disease communicable from person to person by means at present unknown." The fact that the disease was strongly linked with poverty, and clustered in the poorer parts of town where housing and sanitary facilities were sorely lacking, was not considered.

In 1914, Dr. Joseph Goldberger, a physician with the U.S. Public Health Service and an experienced officer in the study of infectious diseases, was assigned to investigate this growing threat. The public health doctor was Jewish, born in Hungary, and raised on New York City's Lower East Side. After graduating from medical school and joining the Commissioned Corps of the Public Health Service, he was dispatched all over the country, to study dengue fever in Texas; yellow fever in Puerto Rico, Mississippi, and Louisiana; and typhus in Mexico, and his research resulted in major breakthroughs in our understanding of the transmission of measles and typhus. He was fighting a diphtheria outbreak in Detroit when the surgeon general sent him to the South.

The forty-year-old epidemiologist spent three weeks in the field, touring several institutions, including a hospital for people with pellagra in Spartanburg, South Carolina, Georgia's state mental asylum, and orphanages in Jackson, Mississippi. It became readily apparent to the veteran disease fighter that pellagra was not communicable. None of these institutions' staff members who were in intimate contact with the patients was stricken with pellagra. In his extensive experience, he had never seen an infectious disease that differentiated between inmates and employees or the rich and the poor.

But their limited diets, which consisted mainly of cornmeal mush, cane syrup or molasses, and gravy and biscuits, immediately attracted his attention. In September of 1914, he began federally funded studies to prove that dietary deficiencies were responsible for the outbreaks. In research on children at two of the orphanages in Jackson, Goldberger provided them with a more varied diet that included fresh meat twice a week, vegetables, and plenty of milk. He began a similar study among inmates of the Georgia asylum. The results were dramatic. By the spring of 1915, pellagra patients in all of these facilities were cured, no new cases emerged, and there were no relapses. (Unfortunately, once federal funds dried up, they returned to the old diet, and by the spring of 1916, 40 percent of the children in orphanages had the disease.) Goldberger was elated by the study's results, and in his report to his superiors, he wrote that he was convinced the disease could be eradicated. His research clearly showed that social and economic factors were responsible for the poor diets that led to the pellagra outbreak. This also illuminates why public health is such a big tent: So many disciplines and professions play roles in it.

Goldberger did a handful of other experiments—which would never be approved today—to prove that pellagra was not infectious. He organized what he called "filth parties": He, his wife, and his associates injected themselves with blood from people suffering from pellagra, and he ground up skin scales, feces, dried urine, and dirt from pellagra sufferers, which they put in capsules and ingested in several doses. All they experienced was nausea and mild diarrhea, but no pellagra.

In 1915, Goldberger began an experiment in which he attempted to induce pellagra in a group of healthy white males in Parchman prison. (Research on inmates in exchange for pardons was common then.) This wildly unethical and callous practice was eventually stopped, but it is indicative of the moral blindness and cruelty of medical research at that time. Starting in the spring of 1915, he fed them a diet of grits, biscuits, and gravy. By November, six of them had full-blown pellagra, and a few couldn't walk. "I have been through a thousand hells," one inmate complained. Others asked to be shot.

Goldberger thought he finally had conclusive proof that pellagra was a nutritional disease. But his findings were greeted with widespread skepticism in the medical community and stirred up a storm of controversy in the South. In 1915, after lectures at the Southern Medical Association and the National Association for the Study of Pellagra, he was roundly attacked and his studies called "half-baked" or outright fraud; his contention that the disease could be prevented by a more nutritional diet that included vegetable proteins, such as beans, was dismissed.

Worse yet, his research ruffled Southern sensibilities in a region still smarting from the defeats of the Lost Cause half a century earlier; they resented the implicit criticism of the state of their economy, especially from a Northerner and an immigrant to boot. "Editorial pages and speeches by congressmen criticized and condemned such insulting inferences concerning the contentment of the people of the

South," noted Dr. Alfred Jay Bollet in *The Yale Journal of Biology and Medicine*. "Furthermore, the suggested remedy of improving the diet of impoverished citizens was clearly impractical."

In frustration, Goldberger finally gave up trying to convince the stubborn naysayers and devoted the remainder of his career to uncovering the nutritional deficiency responsible for pellagra. He died in 1929 before the key element was identified as niacin (vitamin B), which plays a crucial role in cell metabolism. It was later speculated that changes in the way corn was milled, a process called degermination, was responsible for the sudden appearance of pellagra in the United States, mainly among the poor, whose primary source of calories was the denatured cornmeal. Degermination came into routine use in 1901 and removed microbes from the corn's surface, but it removed most of the nutrients, too, resulting in a form of malnutrition that caused pellagra.

The pellagra story is a prime example of what happens when political influences outweigh good science, in this case the Southern politicians downplaying the role of poverty in the development of pellagra, which they saw as an embarrassing social problem that cast the region in a bad light. But this willful blindness hampered the objective study of the disease and the recognition of the actual cause, despite Goldberger's noble efforts, and thus delayed the use of simple preventive treatments that would have saved lives and eased suffering.

It was more acceptable for pellagra to be caused by an infectious agent, which was the dominant disease theory at the time, rather than the result of poverty and a poor diet. This inverse hierarchy, in which laboratory sciences outranked social, environmental, and behavioral sciences, resulted in preventable deaths. When all the different sciences that contribute to our well-being are allowed to come together under the umbrella of public health, they improve community health on a broad scale.

Still, during the early years of the twentieth century, what we know as the modern public health movement did pick up momentum, although it rapidly lost steam because of unfounded political concerns. A coalition of health care professionals, community leaders, and reform-minded activists joined together to spearhead community-based campaigns that tackled many of the underlying social inequities that undermined health. They pushed for better housing and sanitary conditions; sponsored programs to improve maternal and child health, infectious disease control, and workplace safety; dispatched health professionals to improve school hygiene; and advocated laws and policies to ensure that foods weren't adulterated.

Among their leaders were Charles V. Chapin, Jane Addams, Alice Hamilton, and Sara Josephine Baker, the first woman to receive a doctorate in public health and the first director of New York City's Bureau of Child Hygiene. Because of Baker's unstinting efforts in promoting programs to improve maternal and child health, New York had the lowest infant mortality rates of any major American city. Their work reflected the policies of fairness, inclusion, and social justice of the Progressive era championed by politicians like President Theodore Roosevelt; their credo, historians noted, was "public need over private greed."

But all that soon changed. In the wake of the Russian Revolution in 1917, which raised the threat of Bolshevism in the United States, many of these programs were condemned as "socialized medicine" and attempts to "Russianize" the U.S. By the 1920s, a conservative tide had swept across the country and Republicans captured Congress and the White House. A swelling backlash against the reforms of the Progressive era, along with the increased political clout of the medical establishment, accelerated public health's retreat from the community.

In the first wave of attacks, in 1920, the New York Medical Society defeated a proposal for a system of public rural clinics throughout the state. One of the great achievements of the Progressive era was the Sheppard–Towner Act in 1921, which provided funds to the states for prenatal and child health centers staffed by female physicians and public health nurses. The AMA blasted this as an "imported socialist scheme" and, by 1927, had persuaded Congress to axe the legislation. In short order, school-based nursing, outpatient pharmacy dispensaries, and clinics that provided care for pregnant women were all stripped of funding.

This right-wing shift was fueled by clashes that are echoed by the same issues we're grappling with today. Between 1880 and 1920, more than 24 million immigrants arrived in the United States. They faced the same horrific living conditions that earlier generations of destitute Americans had: filthy streets, dangerous workplaces, derelict tenements, and overcrowded schools where germs spread swiftly.

Conservative politicians fanned the flames of resentment and painted this influx of newcomers as perilous threats or "idiots and insane persons . . . likely to become a public charge." The growing "slums of large cities were 'breeding grounds' that were 'seeded' with bacilli waiting to infect the susceptible victim," according to public health historians Elizabeth Fee and Theodore Brown. This new wave of immigrants, who were mostly from poorer regions of southern and eastern Europe, were seen as biologically inferior, and described as "swarthy," "squalid," or of "bad stock," in much the same way people of color were demonized. Instead of creating more healthful environments, it was easier to scapegoat them, and to "otherize" foreigners by painting them as insidious carriers of lethal pathogens and infections. This was the era of the resurgence of the Ku Klux Klan in 1915, and the Palmer Raids, when U.S. Attorney General A. Mitchell Palmer launched attacks on what he called "foreign-born subversives and agitators"; in 1920, federal agents arrested thousands of immigrants (estimates vary between 3,000 and 10,000), most of whom were deported.

Sadly, this politicization of public health would repeat itself time and again in the decades that followed. Over the last century, these politicians learned that their anti-science messaging plays well with their constituents. We saw that most recently when Covid was first labeled as a "Chinese virus" and there were threats against Americans of Asian descent, and with our own generation's anti-science conservatives crusading against lifesaving Covid vaccine mandates—

including some governors who turned their biases into policy. But how many people died needlessly because of these policies? How many succumbed to Covid because they refused to get a shot or wear a mask?

While science is rigorously non-partisan, the facts are inescapable: During the pandemic, more Democrats survived than Republicans, even when they were demographically matched and living side by side in ruby-red states, according to an eye-opening 2022 study conducted by Yale University scientists. Researchers looked at what's called excess death rates—the percent increase in deaths above pre-Covid levels—between those registered as either Republicans or Democrats in counties in Florida and Ohio. Before vaccines, there was a 1.6-percentage-point difference between the red and the blue, with Republicans having a negligibly higher death rate. Once vaccines were available, that divide sharply widened to 10.4 percentage points. This is a stark illustration of just how irrational politicians can be, and how those who blindly follow their rhetoric often pay the greatest price—with their lives.

The early-twentieth-century campaign to undermine public health initiatives also worked only too well. By the 1930s, only 3.3 cents of the medical dollar was spent on public health, with healthy chunks divvied up between physicians (29.8 cents), hospitals (23.4), and medicines (18.4). Public health suffered gravely from these political attacks. "Yet it had been clear, long before," according to historian Paul Starr, "that public health in America was relegated to a secondary status: less prestigious than clinical medicine, less amply financed and blocked from assuming the higher-level functions of coordination and direction." Fee and Brown conclude that "the great public health surge that had crested in the Progressive Era, like the economy, crashed in the 1920s."

Nearly a century later, the field has still not recovered.

CHAPTER FOUR

W.E.B. Du Bois, the Myth of Racial Inferiority, and the Slave Health Deficit

"The slave health deficit has never been made up and today it is euphemistically known as health disparities."

—DR. W. MICHAEL BYRD

I N JUNE OF 1896, W.E.B. DU BOIS RECEIVED A TELEGRAM THAT changed his life. It was from Charles C. Harrison, a retired sugar magnate and provost of the University of Pennsylvania, on behalf of a group of civic leaders and scholars, offering him a job to determine the "present actual conditions" of Black Americans living in Philadelphia's Seventh Ward. They wanted to know why Black residents in Philadelphia weren't doing well economically, and what could be done to improve their situation.

The invitation was a lifeline for the Harvard-educated twenty-eight-year-old social scientist, who had been languishing in a professional wilderness teaching classics at Wilberforce University, a small Black school in rural Ohio. When he was summoned by the cadre of high-profile progressives in Philadelphia, however, Du Bois knew he faced a daunting task because the answer to their questions was blindingly obvious—it was the color line that thwarted the city's Black residents at every conceivable turn. He would be battling gale-force headwinds to combat the deeply ingrained stereotypes about Black Americans and their "savage nature" that had been used to perpetuate white supremacy for hundreds of years.

Susan Wharton, a wealthy Quaker and prominent social activist with deep ties to the university, had done charitable work in the Seventh Ward. In the fall of 1895, she convened a meeting in her family's townhouse not far from the center of the so-called "Negro ghetto," gathering influential members of the city's Black community, prominent white leaders, and a representative from the University of Pennsylvania.

They discussed conducting a full house-to-house investigation into what was causing all the troubles. But their motives were hardly altruistic. Wharton and other Progressives viewed the rampant criminality and venality of the poverty-stricken community as a Black plague, "a virus to be quarantined," according to David Levering Lewis in his Pulitzer Prize–winning biography *W.E.B. Du Bois*. Their real agenda was to use the cover of quasi-science to enact stern measures to contain these deplorable conditions—and presumably the people who lived in them—and prevent them from infecting polite society.

But Du Bois had an entirely different agenda, one that only someone of his prodigious intellect and self-confidence would attempt. He wanted to turn around the racial paradigm and challenge centuries of thinking about the health of Black Americans. In the accepted wisdom of that era—which certainly has its echoes today—the illnesses, vulnerability to disease, and early deaths of Black Philadelphians were their own fault, the result of moral failings and inborn inferiority, not societal forces over which they had little control. This absolved civic leaders of any responsibility for the abysmal state of one of their city's communities. And what better way to prove their case than to have Harvard's first Black PhD make it for them?

Du Bois set out to prove them wrong. The groundbreaking research he did that year rescued him from obscurity and established his reputation as one of the nation's most eminent scholars; he is widely considered the founding father of social epidemiology. His seminal study became arguably the first in the world to meticulously document the effects of racism on health, and it laid the groundwork for our contemporary understanding of how social inequities, and not personal failings, are often largely responsible for communities facing dismal circumstances and poor health.

Data made the difference. In those days, it was convenient for even scientists and doctors to cling to unscientific ways of thinking—not just about race but also in matters of class, gender, ethnicity, and national origin—that were steeped in racism and social Darwinism because of the lack of insight into the reality of the poor's circumstances. In the absence of data, it's easy to look at how poor people were living and blame them for their unhygienic conditions; easy to conclude that somehow it's their own fault and the result of moral failings, or because they're genetically inferior. These attitudes persist to this day, reminiscent of the arguments made by J.D. Vance in *Hillbilly Elegy*, about Appalachian poverty.

But what Du Bois did was revolutionary. He provided a three-dimensional glimpse into the reality of these people's lives and backed it up with the data to illuminate the challenges they faced on a routine basis, in housing insecurity, for example, or because they worked at jobs that kept them from caring for their children in ways that they knew how to because they couldn't afford to miss a day of work to see a doctor. What looks like laziness might be that people aren't getting much sleep because they're working two or three jobs. The well-heeled take such things as sleep for granted because they're insulated from the daily indignities and limitations of poverty. "Othering" happens for all sorts of reasons, but sometimes it's unintentional because there is no chance of ever "walking a day in my shoes." The more removed someone is, the less likely it is for them to see another group as citizens like themselves who merely lack the agency to, say, work from home during the pandemic or miss a day's work to go to a well-baby checkup. This is the fundamental argument of Matthew Desmond's brilliant text *Poverty, by America,* in which he writes that "choice"—possessing that agency—"is the antidote for exploitation." This is why we need public health programs and policies that disrupt, not accommodate, poverty.

This is what differentiates public health from clinical care: It is holistic and gathers the data that looks at the lived experience of the vulnerable. The emergence of social science researchers like Du Bois and their rigorous data collection—all aimed at solving problems and creating the conditions for human thriving—largely put to rest those spurious arguments about moral failings and inherent inferiority that justified racial and social injustices. The truth is the prerequisite to any prevention or healing—but first, the problem must be understood. That required the use of science-driven protocols to make medicine useful, but the science had to be married with an appreciation of the social determinants of health.

Du Bois and his wife, Nina, his bride of three months, arrived in Philadelphia in late summer of 1896 and moved into a one-room apartment at 617 Carver Street in the College Settlement House at the edge of the Seventh Ward. They were immediately struck by the stark contrast between their old neighborhood in Ohio and their new neighborhood, with its diverse and impoverished Black population and the constant threat of violence. "Murder sat at our doorsteps, police were our government, and philanthropy dropped in with periodic advice," he later wrote. They found themselves surrounded by "an atmosphere of dirt, drunkenness, poverty, and crime."

Economic opportunities in the decades after the Civil War had prompted a mass migration of Black Americans to Philadelphia. They were also escaping from Southern violence, and they numbered 43,000 in a city of more than one million. Black residents were relegated to the worst schools and jobs, and even those who were well-educated found themselves limited to low-skilled and low-paying occupations. Because of segregation, and landlords' refusal to rent to them in middle-class communities, they were forced to live in unsafe and unsanitary homes in unhealthy neighborhoods scattered across the city. But many of them were crowded into the dense Seventh Ward, where they were forced to pay relatively higher rents and live in run-down dwellings because of the scarcity of housing available to Black people in the city. Landlords refused to make needed repairs, because they knew their Black tenants had no other choice. Unfortunately, we can draw a direct line from the late-1800s Philadelphia ghettos, through the troubled neighborhoods the writer Richard Wright encountered in Chicago and New York City that he so poignantly described in *12 Million Black Voices,* to Matthew Desmond's recent texts, *Evicted* and *Poverty, by America,* which reflect twenty-first-century impoverishment.

Although he was still in his twenties, Du Bois already possessed a stellar résumé. William Edward Burghardt Du Bois was born just three years after the end of the Civil War, in 1868, in Great Barrington, a bucolic hamlet in the Berkshires, in the southwest corner of Massachusetts in the Housatonic River valley. The area had been settled by colonists in the early 1700s, and his mother's family had lived for more than a century in the predominately white region, which had a population of about five thousand at the time. His father was from Haiti, and on his mother's side, he was a descendant of a West African named "Tom," who was kidnapped by Dutch slave traders. Tom later fought for the Americans in the Revolutionary War, which probably enabled him to gain his freedom.

Although Du Bois was the only Black pupil in his high school and there were perhaps two dozen African American families in the town, he was well liked by schoolmates and became the class valedictorian. But even as a young boy, he was keenly aware that he was not like them. "It dawned upon me with a certain suddenness that I was different from the others; or like, mayhap, in heart and life and longing, but shut out from their world by a vast veil," he wrote in an 1897 essay for *The Atlantic Monthly* that would later become the basis for his book *The Souls of Black Folk.* "The world I longed for, and all its dazzling opportunities were theirs, not mine."

His school's principal, Frank Hosmer, recognized his exceptional talent and raised money from local civic leaders to enable the gifted teenager to attend Fisk University, a historically Black college in Nashville, Tennessee, founded just after the Civil War. He yearned to attend Harvard but had no money, and he worked in construction for a year to earn enough to fulfill his dream. After getting his bachelor's degree at Fisk, he was admitted to Harvard as a junior. He graduated cum laude in 1890, and in 1895, he became Harvard's first Black PhD after completing his dissertation on the United States and the African slave trade. Du Bois was intimately familiar with this long and sordid history, and in his work in Philadelphia, he knew he'd have to find a way to counteract centuries of poisonous lies.

Europeans who hunted and sold human beings and plundered the African continent justified their legalized system of kidnapping, assault, child abuse, rape, torture, and murder under the shroud of religion, namely that God wanted Christians to enslave infidels. But in the supposedly more enlightened era of the nineteenth century, they turned to science. Racial disparities in health, they claimed, stemmed from fixed biological differences—Blacks were inferior intellectually and physically, they argued, and might even be a different species. "Pro-slavery politicians therefore began trumpeting scientific proof of Black inferiority not because they suddenly thought science should rule society," noted Nancy Krieger, a professor of social epidemiology at the Harvard T.H. Chan School of Public Health, in the *International Journal of Social Determinants of Health and Health Services*, "but because science alone could lend a legitimacy and authority capable of offsetting the abolitionists' moral and religious clout."

These debates reached a crescendo in the 1840s and 1850s, when the question of slavery polarized even the medical profession. For Southern physicians, slavery was a cash cow, enabling them to liberally supplement their income by being on retainer at plantations or in the auction houses. But even in the North, physicians made their money treating wealthy merchants and landowners, and there wasn't any financial incentive in siding with the reviled abolitionists and challenging the so-called scientific basis of slavery.

Perhaps the most notorious of these racist apologists was Dr. Samuel Cartwright, a prominent Southern physician in Natchez, Mississippi, whose patients included his friend Jefferson Davis, who would later become president of the Confederacy. While at Tulane University in New Orleans in the late 1840s, he was asked by a Louisiana medical committee to perform an analysis of "the diseases and peculiarities of our negro population."

In examining the anatomical and physiological differences between the Negro and the white man, he concluded that Black Americans, because of their allegedly smaller brains and blood vessels—what Cartwright called "defective hematosis" coupled with a "deficiency of cerebral matter in the cranium"—were unable to take care of themselves. Enslaved Americans' repeated attempts to escape barbaric treatment—which would be the reasonable reaction of any sane person to the savagery of bondage—were actually the result of an illness that Cartwright labeled "drapetomania," which is a combination of two Greek terms, *drapetes,* a runaway, and *mania,* madness. Freedom, he maintained, "was actually poisonous to [the] happiness [of the Negro race]." While these declarations seem ludicrous today, Cartwright was considered a legitimate scientist.

Even John C. Calhoun, the virulently racist senator from South Carolina and former U.S. vice president who favored secession, went so far as to say that Blacks were better off during slavery. Using the 1840 census, he reported that Africans' health deteriorated once they were emancipated and that data indicated that Blacks in the North had higher insanity rates. Calhoun proclaimed this was "proof" that "the African is incapable of self-care and sinks into lunacy under the burden of freedom."

Other physicians, however, like Dr. Samuel Forry, editor of the *New York Journal of Medicine,* demonstrated that the interpretation of the data was fraudulent and that Northern Black insanity rates had been greatly inflated, especially given the Southern tendency to treat insubordination as proof of an enslaved person's madness. In the run-up to the Civil War, the pro-slavery argument seemed to win the day. But there was growing pushback led by the first generation of Black physicians, whose pioneering research in the face of intense resistance laid the groundwork for Du Bois's seminal work.

The most prominent of Du Bois's intellectual influences was James McCune Smith. Brilliant and uncompromising, Smith was a public intellectual with the distinction of being the United States' first university-trained Black doctor. In 1846, in a stinging and exhaustively researched rebuttal, he showed how John Calhoun's racist analysis was spurious. Using the relatively new field of biostatistics, along with demographics, he exposed the Southern senator's questionable claims. Specifically, he did a spatial analysis using latitude coordinates to show that Black people lived longer in states that abolished slavery, like New Hampshire and Connecticut, than in Georgia where slavery was legal. He also stratified mortality rates by age, race, and place to demonstrate that Black people in New England lived longer than those in the South. And finally, he showed that racial differences in longevity were due to socioeconomic factors and were not inherently biological. "There are sufficient grounds for the belief that the slaves . . . under all [their] disadvantages, would, if freed from slavery, attain a longevity not very much below that attained by the Europe-American population."

James McCune Smith was born in 1813 and grew up in the Five Points neighborhood in New York City. He was the son of a South Carolina enslaved woman who fled to New York to escape his father, a wealthy merchant named Samuel Smith who enslaved them both. Young James and his mother lived in constant fear that the slave hunters who patrolled his neighborhood would recapture them. Despite his difficult childhood, his intellectual gifts were obvious.

He graduated from the first African Free School, which was funded by the New York Manumission Society, a wealthy group of progressive white men that included Alexander Hamilton and John Jay, but was denied admission to Geneva Medical College (later part of Syracuse University) and Columbia University because he was Black. So benefactors from his days at the African Free School paid for him to attend the University of Glasgow in Scotland, then one of the premier academic medical institutions in the world. He graduated at the top of his class, earning a BA in 1835, an MA in 1836, and a medical degree the following year. Later, a hall at the school would be named after him.

Throughout his life, McCune Smith was a fierce and fearless advocate for the less fortunate. As a young medical student in Glasgow, he was horrified to discover that a senior physician at the hospital where he was training was treating impoverished women suffering from gonorrhea with silver nitrate. This was normally used in low concentrations as a topical treatment, but his superior, Alexander Hannay, was using it full strength internally, which may have resulted in several deaths. McCune Smith exposed the more powerful physician, in two articles in the weekly science journal, *The London Medical Gazette,* risking his career and jeopardizing his own future. This was certainly not the first, nor would it be the last, time one of our public health warriors took steps toward justice at great personal cost.

McCune Smith never shied away from controversy. In 1859, as the country teetered on the brink of war, he took on one of our most revered founding fathers, Thomas Jefferson, an esteemed intellectual and enslaver who played an early and influential role in the spread of these toxic myths. In 1787, a decade after he helped write the Declaration of Independence, the second president published his widely read treatise *Notes on the State of Virginia,* in which he questioned whether enslaved people could ever be equal to whites, and advanced his theory that Blacks were inherently inferior, fit to be field hands and little else. The book was perhaps the most damaging and enduring instance of scientific racism in American history, according to historian Ibram X. Kendi.

In his own highly influential pamphlet, McCune Smith refuted Jefferson's famous query as to whether Blacks and whites could ever live together, and he even challenged the notion of race as a distinct biological category, an assertion that wouldn't gain common currency for more than a century. Smith began to advance the idea of what we would later call social determinants of health: namely that someone's health status is largely influenced by the strata of society in which they live, and not because of some innate weakness or strength.

In the U.S., James McCune Smith was virtually a lone voice, drowned out by the racism deeply embedded in the medical field. In Europe, however, reform-minded doctors had begun to look at the social origins of illness and the relationship between the social environment and health. Rudolf Virchow, a doctor in Prussia in the mid-nineteenth century, spearheaded the social-medicine movement.

Virchow already had a reputation as a social reformer and outspoken advocate for public health when he was commissioned in 1848 by the Prussian government to investigate an outbreak of typhus in Upper Silesia, an impoverished region in Eastern Europe where mine workers were being ruthlessly exploited. Typhus had ravaged the local population, and tens of thousands of people died because of the twin epidemics of starvation and disease. Virchow was convinced that typhus had been allowed to race unchecked through the community because poor diets, poverty, illiteracy, and squalid living conditions had made the people more vulnerable to illness—and not because of their "sinfulness" or some inherent inferiority.

After surveying the destruction that had orphaned thousands of children, Virchow produced a blistering indictment of the civil servants whose negligence contributed to "the enormous compilations of misery" that were disturbingly reminiscent of what had happened during the previous decade's cholera epidemics. "The plutocracy, which draw very large amounts from the Upper Silesian mines, did not recognize Upper Silesians as human beings, but only as tools," he wrote in his report, which blamed the outbreak on social conditions and the government. Virchow went on to become one of the most influential physician scientists of the nineteenth century, and his pioneering research helped build the scaffolding of his nation's modern public health system.

On the other side of the Atlantic, James McCune Smith would spend much of his career as the physician for the Colored Orphan

Asylum in Midtown Manhattan, which was founded in 1836. He worked tirelessly for his young charges, some of whom were dying from measles, smallpox, and tuberculosis. Some of them were there because their parents had died or because they could not take care of them. McCune Smith wrote rigorous research articles debunking phrenology, a pseudoscience that claimed that an individual's intellectual capacity is determined by the size of their skull, and homeopathy, which he called "the most deadly quackery that curses the nineteenth century." He died shortly after the end of the Civil War, in November of 1865, three years before the birth of the man who would become his intellectual heir and carry on his legacy of social activism: W.E.B. Du Bois.

When Du Bois began his fieldwork in the shadow of post-Reconstruction America, there was a new and even more virulent strain of racism emerging that perpetuated toxic myths about race under the cloak of science: eugenics. The basic premise of eugenics is that racial and ethnic differences are due to genetic differences—and that undesirable traits like "feeble-mindedness" and poverty were inherited. Society would be better served by "thinning the herd," a social Darwinist idea that was used as the pretext for barbaric acts like the sterilization of thousands of poor women of color—the so-called "Mississippi Appendectomies"—and was later championed by Adolf Hitler, whose quest to build an Aryan master race led to the extermination of millions of Jews, Gypsies, homosexuals, Slavic prisoners of war, and other "undesirables" in the 1940s.

This was the context in which Du Bois began his work. He knew that the only way to combat the ideas of inherent inferiority—ideas that even his seemingly progressive sponsors might hold implicitly—was to use the tools of sociological research to document the conditions of the neighborhood. "My vision was becoming clear," he wrote in his memoir *Dusk of Dawn*. "The Negro problem was in my mind a matter of systematic investigation and intelligent understanding. The world was thinking wrong about race, because it did not know. The ultimate evil was stupidity. The cure for it was knowledge based on scientific investigation."

Despite the fact that he wasn't given an office or even an academic title, on August 1, 1896, he started work, canvassing door to door for eight hours each day, talking to local residents about their work lives and families. Although he was initially frightened by the rumors of violence that hung in the air, what he discovered surprised him. Even though the ward was poor, it pulsated with life. There were nearly two dozen restaurants and taverns, thirteen grocery stores, a handful of bicycle shops, three bakeries, a hardware and furniture store, and four mortuaries, including two establishments run by women. There were more than a dozen schools in the ward staffed by sixty-four teachers, and about 86 percent of school-age children attended.

The diminutive scientist—he was only 5'6"—cut a striking figure in his dapper three-piece suit, top hat, and cane. Sitting in the parlors, kitchens, and living rooms of his subjects enabled Du Bois to inspect their residences and witness firsthand the reality of their living conditions. Over a three-month period of field research, he spent more than eight hundred hours and spoke with approximately 2,500 households in his investigation. He augmented his research by combing through background materials from Philadelphia libraries—including the private libraries of some of the more well-off locals—finding colonial records, manuscripts, biographies, legal documents, newspaper articles, correspondence, and other publications to corroborate his work.

His exhaustive research of census data revealed that Black Philadelphians were dying of several common maladies, including pneumonia and tuberculosis, at a rate two times higher than their white neighbors were. The gap in infant and childhood mortality was huge: Black Philadelphians were twice as likely to die before the age of fifteen as their white counterparts. But his greatest achievement was proving that racial differences in health were primarily due to social, not biological factors; they were the inevitable consequence of the "vastly different conditions" of living between whites and Blacks. Only about one in eight of the dwellings in the Seventh Ward had access to bathrooms and toilets or even hot water, because the area was in an older part of the city that lacked indoor plumbing. Families were often crammed into one room, with four or five people sharing the space, and some were forced to take in itinerant borders, many of them newly arrived from the South, to help defray expenses. Residents did the best they could under difficult circumstances, building outhouses or makeshift latrines in hallways that were shared communally.

While tuberculosis was the leading cause of death for Blacks in Philadelphia, the chief culprits behind the excess death rates were primarily environmental, such as bad ventilation and lack of protection against the dampness and cold. Being forced to live in the most unsanitary places in the city was making Black Philadelphians more vulnerable to highly contagious infectious diseases like tuberculosis, Du Bois noted—not some inherent inferiority. Especially significant is that he found that death rates were higher in the Fifth Ward, "the worst Negro slum in the city and the worst part of the city in respect to sanitation," he wrote, than in the predominately Black Thirtieth Ward, which had "good houses and clean streets," a finding that added further weight to the fact that their skin color was not the cause of their poor health.

Even more eye-opening: Du Bois documented that life expectancy for Blacks was between 30 and 32 years in 1900, compared to 49.6 years for whites; poverty, segregation, and lack of access to doctors and health care facilities effectively excluded them from the health-care system. "The most difficult social problem in the matter of Negro health is the peculiar attitude of the nation toward the well-being of the race," he noted. "There have been few other cases in the history of civilized peoples where human suffering has been viewed with such peculiar indifference."

Du Bois's ultimate report was a subversive text because it went far beyond the scope of his original mission, which was simply to provide a quasi-scientific cover for his elite sponsors' barely concealed contempt and their devious plans to subjugate the residents of the Seventh Ward. His vision and execution of a disciplined research plan enabled him to build a holistic and scientific foundation that could upend centuries of structural racism and dehumanization that robbed marginalized groups of their humanity. He didn't just chronicle the miserable aspects of the neighborhood, but offered a reason why the houses were so filthy and their lives sometimes chaotic: Whatever was plaguing the community was a symptom of the despair of racism. What makes his beautiful work so powerful, and what is at the heart of it, is that it not only looks at the historical roots of his subjects' struggles but goes beyond the basics of data science and embraces their deep humanity in all its beauty, culture, possibilities, and messy splendor.

He discovered that these people were hardly down and out. "Behind the veil, you find a city within a city, with its own ecosystems that had different class hierarchies and different occupations, and different educational levels," said Marcus Hunter, a professor of sociology and African American studies at UCLA. "He felt it would be a disservice to that community to not amplify all its diverse dynamics. Essentially, what he was saying is look at what these people are doing without any resources. Imagine if you actually fulfilled your duty of giving them resources, how they could actually live."

Du Bois's groundbreaking work *The Philadelphia Negro,* which was published in 1899, established his reputation as one of the United States' premier intellectuals, a voice for "his people," as commentators would later say. But beyond that, his study is considered a foundational text in the then-nascent field of sociology and statistical research. Du Bois was unflinching in his condemnation of the social forces that created the so-called "Negro Problem." The poverty, disease, crime, and frail family structure that still hadn't recovered from centuries of slavery were largely the result of racial prejudice that cut off opportunities, he maintained: "How long can a city teach its black children that the road to success is to have a white face?"

Despite his prodigious achievement, however, a permanent faculty appointment to the University of Pennsylvania was not forthcoming. Even though his report was warmly received by the intellectual elite, did it make any real difference? And did the studies, conferences, and organizations that followed? In Philadelphia, at least, more investigative reports were commissioned on the plight of the Seventh Ward, which one newspaper called "Hell's Acre," and they only confirmed, decades later, what Du Bois had uncovered: Housing continued to be dilapidated and overcrowded, with leaky roofs, peeling paint and plaster, and no heat; sanitary equipment didn't work; there were no adequate water or toilet facilities, and many rooms were windowless and without ventilation. By 1936, some of the buildings had become so decrepit that one of them collapsed right before Christmas and seven people died. "There were no meaningful interventions or programs developed following his recommendations," said UCLA's Hunter. "But the time he spent in Philadelphia forever changed him and informed and influenced everything he wrote afterwards."

In 1897, shortly after completing his fieldwork, Du Bois accepted a position at Atlanta University, where he taught sociology. In May of 1899, the same year that the publication of his landmark study made him an academic celebrity, in a cruel twist of fate, Du Bois found himself in a predicament similar to that of many of the people he interviewed. His only son, Burghardt Gomer Du Bois, was stricken with diphtheria. Called "the strangling angel of children," the bacterial infection triggers high fevers and a thickening of the throat, which constricts the windpipe and causes death from asphyxiation. An effective diphtheria antitoxin had been developed by a German and a Japanese scientist in 1890, and by 1897, it was available in places like New York.

But in Atlanta, a city that had been a stronghold of the Confederacy, white physicians refused to treat Du Bois's desperately ill two-year-old. Du Bois spent a frantic night searching for a Black physician who could help him. Du Bois's brilliance, his glossy résumé, and his extensive social network didn't matter when it truly counted; he was still just another Black father powerless to save his sick child, whose death may have been preventable. His wife Nina's intense dislike for the racist, sharply segregated city curdled "into bitter loathing," in the words of David Levering Lewis. While she understood his need to earn a living, she never truly forgave him for relocating the family to a place where there were hardly any Black physicians.

In response to the growing violence and deteriorating status of Black Americans in the early twentieth century as Jim Crow tightened its grip throughout the South and scientific racism grew in the North, Du Bois helped found the NAACP in 1909. He remained a fierce and passionate civil rights activist as well as a leading scholar throughout the rest of his long life. Frustrated and disillusioned by America, when his passport was confiscated—he was a victim of the anticommunist witch hunts of the McCarthy era—he accepted the invitation of President Kwame Nkrumah, a University of Pennsylvania alumnus, and moved to the newly independent nation of Ghana in 1961. He died in that country's capital, Accra, at age ninety-five on the day before the historic 1963 March on Washington, which was the decades-long culmination of the movement he helped inspire.

Du Bois's landmark work paved the way for research that has deepened our understanding of the crucial role that social determinants play in our health—not just present-day social determinants, but the ones we inherit. For Black Americans, this means that poor health outcomes are not due to biology or simply an unfortunate circumstantial accident, but the direct result of the legacy of slavery and racism. Aside from momentary periods of reform, during Reconstruction after the Civil War with the short-lived Freedmen's Bureau and in the programs spawned by the Civil Rights era of the 1960s, Black Americans have been subjected to second-class care, if any, since arriving in the United States from Africa.

The concept of slave health deficits—that starting with the trans-Atlantic slave trade, centuries of slavery, institutionalized neglect, and deep disparities in health care have never been corrected—is a term coined by Dr. W. Michael Byrd, a physician and medical historian, and later, his wife, Dr. Linda A. Clayton, a gynecologic oncologist and health-care policy expert, to identify the origins of the vast public health gaps between Blacks and whites. "Trapped in his segregated, inferior health system, the Negro never made up his slave health deficits," wrote Byrd in an editorial in the *Journal of the National Medical Association.* "And he suffers health discrimination to the present day in the bottom half of a 'dual,' unequal, sometimes cruel health system."

The couple's trailblazing research was sparked by their own personal experience. Byrd was born in 1943 in Galveston, Texas, and after earning his medical degree in 1968 from Meharry Medical College in Nashville, he served in Vietnam as a U.S. Army battalion surgeon and was awarded the Bronze Star. But he had learned about the horrors of slavery firsthand through his great grandmother, who was born into enslavement and emancipated in childhood. But, Byrd thought, those days were long in the past, so why were so many African Americans still suffering from poor health? Clayton, who received her MD from Duke University, had similar questions. Her grandfather had also been emancipated as a young boy. However, when she was growing up, she saw serious deficiencies in care for Black Americans, even for middle-class people in her own family who had the resources to pay for adequate care. An aunt perished in childbirth, while two of Clayton's siblings contracted polio and couldn't get decent treatment. Her mother was misdiagnosed and died young of a cancer that might have been controlled if caught earlier.

In 1988, the couple met when they were both on the faculty of Meharry Medical College. Byrd had already spent two decades researching the underlying reasons for what he described as "the shockingly poor states of health of Black America." The two joined forces, and their analysis of the role that race played in medicine in the U.S. resulted in a series of influential papers, published in a two-volume work called *An American Health Dilemma,* which inspired changes in governmental policies.

These deep-seated inequities were rooted in events that had occurred centuries ago, according to Byrd and Clayton. Enslaved people who survived the traumatic and disease-ridden Middle Passage, which exposed Black Africans to dysentery, malaria, scurvy, and typhoid fever as well as tortuous whippings and imprisonment in shackles, were sentenced to a lifetime of enduring unsanitary and cruel conditions with virtually no health care. Byrd and Clayton traced the shocking mortality rates that marked this experience: It started with the coastal African slave trade, with a death rate of at least 25 percent, combined with an estimated 15 to 50 percent slave mortality during the voyage across the Atlantic to the New World, followed by a "breaking-in period" death rate of 30 to 50 percent. "This entire process established the 'slave health deficit' that was perpetuated in America," Byrd said in a 2016 lecture at Boston University. "The slave health deficit has never been made up, and today it is euphemistically known as health disparities."

Their historical overview of how the public health and medical systems have consistently failed Black Americans, coupled with their in-depth statistical analysis of the vast gulf between Black and white health, was an explicit condemnation of the white medical establishment's complicity. Whereas the myth of racial inferiority came from colonialists, slave traders, plantation owners, and their brutal minions like the Ku Klux Klan, the supposed scientific establishment were the ones who helped establish the slave system, added to the pseudoscience of racial inferiority, and created a segregated health system for Blacks and the poor.

Ironically, the movement to professionalize medicine in the early twentieth century solidified and maintained the systemic segregation of medicine that persists to this day. William Welch and his Canadian-born colleague William Osler, who are considered pioneering giants in medicine and helped found Johns Hopkins School of Medicine in 1893, spearheaded the drive to improve and standardize medical education. Their ultimately successful campaign modernized a profession that had been rife with bogus cures touted by incompetent physicians and outright quacks and was responsible for the professionalism that characterizes the practice of medicine today. But their seemingly noble efforts had unintended consequences that reverberate a century later and led directly to our failures to contain Covid.

In the early twentieth century, rapid advances in scientific knowledge about the causes and prevention of diseases fueled growing momentum to improve medical education. Osler and Welch trained in Germany under the famed Rudolf Virchow. At Hopkins, the two doctors instituted the German model of medical education, which required a university education prior to medical school admission and embraced the scientific method. They recruited Abraham Flexner, an educational reformer who had studied at Johns Hopkins. Flexner was an unlikely choice to spearhead a complete overhaul of medical education in this country because he had no medical background. He was also a virulent and unapologetic racist and sexist who thought women and Blacks had no place in medicine. His research reflected his prejudices, and we're still feeling its effects today.

Flexner traveled to all of the 155 medical schools in North America to evaluate the state of medical education, and he published his findings in what became known as the Flexner Report in 1910. The report radically transformed medical education by providing criteria to standardize and improve medical schools. In the aftermath, one-third of American medical schools, which were mostly for-profit enterprises that produced poorly trained physicians, were shuttered, paving the way for medicine to be firmly based on science rather than questionable remedies that often did more harm than good.

This was a welcome improvement, but the transition to a more professionalized medical model accelerated the retreat from the basic tenets of public health, which saw the population as the patient and took a more holistic approach to disease prevention and health promotion. Du Bois, and others before and after him, understood that several factors, ranging from housing insecurity and toxic environments to hazardous workplaces, created the conditions for poor health, which meant that the solutions to improve health across the board for everyone, and for the common good, required working on several fronts. But in professionalizing medicine, we began to define health education and health practice along narrow, rigid, academic disciplinary lines. Clinicians treating infectious diseases, for example, were only battling a single disease-causing pathogen, in direct contrast to social scientists like Du Bois, who were looking at a more holistic web of the root causes of poor health and premature mortality.

That's the key difference between clinical medicine and public health, which emphasizes prevention as much as treatment. Science-driven protocols make medicine more useful and effective, but they need to be augmented with an appreciation and recognition of the importance of the social determinants of health. As the field of medicine has developed, we have undervalued, and under-invested in, the contributions of scientists like McCune Smith and Du Bois. A pecking order has given too much weight to the hyper-specialized and hyper-technical way that medicine has evolved. In this way, we have become less effective, less aware, and less incentivized to support the work that Du Bois and others knew to be real.

Closing dozens of medical schools also turned out to be a grievous development for Black Americans, and we continue to experience the fallout from this seismic shift. All but two of the seven medical schools that trained Black Americans—Howard and Meharry—were shut down. Most Black medical schools of that era educated students from rural, low-income communities, and they did not have the resources or philanthropic backing necessary to implement the rigorous standards that Flexner called for in his report.

Historically, white physicians barred Black doctors from practicing and training in their facilities. This meant that Howard and Meharry were forced to produce enough doctors to serve the ten million African Americans living in the country at the time, which drastically reduced the number of Black doctors in the training pipeline. More than a hundred years later, we're still trying to make up for the ripple effects of this. Today, Black physicians comprise only 7 percent of the workforce, even though Black Americans account for 13 percent of the population. "The Flexner report was a catalyst," Dr. Wayne Frederick, president of Howard University, said in a recent interview. "It started us down a road that is hard to undo."

Hospitals and doctor's offices are no longer segregated, but the shortage of Black physicians is an ongoing crisis and contributes to the stubbornly persistent health inequities. That's because when Black people are treated by Black physicians, they live longer, healthier lives and their mortality rates plummet, according to a groundbreaking national analysis in 2023 that appeared in the *Journal of the American Medical Association* (*JAMA*). Experts say this finding provides the strongest evidence yet that a diverse workforce may be key to ending the racial health disparities. This study comes on top of previous research showing that when Black patients were treated by Black physicians, they were more satisfied with their health care, more likely to receive preventive care, and more willing to follow doctors' orders about tests and vaccinations.

There are numerous reasons why this happens. Black physicians are more likely to work in underserved areas, the *JAMA* study showed, and a more diverse workforce improves community level access. But perhaps the most important factor, researchers found, was something W.E.B. Du Bois uncovered more than a century ago: When doctors, or scientists for that matter, have skin in the game, when they come from similar backgrounds and have had similar life experiences, they're more sensitive to the challenges their patients face, and they listen more closely and sympathetically to their complaints. Although Du Bois was Harvard-educated, he was keenly aware that he faced discrimination in his daily life, most notably in the poignant and untimely death of his son, and this made him better able to recognize and appreciate the humanity of the less fortunate.

In my own experience, medical professionals from more diverse backgrounds have a more holistic grasp of what the drivers of health are, and they bring a certain compassion and understanding that doesn't blame the vulnerable for the conditions they ended up with because of forces outside their control. And in listening to the complaints of my colleagues of color, I heard a strikingly familiar litany:

Many of them went into medicine because of the poor treatment or misdiagnosis that their mother/father/brother received at the hands of insensitive or even callous white male doctors who dismissed their very real symptoms, which often resulted in unnecessary suffering and death.

But even today, the shortages continue because aspiring young Black doctors face significant structural barriers throughout the educational pipeline. They start with inferior schools, and continue with a dearth of mentors, role models, and science-preparatory experiences once they are in high school and college. Also, increasingly high costs put a medical school education out of reach for many Black Americans.

Moreover, racism remains a real part of medical school experiences for students of color who attend predominately white institutions, and many choose to attend historically Black institutions to avoid these prejudices. Major philanthropists such as Michael Bloomberg, who donated $600 million to the nation's four historically Black medical schools in 2024, recognize the need to invest in training Black doctors. But that alone isn't enough, because the ecosystem must become a place where there is belonging and equity in educational and practice spaces.

There have been some gains in medical school education for physicians of color, but they have come at a glacial pace. In 1985, the Morehouse School of Medicine in Atlanta became fully accredited. Nearly forty years later, in 2023, Los Angeles's Charles R. Drew University of Medicine and Science welcomed its first sixty-member medical-school class, who were recruited heavily from the surrounding Black and Hispanic communities. Many of the students were the first members of their families to attend college. "We just had our white-coat ceremony," which is a rite of passage for medical students that marks their entrance into the medical profession, said Dr. Deborah Prothrow-Stith, dean and professor of medicine for the College of Medicine at Charles R. Drew University of Medicine and Science, in an interview in June of 2023. "There were over a thousand people here. The students, some of them had thirty and forty family and friends. It was just this amazing feel-good celebration for the community."

Unfortunately, the continued lack of physicians of color has contributed to the stubbornly enduring Black health crisis that was reflected in shameful numbers that shocked even Byrd and Clayton. Black people in this country suffer a grave loss in quality and length of life because of a lack of access to decent medical care and the structural racism that endures in medicine. In an analysis they conducted in the early 1990s, they discovered that Black people live five to seven years less than whites; they are stricken with cancer more frequently and die at higher rates; heart disease is twice as common in Blacks; they suffer almost half of the nation's maternal deaths, experience infant mortality rates that are as high as those in developing countries, and suffer from more than 59,000 excess deaths annually. The list goes on and on. These inequities became starkly apparent during the pandemic.

Lack of access to quality care and easy-to-see structural racism are major parts of the health-disparity equation, but there's another factor: hidden biases in our medical system. Take the high rate of kidney failure in Black Americans, which is three times that of their white counterparts. Black people do suffer from much higher incidences of hypertension and diabetes, two of the leading causes of kidney failure, but that doesn't fully account for the disparities. For decades, a key measure for calculating kidney function was the estimated glomerular filtration rate (eGFR), which measures how well the kidneys are filtering toxins. This metric had been automatically adjusted to give a higher number for Black patients because of their race. But we now understand that so-called "race" is a social construct, not a biological distinction, and that using this incorrect algorithm meant that perhaps hundreds of thousands of Black Americans' kidneys seemed healthier than they really were.

This translated to critical delays in referrals to kidney specialists and counseling to manage this chronic disease and prevent its progression to kidney failure, which can only be remedied with dialysis or a kidney transplant. In the past few years, the medical profession has agreed not to use these bogus race modifiers to calculate a patient's kidney function. But how many tens of thousands of Black Americans were misdiagnosed over all those years?

Even when something like the incidence of cancers is the same, according to Dr. Otis Brawley, former chief medical and scientific officer for the American Cancer Society, there can be a widening gap in mortality once new technologies are introduced that aren't available to poorer populations. Breast cancer is a prime example. In 1975, breast cancer mortality was the same for Black and white women. But once mammography and better treatments were developed, white breast cancer mortality dropped dramatically while the deaths of Black women, even educated middle-class women, rose for decades. It's only recently, noted Brawley, who is currently on the faculty of Johns Hopkins University, that the mortality rates of Black women have slowly dropped.

In contrast, a recent experiment conducted by Kaiser Permanente illuminated in stunning clarity how even relatively minor changes that remove racial biases and barriers can save countless lives. The health-care giant, which has twelve million members in eight states, is a closed system: Members go to Kaiser hospitals, get their prescriptions filled at Kaiser pharmacies, and are treated by health-care professionals who are on salary. There is no fee for services rendered and no insurance-company middleman—Kaiser makes its operating expenses through members' premiums. As a consequence, there is no financial incentive to perform unnecessary procedures, and there is a strong emphasis on prevention and keeping members healthy.

Research scientists in their Northern California region wanted to find out why there was such a disparity in death rates from colorectal cancers between their Black and white members. In 2009, the death rate (per 100,000) for Blacks was 54.2 versus 32.6 for whites. That same year, they instituted an organized colon cancer screening outreach program that eventually doubled the number of members getting regular colonoscopies. When detected early, colon cancer is quite treatable. The study, which was published in 2022 in *The New England Journal of Medicine,* found that within ten years, by 2019, death rates had plummeted, and disparities were virtually erased: For Black members, death rates had dropped to 20.9 compared to 19.3 for white members. The study, one of the authors noted, demonstrates that "delivering care in an equitable manner can eliminate health disparities."

Recent research has advanced our understanding of what's perpetuated these wide gulfs in health. These studies underscore public health's failures to protect vulnerable populations when they gradually moved away from implementing the costly social reforms and infrastructure projects that are crucial factors in preventing disease. The catchphrase today is that your zip code is a better predictor of your health than your genetic code. What this means in practice is that where we live, work, and play and the places that we spend most of our time, in our neighborhoods and our workplaces, have the most influence on our health. "Health is not just our biological endowment or our access to high-quality medical care, which is important," said my colleague and good friend David Williams, of the Harvard T.H. Chan School of Public Health, "but how that interacts with the conditions in which we live and work and how that shapes our opportunities to be healthy."

In simple terms, it's the difference between living in a quiet neighborhood with tree-lined streets where people are out walking their dogs before dinner, with a vibrant street life and a convenient access to doctors and hospitals, and residing in a harsh, unsafe environment with little vegetation, derelict housing, and street violence. This is compounded by long commutes to low-paying jobs, often in areas without adequate public transportation, and a lack of ready access to decent medical care or nutritious food ("food deserts"). Facing each of these stressors day in and day out has a cumulative effect over decades, resulting in high blood pressure, strokes, diabetes, obesity, and an array of other chronic illnesses that needlessly worsen because they are neglected or inadequately treated.

David Williams's own research took this one step further and drilled down to how even the routine, everyday indignities of racism can seriously undermine health. Williams, who grew up on St. Lucia in the Caribbean before emigrating to the U.S. as a young man, is intimately familiar with what a truly healthy lifestyle in a supportive social environment looks like. The differences between that and what's typical for many Black Americans could not be starker. As a Seventh-day Adventist, he did some of his early training at Loma Linda University in Loma Linda, California, an Adventist stronghold, which is about sixty miles due east of Los Angeles.

Loma Linda is a high-desert Shangri-la known as America's longevity capital and a veritable living laboratory on how to live longer, where sixty—or even eighty—is genuinely the new forty. They call this region "the other California," far removed from the sparkling beaches and glitzy sheen of the affluent coastal cities, because it is comprised of flat patches of dusty farmlands and hardscrabble suburbs covered with strip malls, cookie cutter subdivisions, big-box stores, and fast-food outlets. But Loma Linda, which was settled in the late 1800s, is an oasis of tranquility with the soothing, placid rhythms of a small town, reminiscent of Norman Rockwell's 1950s America. It's a place where centenarians can be found hiking two miles a day in the town's gently rolling hills, which are covered with desert scrub brush and tall grasses. Perhaps not surprisingly, among the first people to come here in the early twentieth century were tuberculosis patients seeking a cure in the hot, dry desert air.

Many of the residents live as much as a decade longer than their counterparts in surrounding communities, and it's not unusual to find people in their seventies and beyond doing jobs we normally associate with people half their age. The reason Loma Linda residents enjoy such longevity seems to be because of their religion: About 9,000 of Loma Linda's 22,000 residents are Seventh-day Adventists, a conservative denomination of Christianity founded in the mid-1800s that advocates cultivating a culture of healthy living.

One of the basic tenets of their faith is to treat their bodies as temples: They eat little or no meat or fish; shun smoking, alcohol, and stimulants like caffeine or even spicy condiments; get plenty of exercise; avoid stress; and live a purpose-driven life. Loma Linda University scientists have been collecting data on the benefits of the Adventist lifestyle for more than fifty years. Their early results confirmed the hazards of smoking tobacco and later on provided much of what we now know about the benefits of plant-based diets.

Williams subsequently moved to Battle Creek, Michigan, and worked at the very first Adventist Hospital, whose original medical director was Dr. John Harvey Kellogg, a self-styled health nut who invented corn flakes to provide a healthier alternative to bacon and eggs for breakfast. Williams began working with local Black residents as a community educator, but he realized that he needed to go beyond the basic bromides of health education—stress reduction, eating right, getting plenty of exercise, not smoking—and "understand the stressful circumstances, the living and social conditions that people face," he recalled. "I needed to be better able to address their social conditions."

But even in his early research, it quickly became clear that at every level of income and education, race still mattered. Even the best-off Black Americans, who are educated and successful, have a lower life expectancy than whites who only graduated from high school. Studies of the most advantaged Black women in the U.S. show that they experience higher levels of infant mortality, obesity, and hypertension than poor white women who are high school dropouts. But how do you measure racism? Or quantify its effects?

To capture these metrics, Williams devised the Everyday Discrimination Scale, which is now a widely used research tool and tracks not just the most blatant incidences of racial discrimination—being harassed or physically assaulted by police, or denied housing or a job—but the routine and often subtle indignities that can have a cumulative impact on health. The questionnaire inventories the mundane details of life—whether people dress differently because of experiences of racism, are exceptionally careful about where they go, or map out a special route driving to work. A high score on the questionnaire translates into a state of almost constant hypervigilance to guard against perceived threats.

Because of the reality of their lives, Williams's later research revealed the complex pathways by which racism adversely impacts health, even among those who enjoy a comfortable standard of living. He found that for both Black Americans and U.S.-born Latinos, chronic stress is simply a fact of life, and they encounter more stressful life events than their white counterparts: They're more likely to experience the death of a loved one, unemployment, difficulties making ends meet at the end of the month and other financial anxieties, troubles at work, and problems in relationships. "Stress is a normal part of life, but when it is a persistent daily experience, it exceeds our ability to cope," Williams observed. "The result leads to increased high blood pressure, heart disease, obesity, diabetes, and other health problems."

This ongoing, chronic onslaught of psychosocial stressors ages Black Americans prematurely. Research shows that the bodies of Black Americans at midlife, in standard measures of health such as blood pressure and cholesterol, have aged the equivalent of ten years faster than those of their white counterparts. Black Americans also contract serious diseases sooner, resulting in 96,800 annual deaths that would not have happened if they fell ill at the same rate as white Americans, according to research conducted in the late 1990s. To put that kind of excess loss into perspective, Williams compares it to a jumbo jet with 265 passengers and crew crashing, killing everyone on board. Every single day for a year. Year in and year out.

Behind these cold statistics are real people and real families haunted by unnecessary grief that reverberates through generations. Like W.E.B. Du Bois and his wife, Nina: The death of their son, and the circumstances surrounding his likely preventable premature death, caused a rupture in their marriage that was never repaired. These excess deaths have a ripple effect that create inestimable losses throughout the larger society and across generations.

"It is the loss of breadwinners, the loss of role models in the community, the loss of social ties and social support, and the community fabric and the family fabric that is so important to all of our good health," Williams observed. "We often think of these losses as just a higher death rate, but we haven't paid enough attention to what that means for the fabric of the community. We need to realize that these racial disparities in health means the loss of supportive social resources across our lifetimes."

But there are some hopeful developments. We are at the threshold of a new era with the computational capacity that we have with generative AI tools, and we cannot let this advancement broaden the divide. We have to find ways to enable data scientists of the future, like Du Bois, to have the resources to identify vulnerable populations with early monitoring, and then we must design and implement interventions that can be evaluated and shown to actually close disparity gaps.

We must never forget the equally important tragedy of the loss to humanity of the lives that are short-circuited by disease, discrimination, and premature death. In a conversation at the Harvard T.H. Chan School of Public Health, Isabel Wilkerson, a Pulitzer Prize winner and author of the bestseller *Caste: The Origins of Our Discontents*, talked about wasted lives and used the examples of John Coltrane and Toni Morrison. "Their ancestors could have been just as magnificent in music and in literature, but they were held in a fixed place," she said, mournfully. "All the waste in genius and brilliance that can never be recovered."

Dangerous Trades: From the Triangle Shirtwaist Factory Fire to the World Trade Center Collapse

Occupational safety and the long struggle for the rights of working people to a safe and healthy workplace must be embraced as an integral part of the public health movement.

IT WAS ALL OVER IN LESS THAN TWENTY MINUTES OF SHEER TERror. Just before closing time at the Triangle Shirtwaist Factory, on an unseasonably warm Saturday afternoon in March of 1911, a container filled with fabric scraps burst into flames. The company was located in a building in Greenwich Village in New York City, and more than five hundred seamstresses worked in the sewing factory, toiling fourteen-hour days with no breaks for low wages in unsanitary conditions. Telephone operators on the first floor alerted the factory owners and clerical staff sequestered on the tenth floor about the fire, and they fled through the roof.

But they failed to warn the seamstresses on the eighth and ninth floors. By the time the women smelled smoke, it was too late. The blaze spread so fast that 146 workers, mostly young Jewish and Italian immigrant women and girls, perished because they had no way to escape. One of the exit doors was locked to prevent theft, the fire escape collapsed, the elevator stopped working, and fire ladders couldn't reach them. Many fell or jumped to their deaths.

The Triangle Shirtwaist disaster sent shock waves throughout the city, especially in the immigrant communities of the Lower East Side. Grief-stricken families struggled to identify their lost family members' charred remains—often, they could be identified only by a cherished piece of jewelry, unusual stitching on a stocking, or dental work—in makeshift morgues that had been set up at the nearby 26th Street Pier. On April 5, 1911, 400,000 mourners—one out of every ten New Yorkers—lined the streets as the funeral procession passed by. Shielded under a sea of umbrellas, they crowded the rain-drenched sidewalks to pay their respects. Ashen-faced police lined the streets as an empty horse-drawn hearse slowly traversed the narrow cobblestone streets of the garment district on the Lower East Side and headed up Fifth Avenue toward the gleaming skyscrapers of Madison Square.

The Triangle fire was an accident waiting to happen. Garment workers had been complaining for years about brutal working conditions in cramped quarters that were veritable fire traps. But it was only because of the public outcry in the aftermath of the Triangle fire that the conditions in the city's sweatshops were finally addressed. The Triangle Commission, created to investigate the disaster, held a series of inquiries around the state, interviewed 472 witnesses, and dispatched field agents to do on-site inspections of factories; they visited 359 chemical plants and found horrific conditions in many of them. Their findings led to thirty-eight new laws regulating labor in New York state. Provisions covered fire safety, factory inspection, and sanitation and employment rules for women and children. This legislation was considered the most progressive in the nation, and these workplace safety standards and reforms became the template for similar laws that were soon adopted across the country.

The Triangle factory fire remained the deadliest workplace tragedy in New York's history until the terrorist attacks on the World Trade Center ninety years later. It was an inflection point in the crusade for industrial safety and better conditions in the dangerous and often lethal environments that millions of Americans across industry were forced to work in. But as one historian acidly observed, "Women had to burn to death for this to happen."

The perils of the workplace, the horrendous working conditions in industrial states, and the human costs of industrial capitalism had finally caught the attention of a national audience. In 1912, 18,000 to 21,000 workers died from work-related injuries, according to estimates by the National Safety Council. In 1913, the Bureau of Labor Statistics confirmed these high rates of fatalities and documented about 23,000 industrial deaths among a workforce of 38 million. From the turmoil of the early 1900s, and throughout the twentieth century, we saw a growing coalition of reform-minded activists, public health officials, progressive politicians, journalists, social workers, medical clinicians, and leaders in the nation's emerging labor movement lead the struggle to make workplaces safer, and to improve the lives of working people, their families, and communities, in a fight that would save countless lives.

Occupational safety and the long struggle for the rights of working people to a safe and healthy workplace were embraced as integral parts of the public health movement. We now know that so much of our well-being is determined by where we live, yet many of us scarcely have control of our environment because of the restrictions imposed by capitalism and racism, which make it difficult to live in healthful neighborhoods. And while our jobs are central to our lives, we have even less control over our workplaces, which historically have been even more dangerous. The fight for healthy workplaces is the fight for health—and another key marker of a society that enables its people to thrive.

But many experts believe that we're now losing ground in the battle for improving working conditions with globalization, the decline of unions, and severe cutbacks at federal watchdog agencies, and with rollbacks in worker protections and even a gutting of child-labor laws. In the early days of the Covid pandemic it wasn't a coincidence that up to 8 percent of Covid cases in the United States were tied to outbreaks in meatpacking plants, which employ the most vulnerable, defenseless, and marginalized members of society. When the shock of the pandemic hit, we were rudely awakened to the fact that so much of our health was not under our control. The pandemic laid bare the deficiencies and vulnerabilities that have existed and festered for decades in our workplaces. Our disastrous response to Covid and our failures to protect not only essential workers but frontline health-care professionals are only a piece of a much larger, troubling picture.

IN THE DECADES BEFORE THE Triangle fire, it was already evident that workplaces had become hellish death traps for the nation's mostly immigrant labor force. Unable to speak English, and fearful of losing their jobs and becoming blacklisted if they complained, workers were ruthlessly exploited during the second wave of the Industrial Revolution. After the Civil War, the United States underwent explosive growth that triggered huge waves of immigration in the late nineteenth century, as tens of millions of Europeans flooded into America in search of a better life. By the century's end, America had become the world's foremost industrial powerhouse. But the 1890s were a "period of savage inequality, rapid technological disruption, pervasive political dysfunction, and controversial waves of immigration," David Brooks noted in *The Atlantic*. "Unemployment surged from 3 percent to almost 19 percent among working-class Americans, as populism rose and spread, as class conflict and horrendous poverty became more rampant."

Factories became killing grounds. Industrial accidents were commonplace, and thousands of workers died or were permanently harmed every year because of hazardous conditions in unventilated plants and constant exposure to poisonous chemicals. Few paid attention to these largely invisible assaults on the army of anonymous workers in factories, steel mills, smelters, mines, and munitions plants. These workers brought deadly substances home to their families in their poison-saturated clothing. Safeguards were virtually nonexistent because the endless supply of mostly destitute immigrant laborers were viewed as collateral damage, not worth the cost of protection.

Alice Hamilton, a pioneer in the field of industrial medicine and among the first scientists to demonstrate the dangers of industrial toxins and the severe toll they were taking on human health, had a name for this gilded era of unbridled capitalism. She called it an age of "triumphant ruthlessness" in the corporate class. Workers, Hamilton said, were seen as expendable.

Throughout her long life, Hamilton fought courageously for better working conditions. Her struggles echo the battles faced by those toiling today in the sweatshops spawned by globalization, the farmworkers laboring in hellscapes, and the alarming numbers of meatpacking workers who perished from Covid-19 because of a failure to institute even rudimentary safeguards.

But the self-effacing physician, shy and modest to a fault, was an unlikely champion of the working class. Nothing in her upbringing would suggest she would become an implacable social reformer who would lead the scientific crusade to make workplaces safer. Born in 1869 to a wealthy Indiana family, she was mostly homeschooled, although she did attend Miss Porter's in Farmington, Connecticut, for two years, and rarely ventured beyond the confines of her family's expansive estate in Fort Wayne until she attended college. She chose to go into medicine because it offered her independence as a woman—it freed her of the societal constraints of women at that time, who were expected to marry and have children—and it was a way to be of service. She received her medical degree in 1893 from the University of Michigan, becoming one of only about 4,500 women doctors in the United States (of about 105,000 doctors in total). After internships at hospitals in Minneapolis and Boston, she studied bacteriology and pathology at universities in Munich and Leipzig before she accepted a job teaching pathology at the Woman's Medical School of Northwestern University in Chicago in 1897.

It was here, in Chicago, that the young doctor began what became her life's work, in industrial toxicology. She moved into Hull

House, which was then the most famous of the more than four hundred settlement houses in the United States in the early twentieth century. Settlement houses provided social services for people who had nowhere else to turn—they helped new immigrants and alleviated the miserable housing conditions for the poor. Hull House was founded by Jane Addams, who was on the front lines of the settlement-house movement and, in 1931, became the first American woman to win a Nobel Peace Prize. Hamilton, who lived at Hull House for twenty-two years, became her personal physician and the two women became lifelong friends.

Shortly after settling in Chicago, Hamilton opened a well-baby clinic, where she had her first encounters with impoverished immigrant mothers. She listened to their stories about nightmarish working conditions; for instance, of husbands who toiled fourteen hours per day or suffered from palsy from brain damage because they worked in paint factories. She couldn't help but notice how many of them had been driven into impoverished widowhood when the family breadwinners were killed in factory mishaps or died from carbon monoxide poisoning in steel mills. She began seeing the garishly clear connection between working conditions and occupational illnesses.

Hamilton went searching for scientific literature on the subject and quickly discovered that there was a paucity of research on basic safeguards for workers in the U.S.—and even less interest in implementing them. Like Du Bois before her, Hamilton intuitively understood that she needed the data and research to promote lasting, broad-based societal changes. European countries, in contrast, had long recognized the inherent dangers of mechanization and mass production. There was a substantial body of research in European countries on hazardous working conditions and industrial diseases—and that research in turn led to reforms. In some nations, meaningful regulations had already been in place for a generation.

The use of white phosphorus, for example, was banned in six nations, including Finland and Denmark, by 1909. The fumes from white or yellow phosphorus, which was used to make matches, caused "phossy jaw" in the young women who worked in the factories. The chemical penetrates the teeth and travels down their roots to the jaw-bone, causing tissue necrosis that steadily disintegrates the bone. Those afflicted with the disease were severely disfigured, and these deformities led some women to commit suicide. If the infection spread, they could also lose an eye or suffer from brain damage, so in some cases their upper and lower jaws needed to be removed to save their lives. Many of these survivors were forced to live on a liquid diet. In response, European match factories were required to have desig-nated wash and lunch areas, protective clothing, medical doctors as factory inspectors, ventilation rules, and prohibitions against child labor. In 1910, nearly a dozen countries outlawed the use of the wax-like chemical substance altogether. Here in the United States, on the other hand, the industry went unchecked. A federal investigation of match factories in 1908 uncovered more than 150 cases of phossy jaw, and it was finally outlawed here in 1912.

Phosphorus wasn't the only industrial toxin. Workers who made felt hats often suffered from mercury poisoning, which caused uncon-trollable jerking of arms and legs and mental illness (the origin of the phrase "mad as a hatter"). Lead, however, was the worst offender. The toxic metal can insidiously accumulate in the body virtually un-detected over long periods until there are sufficient amounts to trig-ger serious damage. Workers in dozens of industries were vulnerable to lead poisoning, from pottery and the enamel trades, to lead smelt-ing and refining, to paint manufacturing and making storage batter-ies. Lead exposures were the culprit behind a broad range of illness symptoms, including weight loss, high blood pressure, anemia, fa-tigue, miscarriages, and stillbirths. Lead also affects the nervous sys-tem and causes paralysis, loss of mental acuity, and premature senility.

In the U.S., research into industrial safety consisted mainly of fa-tality reports in major industries and scattered newspaper accounts of grisly deaths in mines or factories. The difference was stark between what Hamilton called conditions of "neglect and ignorance" here in the U.S. and "intelligent control" in Europe. When Hamilton went to England in 1910, she visited a factory that produced white and red lead and employed ninety men. There hadn't been a case of lead poisoning in five years. At a U.S. factory, in contrast, where eighty-five men worked, thirty-five employees had been stricken with lead poisoning in the previous six months.

Industrialists' attitude in the United States, she later wrote, was that if workers thought their jobs were too hazardous, they could quit.

Hamilton decided to investigate. She tracked down the causes of a typhoid outbreak that hit especially hard in the community surrounding Hull House in Chicago in 1902. She later looked into tuberculosis in the poor immigrants whom Hull House served. She discovered that bad working conditions, including unsanitary environments, low wages, exhaustion, and long, unpredictable work hours, accounted for their higher susceptibility to the disease. Like Snow and Du Bois before her, Hamilton took it upon herself to gather strong evidence— and carefully document the health risks—and use that to encourage public health action. Good public health policies and actions begin with active surveillance of factors and conditions that are harmful. Armed with that information, the next step is to take action and to ensure that the most vulnerable are protected.

These investigations cemented her reputation as an expert in industrial diseases. In 1910, she was appointed by the Illinois governor to examine the high mortality rates in lead and other industries, such as enamelware, rubber production, painting manufacturing, and explosives and munitions. Her research into pollutants in Chicago's factories led to some of the nation's first workplace safety laws. Later, the U.S. Department of Commerce asked her to undertake a similar survey nationwide (the United States Bureau of Labor Statistics was a part of the Department of Commerce until 1913).

She spent the better part of the next decade traveling throughout the country, working for a variety of state and federal health agencies, and generating reports that often led to new laws and improved safety conditions. She visited copper mines in Arizona, steel mills in

Pittsburgh, and factories in just about every major city. She and her assistants employed the basic techniques of public health and "shoe-leather epidemiology," reviewing hospital records to connect specific illnesses and occupations, and carefully observing industrial processes to decipher which ones were hazardous and produced lethal chemicals. Hamilton was intrepid—with steely gentility, she persuaded reluctant factory owners to allow her to inspect their plants and gathered information from locals in the close-knit immigrant communities by joining workers at their favorite pubs after their shifts, or talking to druggists, doctors, and labor leaders in working-class neighborhoods.

In a plant inspection that Hamilton conducted as part of a study of industrial toxins for the U.S. Department of Commerce, she recalled with chilling clarity how the severe injuries workers sustained in the sanitary-ware trade were callously dismissed. One step in the manufacturing process involved coating bathtubs with lead-laden porcelain enamel, which had been ground into a fine powder. The tubs were heated to red-hot temperatures while workers quickly dredged the powdered enamel on the surface where it melted, forming an even coating. At this step in the process, the men, who were breathing heavily because of the exertion and extreme heat, were enveloped in a thick cloud of enamel dust that saturated their lungs in lead. Her research suggested that this was as dangerous as lead smelting, oxide roasting, and corroding white lead, all of which release toxic metals that cause permanent disability and even death.

"Because enameling was notoriously hard, hot, and dangerous work American men shunned it," she noted in her autobiography, *Exploring the Dangerous Trades*. "I found in Pittsburgh and the surrounding towns, in Trenton and Chicago, foreign-born workmen—Russians, Bohemians, Slovaks, Croatians, Poles. I remember a foreman saying to me, as we watched the enamellers at work, 'They don't last long at it. Four years at the most, I should say. Then they quit and go home to the old country.'

" 'To die?' I asked.

" 'Well, I suppose that is about the size of it,' he answered."

At a giant smelter-refinery on the Atlantic Coast, it was the same story. Lead poisoning, Hamilton noted, "was rife among the immigrants who made up the poorly paid force." Labor turnover was high because so many were sickened from inhaling the toxic dust. "But that made little trouble: all the manager had to do was to go to the gates in the morning and pick out from the eagerly waiting crowd the number he needed," Hamilton observed. "He took the company doctor with him to make sure of getting the healthiest men."

Sometimes, the working conditions were so dangerous that lead poisoning wasn't even particularly high on the list of complaints. When she visited smelter plants in Utah, she was shocked "to see how lightly lead poisoning is taken here," she wrote in her autobiography. "One would almost think I was inquiring about mosquito bites." But when she read through hospital records, it became readily apparent why lead didn't seem that important.

> The accidents are so terrible and so numerous that a little thing like lead colic attracts no attention. My hair almost stood straight as I read of the burnings and crushings and laceratings, the amputation of both arms, the loss of eyes, the deaths from ruptured livers or intestines. And there is no system of workmen's compensation in Utah, and the men themselves contribute all the money that their surgical and medical care costs.

When World War I broke out in Europe, pressure from America's allies—Britain, France, and Russia—prompted the creation of munitions plants all along the Atlantic seaboard, especially after their enemies began using chemical weapons. The U.S. became a key supplier of munitions for the war-torn Allied nations. These plants produced shells and mines, as well as the highly toxic and volatile chemicals needed for explosives, including picric acid, mercury fulminate, and TNT. The U.S. had little experience in refining these lethal raw materials or manufacturing explosives, and there weren't even rudimentary safeguards at munitions factories, which became poisonous death traps.

Because these plants were top secret, Hamilton had to ferret out these places on her own using the trusty tools of "pioneer exploration . . . visit the plants I knew and pick up gossip about the others." But they weren't hard to find. Refineries belched out billowing clouds of bright yellow and orange plumes, the waste products of the crude production of picric acid and nitrocellulose. "It was like the pillar of cloud by day," Hamilton noted, "that guided the children of Israel."

On one of her first trips to New Jersey, where many of these top-secret installations were located, she was in a small railway station when she noticed two men who were covered with smears of orange and yellow stains caused by refining picric acid. The men told her they worked in a nearby munitions factory—locals called them "canaries"—and many died from inhaling the toxic fumes. During a visit to the plant, she witnessed at least eight accidents in one day, with men running to escape the clouds of deadly gases, which had withered and blackened all the trees, grasses, and other vegetation in the surrounding countryside.

Black American workers at the plants were especially susceptible, Hamilton reported, because many of them had suffered from tuberculosis, which weakened their lungs. Because a plant owner's mind is "fixed only on profits," Hamilton observed, "he can hire Negro field hands from the deep South and, if the fumes are too heavy and some of the men choke and die, he can see to it that the coroner realizes what an advantage it is to the county to have this huge plant, and that he pronounces such deaths as due to 'natural causes.'"

In the summer of 1917, when a mysterious illness swept through another munitions plant in New Jersey, killing several workers, the army did ask Hamilton to investigate. When the physician arrived at the munitions plant, she spotted the telltale signs of the probable cause: The landscape of the countryside surrounding the facility was blackened and decayed from the clouds of noxious gases, the waste products from making explosives that the factory's smokestacks pumped into the sky.

Like a homicide detective systematically gathering evidence, Hamilton toured the plant, interviewed the affected workers who'd recovered, and combed through hospital and dispensary records to distinguish what was different about the victims and the workers who seemed to escape unscathed. Epidemiologists are often likened to detectives. Hamilton essentially used epidemiological investigative methods to elucidate the risk factors that caused this mysterious illness.

Hamilton discovered that men would leave at the end of their shift, seemingly fine, eat dinner with their families and go to bed, only to awaken in the middle of the night gasping for air, their chests tightening as if they were in the throes of a heart attack. In the worst-case scenario, they'd never fully catch their breath. Their lungs would fill with phlegm and they'd literally drown in their own fluids. The only clue physicians had as to the culprit behind the poisoning was the fact that many of the workers had been exposed to heavy fumes in the plant, causing them to choke at the moment of exposure. But once they were in the open air, this would often pass—until they got home. From these accounts, however, she was able to identify the perpetrator.

The workers who became sickened and, in particular, those who died, were involved in the part of the production process that required them to have daily contact with the explosive TNT (trinitrotoluene). And despite the bouts of coughing that preceded the sometimes fatal episodes of breathing difficulties, blood tests revealed that the lethal poisoning mainly occurs from contact with the skin, not from breathing vapors; repeated exposure to the toxic chemical killed off red blood cells, which ferry lifesaving oxygen to the lungs and other vital organs. The chemicals also ate away at the tissues of their lungs, until the victims no longer had enough lung capacity to breathe.

The remedy was simple and clear: Men working with TNT should wear protective clothing and remove it when they leave the factory, and then bathe to wash off any TNT residue that may be on their skin. Once these protections were put in place, the deadly poisonings stopped. A lifelong pacifist, Hamilton later wrote of her successful efforts to improve conditions in plants making weapons of war that "it is good to have one cheerful feature in this dark picture of a return to barbarism."

In 1919, Harvard Medical School expanded its fledging public health department—which would become a separate school in 1922—and added a section on industrial hygiene. After a lengthy search for a leader in occupational health, they reluctantly realized that the best candidate, by far, was a woman. At age fifty, Hamilton became the first female faculty member at Harvard University. Despite the constant drumbeat of indignities both large and incredibly petty that Hamilton was forced to endure during her nearly two decades at Harvard—she was never granted tenure; she was not allowed to use the faculty dining hall, obtain faculty tickets to Harvard football games, or march in commencement processions—she continued to make necessary trouble.

Hamilton played a prominent role in investigations of the harmful effects of a range of toxic chemicals. They included aniline dyes, carbon monoxide, tetraethyl lead, radium (which was used in wristwatch dials), benzene, mercury, and hydrogen sulfide gases created in the manufacture of viscose rayon. Her research formed the foundations for the field of industrial medicine that improved working conditions and eventually led to the passage of the federal Occupational Safety and Health Act, which became law in 1970 three months after she died at age 101.

After her retirement from Harvard in 1935, Hamilton returned to the Department of Labor. In the face of stiff industry opposition, she worked closely with FDR's labor secretary, Frances Perkins, to expose the dangers of silicosis caused by workplace exposures to silica dust in mines, tunnels, and factories. A kindred spirit, Perkins had been part of Hamilton's social-reform network, and she had personal experience of what happens when a family loses their breadwinner through disability or death. Her husband suffered from bipolar disorder, and she became her family's primary support. Both women had become involved in workplace safety at around the same time; Hamilton through her work in Chicago in the early 1900s, and Perkins in 1911, when she was galvanized by witnessing the Triangle Shirtwaist Factory fire.

At the time of the fire, Perkins was a thirty-one-year-old social worker. She hailed from an old-line Maine family that had been there since the American Revolution, and she graduated from Mount Holyoke, where she majored in chemistry and physics. On the day of the fire, she was having tea with friends at her family's Greenwich Village townhouse off Washington Square Park when they heard the clanging of fire trucks. They rushed out and ran to the nearby Asch Building. Staring up as smoke and flames billowed out of the eighth and ninth floors, they joined the crowd of horrified onlookers on the street. They watched in disbelief as these young girls and women, trapped by the fire, chose, one by one, some alone and some holding hands, to crawl onto the window ledges and jump to their deaths rather than be immolated. "I shall never forget the frozen horror that came across as we stood with our hands on our throats watching that horrible sight," she later recalled, "knowing there was no help."

Perkins was fueled by a moral outrage that transformed her from a modest, genteel do-gooder who worked among the poor in settlement houses into a fire-breathing champion of the working class. Perkins, who was the first woman to hold a presidential cabinet post, is widely credited as the architect of the social legislation known as the New Deal. March 25, 1911, said Perkins, was "the day the New Deal was born."

Perkins resolved to change the conditions in New York City's sweatshops to prevent another tragedy of this magnitude. Two years before the factory was engulfed in flames, in 1909, an industry-wide work stoppage known as the "Uprising of 20,000" was sparked by the horrific working environments. Many of these garment shops were located in damp, dark, and crowded basements where women labored for pennies a day in cold, unventilated rooms. They constantly breathed in toxic dust from fabric cuttings that lingered in the air and fumes from the oily sewing machines and the coal stoves that kept them warm. The conditions aged them prematurely, and even teenagers as young as fourteen looked like old women, with sallow, gray complexions, hanging skin, and the hollow cheeks of someone on the edge of starvation.

"Women often had their fingers punctured by the machines themselves because they were paid by the piece and they're working as fast as they can," said Robyn Muncy, a labor historian at the University of Maryland. "But the biggest threat was fire. There were fabric and open flames everywhere. They were constantly putting out these small fires that catch in these baskets of fabric, or on the floor where there are piles of flammable fabrics blocking overcrowded aisles."

The strike lasted nearly three months. Throughout a long and cold winter, strikers were harassed and beaten by industry thugs and arrested by local police. In those days, Jewish and Italian immigrants were seen as different and inferior races from the earlier waves of northern Europeans. But young, progressive middle- and upper-class suffragettes—"that first generation of college-educated women wanting to make the world better," according to Annelise Orleck, a labor historian at Dartmouth College—saw these women as natural allies. They joined forces with strike leaders including Clara Lemlich, Rose Schneiderman, and Pauline Newman, and held rallies and fundraisers on their behalf at venues like the Metropolitan Opera House and Carnegie Hall. Anne Morgan, daughter of the famed financier J. P. Morgan, joined the picket lines and recruited her socialite friends into what was dubbed the "Mink Brigades," a reference to the costly coats the wealthy young women wore on those frigid days.

"This made a strike that was predominantly immigrant on the fringes of the city visible to the middle class because it became newsworthy," said Richard Greenwald, a historian at Fairfield University in Connecticut. "When Sarah Lawrence or Smith College undergrads walked the picket lines and faced the same violence and brutality and got arrested the same way strikers were treated, it became front-page news."

The women ultimately won some concessions. But the union's male leadership that negotiated the settlement ignored the women's most pressing issue—improving their treacherous working conditions—so nothing was done. The same scenario that we've seen countless times before and afterward played itself out, only this time it wasn't racism as much as sexism, and women were left behind. There was resistance to truly fundamental changes until a catastrophe resulted in the dramatic and entirely preventable loss of life.

After the fire, Frances Perkins realized that voluntary organizations simply didn't have the kind of clout needed to better workers' lives. Government intervention was needed to counteract the harsh conditions of industrialization. She teamed up with two stalwarts of the corrupt Tammany Hall political machine, Robert Wagner, a Prussian immigrant who was majority leader in the New York State Senate, and Perkins's mentor, Al Smith, head of the state assembly in Albany, to push for reforms.

Both men represented immigrant communities and understood what working families needed to survive. Wagner was later elected to the U.S. Senate, and during the Roosevelt administration authored the Wagner Act, which established the National Labor Relations Board. Rose Schneiderman and Pauline Newman became their confidants. Schneiderman later served in Roosevelt's brain trust, and as secretary of the New York State Department of Labor under Governor Herbert H. Lehman. "Wagner and Smith saw political capital in an alliance with the new working class, the Italians and the Jews who had supplanted the earlier generations of Irish immigrants," said Greenwald. "Their thinking was that if we can do something for them, then we can stay in power as Tammany Hall Democrats."

Smith and Perkins were appointed to the Triangle Commission that investigated the crisis. The goodwill generated by the commission propelled Smith into the governor's office in 1919, and he appointed Perkins to his industrial commission shortly after taking office. Perkins threw herself into the job, traveling from the state capital in Albany to factory towns across the state, where she would find herself mediating bitter labor disputes between aggressive union organizers and resolute corporate executives whose jobs depended on healthy profit margins, the lone woman surrounded by a sea of angry men. On occasion, she also worked with another rising political star, the handsome, charismatic—and entitled—scion of one of New York's richest, oldest, and most powerful families: Franklin Delano Roosevelt. Initially, she was not impressed. He struck her as shallow and arrogant. But all that changed after he contracted polio, which wiped away his upper-class hauteur and put the steel in his soul. Perkins was moved by the humility, stoicism, and grace he displayed when he embarked on his political comeback despite his considerable physical disability.

In 1928, when Roosevelt succeeded Smith as New York's governor, Perkins became his industrial commissioner. Four years later, when FDR was elected president, he summoned her to his townhouse on East 65th Street and asked her to be his secretary of labor. But Perkins drove a hard bargain and presented him with a series of demands before she would take the job. Her wish list included a vast array of public-works programs to put people back to work in the depths of the Depression, like the Civilian Conservation Corps and the Public Works Administration, and laws to improve the workplace, end child labor, establish a minimum wage and regular work hours, and create unemployment insurance and "old age insurance" that became known as social security, which would lift millions of the elderly out of abject poverty.

"I suppose you're going to nag me about this forever," Roosevelt reportedly told her. She nodded vigorously in response, and later recalled, "I remember he looked so startled, and he said, 'Well, do you think it can be done?' "

Historians have called this one of the most consequential job interviews in American history.

Working conditions in the United States have dramatically improved since those dark days, but sweatshops never really went away. My father, Noel Alexander Williams, worked in similar sweatshops in the late 1960s and '70s on New York's Delancey Street in the heart of the Garment District, saving every penny he made until he was able to bring my mother, my siblings, and me over from Jamaica. By then, immigrants from Asia and the Caribbean had replaced the seamstresses from eastern and southern Europe, but the local garment industry had experienced a precipitous decline. The days when more than 100,000 workers would flood the streets on any given morning rushing to their jobs on the Lower East Side were long over. The big factories had largely moved out of Manhattan, starting in the years after the Triangle fire when their owners found cheaper, non-unionized labor in rural regions—first in the American South and finally overseas.

When capital fled and started doing production abroad, the smaller outfits that were left behind were often bootleg businesses that flew under the regulatory radar. "*Sweatshops* is a term that refers to sweating labor, when you're squeezing as much as you can out of labor," said Richard Greenwald. "It's all about speed and production. So when you're talking about sweatshops you're talking about inhumane conditions. Mostly, you're referring to places that are unregulated, ostensibly operating or zoned as retail outlets when in reality they were factories. These are shops that are underground really, writing checks or paying bills under one name and renting under another name."

It's entirely possible that my father worked in one of these fringe operations that Greenwald describes, where tons of scrap materials littered the floor, the electrical wiring was not up to factory-required standards, with equipment jacked into multiple extension cords, and no sprinkler systems or properly labeled exits. Like so many others before and since, my father did what he had to do to gain an economic foothold for his family.

But he never complained or talked about the everyday perils he faced, and rarely even slept much, because he was constantly working. He'd be up early and gone before we left for school because the commute on the subway from Queens was about an hour each way. He'd come home late, grab dinner, and disappear into the basement, where he'd spend his evenings making garments for clients off the books. In one corner, he had a workstation set up with a sewing machine, and a flat counter built into the wall where he could do all his measurements and use it as a cutting board. His commission work provided supplemental income, which, combined with his paycheck, allowed him to accumulate the funds he needed to put a down payment on a dry-cleaning business, which enabled him to stop working downtown and gain some independence as a small-business owner. But even after he began operating the dry cleaner, where he and my mother worked sixteen hours a day, six days a week, he would still work in the evenings and on weekends, custom-making clothing for people. And he was admittedly one of the lucky ones. But like so many others, he had to do unacceptable work to bring home the wage that would allow his children to advance in society. What jobs are people doing right now to help their kids?

Sweatshops still exist across America, with probably half of them in Los Angeles and New York. In the garment industry, there are some 22,000 registered contractors; a large majority of them are subcontractors that employ a few dozen workers apiece and often close up shop overnight, vanishing with no advance warning and stiffing their workers. Labor officials estimate that more than half of them pay under the minimum wage and fail to pay overtime, and three out of four garment shops violate health and safety regulations.

Conditions overseas are even worse. The Rana Plaza catastrophe in Bangladesh is just one tragic example. Rana Plaza was an eight-story building in Savar, an industrial city just outside the nation's capital, Dhaka. On April 23, 2013, deep structural cracks were discovered in the building, prompting the shops and a bank on the lower floors to shutter immediately. But managers at the five garment factories on the upper floors insisted that their workers come to work the next day, even though many begged to be excused. Early that next morning, at 8:45, there was a power outage, and diesel generators at the top of the building were fired up. The intense vibration from the generators split open the fissures, and within ninety seconds, the entire building had collapsed. More than 1,100 people perished and another 2,500 were critically injured; many of the survivors are severely disabled and have received little or no compensation for their life-altering injuries.

Local unions called it a "mass industrial homicide." In the wake of this disaster, which was the deadliest garment-industry accident in modern history, the international fashion brands who sourced in Bangladesh—"after a month of highly embarrassing media coverage," according to the head of one workers' rights organization—finally pushed for a package of safety regulations for their suppliers. Over the next five years, more than 97,000 workplace hazards in 1,600 factories were rectified, and 900 factories that did not meet standards were shut down by the government; more than 2.5 million workers now toil in safer conditions, which has saved lives, according to a 2018 study by the Center for Global Workers' Rights.

"Like the Triangle fire, Rana Plaza was a turning point," said Orleck, in that it coalesced the organizing efforts of the Bangladeshi women. Numerous strikes about working conditions, involving hundreds of thousands of women, had taken place in the years preceding the Rana Plaza disaster. "They shut down the port, they shut down streets in major cities, they blocked ships and trucks," said Orleck. "They even set fire to a couple of factories because all of them had lost people to industrial fires."

Here again, we act only after a dramatic loss of life even though it was obvious long before that something needed to be done. Unfortunately, plenty of unsafe sweatshops continue to operate under the regulatory radar in Bangladesh, and many garment makers that didn't want to pay for these costly safety measures simply moved their operations to Vietnam, which is now the world's third-largest producer of clothing. Even though sweatshops in the United States are no longer as active as they once were, we are still, through our consumption, contributing to the global sweatshop economy.

But globalization has hurt American workers in other ways. Exporting manufacturing jobs overseas shuttled the working class into the service sector, mostly to fast-food chains and retail outlets, that are notoriously difficult to organize. As a result, unionization rates plummeted from roughly 20 percent of the entire workforce in 1983 to less than 10 percent in 2024, a sharp decline that not coincidentally parallels the hollowing-out of the middle class, especially in the Midwest, which was once a highly unionized industrial stronghold.

In the past several decades, in the absence of union and regulatory watchdogs, working conditions have arguably become worse. "Right to work" laws, designed to hamstring unions and keep wages low to attract corporate investments, broke out of the South where they began and were passed in states such as Michigan and Wisconsin that were former union mainstays. Under the Trump administration, the National Labor Relations Board, which oversees unions, was stocked with industry appointees and transformed into a toothless tiger. "This agency was crucial to the ability of workers to organize and bargain collectively," said Muncy. "But there was no longer federal support for that."

The federal oversight agency charged with workplace safety, the Occupational Safety and Health Administration (OSHA), was gutted, too. OSHA's contribution to American well-being can't be overstated: Since its launch in 1970, the number of people who die on the job every day has been cut in half thanks to strict federal standards and on-site inspections. But that record of protecting the public is in grave jeopardy.

During the first three years of the first Trump administration, the number of OSHA compliance officers was cut by two-thirds. When the pandemic began, there were about 870 inspectors for the entire country, which translates to one inspector for every 59,000 workers at 8 million job sites across the country. With that number of inspectors, it is estimated that it would take 165 years to adequately police worksites. Out of more than 23,000 employee complaints about workplace hazards that were filed during the first year of the pandemic, the agency issued only one citation, to a company accused of covering up their employees' Covid-related hospitalizations. The other grievances were dealt with "informally" by the agency, which entrusted employers to do their own investigations.

When the pandemic hit, workers deemed "essential," who could not work from the protective confines of their homes—farmworkers, bus drivers, janitors, fast-food workers, health-care aides, and retail clerks—were vulnerable. Many of them were undocumented, with no access to health care or paid sick leave, and they feared reprisals, even deportation, if they complained. They sickened and died at higher rates, and the virus ran rampant through the nation's agricultural heartlands, in California, Florida, Arizona, and Texas, where farmhands ate and slept in overcrowded bunkhouses, and in supermarkets, nursing homes, hospitals, and warehouses. "It's like I'm risking my life for a dollar," said one Amazon worker after she learned that one of her co-workers in his twenties had died of Covid-19.

In the early stages of the Covid-19 pandemic, the severe shortages of personal protective equipment (PPE), such as disposable gloves, gowns, and masks, for frontline health-care professionals was yet another instance of our nation's continued failure to protect workers. Several factors contributed to this crisis, including the sudden explosion in global demand, our reliance on supplies made in China rather than investing in domestic manufacturing, the collapse of the overseas supply chain, and our failure to replenish the Strategic National Stockpile (SNS).

During the 2009 H1N1 pandemic, the Obama administration depleted the Strategic National Stockpile (SNS), which is a set of government-run warehouses that, in emergencies, serve as a fallback supplier of crucial medical supplies, such as ventilators, N95 respirator masks, gloves, and protective gowns. No effort was made to replace these stocks. The Trump White House's neglect of production and distribution of PPE worsened the crisis, forcing desperate states, hospitals, nursing homes, and small rural facilities to compete for limited supplies. Profiteering and price gouging became commonplace, and counterfeit products flooded the market.

But the real toll was on the frontline health-care professionals, who were forced to ration or reuse N95 masks and gloves and in some cases use garbage bags instead of gowns as protective coverings. During that first horrific year, more than 3,600 health-care workers perished, according to a report called "Lost on the Frontline," by *The Guardian* and *Kaiser Health News*. Nurses accounted for one-third of the deaths, 20 percent of the fatalities occurred among the support staff, and 17 percent of those who died were doctors. Two-thirds of the deceased health-care workers identified as people of color, the report discovered, "revealing the deep inequities tied to race, ethnicity, and economic status in America's health care workforce."

Their investigation also found that the Labor Department under the Trump administration "took a hands-off approach to workplace safety" during the pandemic. Even though 4,100 safety complaints were filed by health-care workers to OSHA, mostly about PPE shortages, nothing was done and workers continued to die. While it is difficult to calculate how many of these lives could have been saved if there had been adequate supplies of PPE, this staggering loss of life among our nation's health-care workers is unacceptable in a country as rich as the United States.

"The total disregard for our safety has been unconscionable," Mary Turner, an ICU nurse and president of the Minnesota Nurses Association, told *The New York Times*. "They call us heroes but we're not being treated like soldiers at war because if we were, the federal government would make sure we have everything we need."

The pandemic had other surprising consequences for American workplace safety—including deteriorating conditions in the food-production industry and the erosion of prohibitions against child labor that workers fought and died for a century ago. As the pandemic wound down in 2023, states such as Ohio, New Jersey, and

New Hampshire passed or introduced legislation that would make it easier for minors to work, ostensibly because of the tight labor market. The legislation included expanding work hours and the types of jobs minors can do. But immigration activists contend that there is already a shadow workforce of minors working in deplorable conditions in places like sawmills, toiling in hazardous jobs at slaughterhouses and plants, and operating and cleaning meat-processing and -packing equipment. Between 2015 and 2022, in fact, there has been more than a 50 percent increase in cases involving child-labor violations, according to Labor Department statistics.

In one horrific incident in July of 2023, a sixteen-year-old boy died on the job at the Mar-Jac Poultry plant in Hattiesburg, Mississippi. The teenager, Duvan Tomas Perez, was an indigenous Guatemalan who had emigrated six years earlier with his family, who were fleeing that nation's violence and bone-crushing poverty. He was fatally injured when he "became entangled" in one of the machines he had been cleaning, according to a press release issued by the company, which maintained they weren't aware he was underage. OSHA launched an investigation. But no matter how this all eventually plays out, a middle schooler who had his whole life ahead of him died on a factory floor, noted Caitlin Flanagan in *The Atlantic,* "in what must surely have been an event of overwhelming terror and pain, dying in the same pitiless place where the chickens are killed."

One of the more egregious failures of workplace safety happened not in a remote factory in a rural area that employed undocumented workers, but in our most populous city, in plain sight of the nation's media headquarters and witnessed daily by millions. The death toll from this calamity, which is already in the thousands, continues to climb. It is the aftermath of the attacks on New York's World Trade Center on September 11, 2001, when terrorists hijacked two planes that brought down the center's twin towers, along with two other commercial jets that crashed into the Pentagon and a field near Shanksville, Pennsylvania.

The suffering of those who worked in the rubble of the World

Trade Center brings this story full circle, in the kind of synchronicity we don't often appreciate in the seemingly random disorderliness of the real world. We're almost thrust back in time, in the heart of lower Manhattan, with the modern-day equivalent of the hellish sweatshops with workers forced to toil under hazardous conditions with no regard for their safety. But in this instance, it was the first responders, the firefighters, the cleanup crews, and the demolition teams who were giving their lives in service to a nation that failed them, in the same way we failed the first responders, doctors, nurses, and medical professionals who died during the pandemic, because we disastrously underestimated what it meant to take care of them in the middle of an emergency.

A well-functioning public health system protects all of us. The fundamental principle of public health is that no vulnerable population is left behind, and that we're responsible for creating a work environment that is safe for all people. In the Triangle fire, we were talking about employees in a workplace; in the Covid pandemic and in the World Trade Center, these were the people we rely on to help us, but we did not fulfill our end of the social and moral contract to help and protect them.

Within seconds of the skyscrapers' collapse, the air was filled with the pulverized remains of tons of building materials, office furniture, electronic equipment, and the toxic fumes from thousands of gallons of unburned jet fuel from the aircraft. "If you look at the initial photographs after the first tower came down, you can see that dense cloud of smoke and dust rolling through the streets of lower Manhattan," said Dr. Philip Landrigan, pulling up the searing images on his computer screen. He's the former chair of the Department of Preventive Medicine at Mount Sinai School of Medicine in New York (now the Icahn School of Medicine at Mount Sinai), which became the nerve center of the World Trade Center Health Program, a consortium of five medical institutions that tested, tracked, and treated the thousands of people sickened in the aftermath of 9/11.

"Anyone who was caught in that cloud and survived was intensely exposed to that dust," said Landrigan, now the director of the Program for Global Public Health and the Common Good and Global Observatory on Planetary Health at Boston College. "The concentrations of dust in the air were so high that they overwhelmed the normal defenses of the human respiratory tract, and people inhaled ounces of dust into their lungs."

There was a massive plume of poisonous vapors, too, that smothered lower Manhattan for days and included PCBs, black soot, lead, a toxic soup of volatile organic compounds, and the highly carcinogenic chemical benzene, from the jet fuel. The lingering toxic cloud was thick with plastics, metals, millions of tiny particles of cancer-causing asbestos, microscopic shards of glass that can become embedded in the air sacs of the lungs, and tons of crushed concrete, which is intensely alkaline and caustic—like breathing Drano—that causes burns in the lining of the throat and trachea.

Yet less than two days after the attack, based on no data whatsoever, Rudy Giuliani, then New York City's mayor, told reporters that the financial district was open for business, and urged everyone "to go back to normal" because the air around Ground Zero was "safe as far as we can tell, with respect to chemical and biological agents." A week later, on September 18, EPA administrator Christine Todd Whitman, presumably in an effort to get the traumatized city back to some semblance of normalcy, assured New Yorkers that "their air is safe to breathe and their water is safe to drink."

Nothing, of course, could have been further from the truth. Whistleblowers from the CDC and the EPA, who fired off repeated warnings that the air was toxic, were largely ignored by George W. Bush administration officials. Based on these erroneous guarantees, employees working in the financial district surrounding Ground Zero were summoned back to their workplaces within a week of the attack, even though the collapsed skyscrapers were still burning, and the streets were covered with mountains of debris.

Mount Sinai was home to the largest occupational health program in the tristate area. Medical professionals there knew right away that workers at Ground Zero were in grave jeopardy and that they were going to be seeing thousands of sick people as time passed. Landrigan watched in horror as cleanup crews at Ground Zero worked twelve- to fourteen-hour days for weeks clearing the smoldering wreckage without proper respirators or other protective gear. "Emergency responders at the Pentagon were fully wrapped up in Hazmat gear from day one, which prevented a lot of disease," he recalled. "We would've had fewer illnesses and premature deaths in the New York City 9/11 workers if they'd been fully protected from the beginning, and if we'd paid attention to the data and not just made impulsive comments. Whitman and Giuliani should never have told people that the dust was safe. That was just a huge mistake."

Fortunately, Mount Sinai had the resources to respond swiftly to a calamity of this magnitude with an experienced staff of occupational health doctors, nurses, industrial hygienists, and environmental specialists who instantly swung into action. The hospital's leadership quickly approved plans to provide medical care to these men and women free of charge. "That was a good and noble thing that they did," said Landrigan. "Within forty-eight hours, we reached out to all the unions—the firefighters, the police, transit workers, the construction workers, the crane operators who were trying to pull people out—and we told them if you're experiencing any symptoms, come up to Mount Sinai and we will take care of you."

In the intervening decades, as long-gestating illnesses like cancer and respiratory diseases continue to emerge, the toll has grown dramatically beyond the nearly three thousand people who lost their lives on 9/11. By the twentieth anniversary of the attacks, more than 4,600 responders and survivors enrolled in the World Trade Center Health Program had died, according to the program's tallies. However, not all these deaths can be attributed to Ground Zero exposures, since all fatalities for any reason are included. Still, the actual numbers may be far higher because only about 112,000 people are members of the program, which is roughly one quarter of the estimated 410,000 who were exposed to the toxic environment and emotionally stressful conditions in the months following the attack.

More than 65,000 people enrolled in the program have at least one of the huge number of health conditions associated with the aftermath of this tragedy. These include digestive issues like gastroesophageal reflux disease (GERD), sleep apnea, asthma, chronic obstructive pulmonary disease (COPD), and other respiratory illnesses, as well as profound psychological trauma, resulting in high rates of persistent anxiety, major depression, and post-traumatic stress disorder (PTSD). Roughly one-quarter of those enrolled in the program (23,000) have at least one type of cancer that includes tumors of the blood and lymphoid tissues (lymphoma, myeloma, and leukemia), as well as breast, head and neck, prostate, lung, and thyroid cancers, and even mesothelioma, an aggressive form of cancer caused by exposure to the asbestos used in the early construction of the north tower.

In 2001, the September 11th Victim Compensation Fund was established to provide health benefits to those who worked in the rescue and recovery efforts, along with their families. However, the program was allowed to expire in 2004 and wasn't reauthorized until 2010 with the passage of the James Zadroga 9/11 Health and Compensation Act, named after a New York City police detective who died of respiratory failure after working for months at Ground Zero. The bill finally became law after years of lobbying by rescue workers, activists, and surviving family members, and after comedian Jon Stewart shamed recalcitrant lawmakers when he interviewed several first responders on *The Daily Show*. (Stewart would later champion "burn pit" legislation to provide health benefits for veterans exposed to toxic chemicals.) "There was a lame-duck session of Congress at the end of 2010, and [President] Obama brought the Congress back in and said, 'You're not going home until you pass this legislation,'" Landrigan recalled. "Three nights in a row, Jon Stewart had a cop, a firefighter, and a construction worker on the show talking about their health problems. He just finally embarrassed [Senator] Mitch McConnell and those people to do the right thing. But it was not a sure thing—it was close."

CHAPTER SIX

The CDC: A Checkered History

The founding of the Centers for Disease Control ushered in a new
era in public health, and established the CDC as the world's flagship
disease prevention agency.

T HE POLITICIZATION OF THE CENTERS FOR DISEASE CONTROL
and Prevention that we saw during the first Trump administration, when public health officials were vilified and their
lives threatened, and communities of color were marginalized, sabotaged our response to the Covid pandemic and resulted in countless
preventable deaths. But this wasn't the first time that public health
was caught in the political crossfire, and it had the same disastrous
consequences.

When Dr. David Satcher was appointed director of the CDC in
1993 by President Bill Clinton, he was taking the reins of a "demoralized" and "fragmented" agency, according to the *Los Angeles Times*,
and he was faced with two deeply entrenched problems that still plague
the agency today. The CDC had been sharply politicized during the
Reagan White House years, and the agency had consistently failed
to protect vulnerable communities because of the institutional blind

spots of the well-meaning but largely white male leadership. These two issues played key roles in the botched public health response to the AIDS crisis, which was raging when Satcher took the reins of the CDC, and prefigured our later failures during the pandemic.

As the first Black American to head the CDC and a lifelong social activist, David Satcher was committed to turning the agency around and restoring its once-lofty reputation. The bearded and bespectacled physician, whose folksy manner hid a will of titanium, already had a stellar résumé when he arrived in Atlanta at CDC headquarters. He was born and raised in segregated rural Alabama, and a nearly fatal bout of whooping cough and pneumonia when he was two years old set the stage for the rest of his life. Even though he was near death, Satcher recalled in his book *My Quest for Health Equity*, his doctor "could not admit me to the hospital because the only hospital in the area did not admit black patients or allow black physicians to admit. Black kids with illnesses like mine usually died at home, without the benefit of hospital care."

By age eight, he knew he was going to become a doctor. He attended Morehouse College in Atlanta and had been arrested and jailed on at least five different occasions because of his involvement in the Civil Rights Movement. He received his MD and PhD in cytogenetics from Case Western Reserve University, and he later served on the faculty of the UCLA schools of Medicine and Public Health. He chaired the family medicine department at the King-Drew Medical Center, where he directed sickle cell research and helped open and operate a free clinic in Watts, a poor section of Los Angeles that had been the epicenter of the Watts rebellion in 1965.

In 1979, Satcher joined the faculty of the Morehouse School of Medicine, which was the newest of the three historically Black four-year medical colleges in the United States, where he was able to train the next generation of Black doctors. But his stint there was brief. In 1982, he was called upon to take over Meharry Medical College in Nashville, which was drowning in debt, with a severe staffing shortage. His team's turnaround of the troubled institution was considered miraculous. They added more than forty faculty members, raised more than $35 million in donations and pledges, and engineered a merger of Meharry's teaching hospital with a larger but struggling all-white Nashville hospital that saved both hospitals and the school.

This consolidation—which happened only after years of political struggles—was in progress when Satcher was tapped to lead the CDC. One of his first actions was to clean house at an agency that had become hidebound. He quietly encouraged veterans to retire and appointed women and members of minorities to key positions to replace some of the conservative ideologues that had served under the previous administrations. This was especially the case during the Reagan years, when interference by the religious right and the Republicans' big corporate donors stymied good public health initiatives.

But the Reagan White House's most egregious failure was its glacial response to the AIDS epidemic, which allowed the outbreak to escalate out of control, killing off nearly an entire generation of young gay men. President Reagan never even mentioned the word AIDS until September of 1985, more than four years after the first cases emerged, and he didn't address it publicly until 1987.

Bowing to the political pressure of the right-to-lifers who ushered him into office, Reagan appointed right-wingers in key health-care posts, including Dr. James O. Mason, a Mormon who became CDC director in 1983. He suppressed research on the efficacy of condoms in preventing AIDS transmission, a finding that could have saved countless lives. In fact, any research that had a whiff of sexuality was suppressed by the religious right, even during an epidemic of a fatal sexually transmitted disease.

Every one of the surveys on sexuality that CDC researchers suggested was canceled. Consequently, in the absence of data, there was no way to get a handle on the magnitude of the problem. Apparently, the fear was that if pregnant women found out they were HIV positive, they might choose to get an abortion. We're talking about preventing AIDS in children, yet they refused to deal with it.

Naturally, the casualties of these cumulative failures were the most vulnerable members of society who were at the highest risk for contracting AIDS: women, minorities, hemophiliacs, the poor, and members of marginalized and stigmatized groups (Haitians, heroin addicts, and homosexuals). The stigma was real and harmful, and many doctors refused to treat AIDS patients for fear of becoming infected. (It wasn't until 1987, more than six years into the epidemic, that the American Medical Association declared that doctors had an ethical obligation to treat AIDS patients.) By 1984, AIDS had claimed more than two thousand lives, and dozens of new cases were being diagnosed each week. The gay community was under siege and outraged activists were holding candlelight vigils by the White House.

However, while media accounts about the disease overwhelmingly focused on white gay men, the reality was that AIDS was devastating Black communities. By September of 1983, CDC surveillance data revealed that AIDS was disproportionately affecting Black Americans, who accounted for 26 percent of AIDS cases even though they represented 13 percent of the population. By 1986, the incidence of AIDS among Blacks and Hispanics was three times the rate among white Americans.

Efforts to contain the epidemic were hampered by the profound mistrust of the medical system within the Black community. "Bizarre as it may seem to most people, many Black Americans believe that AIDS and the health measures used against it are part of a conspiracy to wipe out the black race," according to an incredibly tone-deaf editorial in *The New York Times* on May 12, 1992. The editorial cited a 1990 survey of Black church members that revealed "an astonishing 35 percent believed AIDS was a form of genocide."

But these legitimate fears were "bizarre" only to insulated white observers. Black Americans saw AIDS through the prism of three centuries of oppression, exploitation, and abuse, from slavery to Jim Crow, from lynchings to disenfranchisement and residential segregation, from second-class treatment, at best, at the hands of the racist medical establishment and the revelations about the Tuskegee study, which came to light in 1972.

When he arrived at the CDC, Satcher made it clear that closing these longstanding health-equity gaps was at the top of his agenda, and he looked to eliminate or at least curb many of the social inequities that contributed to the disparities. Under his watch, childhood immunizations increased, we improved our ability to respond to emerging infectious diseases, and preventive screenings for breast and other cancers jumped. However, whereas he assured veteran staffers that he wasn't abandoning the CDC's historic role in combating infectious diseases, he embarked on aggressive plans that would go back to public health's roots in community-based initiatives and increase the emphasis on health promotion and disease prevention.

After all, mounting evidence was clear—including in the CDC's own data—that social factors, including guns, tobacco use, and substance abuse, were the root causes of premature mortality among Americans. "I think what we're talking about doing in this country is providing incentives for health care providers, physicians, and others to work to keep people healthy," Satcher told *The New York Times,* "whereas today most of the incentives are toward treating people when they're sick or in bringing to bear the greatest levels of technology that we can."

At the dawn of his tenure, the CDC launched an $800,000 campaign to promote condom use to prevent the spread of AIDS, a controversial and long-overdue program that had been verboten when the agency was controlled by conservatives who refused to recognize that teenagers were sexually active and who advocated completely ineffective "Just Say No" campaigns. Satcher was also keenly aware of the profound skepticism within the Black community about the medical establishment, which fueled the conspiracy theories that revolved around AIDS when the plague ravaged the country in the 1980s and '90s. To counteract this, the CDC director spearheaded the adoption of broad community-based initiatives that partnered with churches, schools, and neighborhood groups, whom he viewed as natural allies and extensions of the public health system.

Through these informal networks, especially Black churches, which are the backbone of the Black community, the CDC spread positive messages about preventive strategies that dealt with the major health threats that plagued most Americans, like gun violence, substance abuse, mental illness, suicide, teenage pregnancy, routine immunizations, and the self-destructive consequences of such poor lifestyle habits as cigarette smoking, stress, lack of exercise, alcohol consumption, and unhealthy fast-food diets. "As early as you can get to people in terms of diet, exercise, and avoidance of toxics, you do it," he told *The New York Times*. "We're going to try to find every successful program we can in this country."

Through these community ties, public health officials were also finally able to break through some of the resistance within the Black community and identify the reasons why AIDS spread so stealthily among Blacks and why the disease seemed to be infecting both sexes equally, and not just gay men. In another vestige of racism, Black people were reluctant to discuss their sexuality because of all the taboos and historical bigotry and perverse attention paid by white supremacists to Black sexuality, dating back to slavery when Black men were portrayed as savage brutes who raped white women. Furthermore, Black and Hispanic men who had sex with other men did not identify as homosexual, per se. As a consequence, public health messages were not tailored for these populations.

It took years to fully realize the epidemiological characteristics of heterosexual AIDS transmission among Black Americans. Because this population was unseen, understudied, and possibly misunderstood, this distinction came very late in the epidemic, when public health people finally realized how AIDS had spread through the Black community and started asking Black men if they had sex with other men. This seemingly obvious admission opened the door to then understanding the behavioral dynamics that contributed to why so many Black women ended up being infected with HIV when there were relatively few infections among white women (outside of high-risk groups, like intravenous drug users). That's why the epidemiology of

HIV looked so different in the Black community, and why there was such a delay in the recognition of this invisible epidemic.

Satcher worked tirelessly to mobilize the Black community's response to the growing crisis. The CDC partnered with local groups to ensure that all people at risk had access to early testing, treatment, and effective prevention programs. Unfortunately, the explosion of AIDS among Blacks and Latinos, he would later say, was a "public health emergency . . . the complexion of the epidemic has changed. Increasingly, it is becoming an epidemic of color."

Despite the strides the CDC made in the fight against AIDS, there was one key area that Satcher failed to make progress on, even though he was keenly aware that this was what was killing young Black men: gun violence. "Violence is the leading cause of lost life in this country today," he said to *The New York Times* in 1993. "If it's not a public health problem, why are all these people dying from it?"

However, any meaningful studies about the causes of gun violence and research into effective strategies to prevent it were derailed for more than a generation with the passage in 1996 of the Dickey Amendment, which banned the use of federal funds to do research that would "advocate or promote gun control."

Back to Basics

When Satcher took over in 1993, the CDC had already become a globe-girdling behemoth. But he pushed hard to get the agency back to its original mission, from dispatching public health officers to disease hot spots and forging deep ties with communities, to collecting and tracking the surveillance data that is fundamental to monitoring the nation's health and identifying outbreaks before they spiral out of control. Boots on the ground and data collection were the twin pillars of the CDC that were established in 1949 by Alexander Langmuir, who became the CDC's chief epidemiologist. In guiding the CDC's core mission of community assessment and high-quality data collection, Langmuir institutionalized for the nation what W.E.B. Du Bois did in Philadelphia when he launched his study of the determinants of health among residents of the Seventh Ward.

The CDC had begun life as a tiny government agency charged with vanquishing one of humanity's most formidable predators: the lowly mosquito, the anopheles mosquito to be exact, the tiny cargo ship that transmits malaria, the fearsome killer that has ravaged continents, crushed armies, and triggered the downfall of empires. The bug-borne illness had plagued the American South since colonial times and was a major cause of death in both the Union and Confederate armies during the Civil War. During World War II, military officials considered malaria to be an even graver threat than Hitler's legions because hundreds of military bases and industrial installations were spread across the South.

But how to intercept this deadly courier? Enter the incredibly effective DDT in 1943, which exterminated adult insects as well as larvae. Because of the eradication campaign's success, the Office of Malaria Control in War Areas, which had been launched in 1942 and was headquartered on one floor of an office building in downtown Atlanta, expanded into a formidable government operation. After the war, when demand for malaria control spread to civilians and businesses, the wartime operation was transformed into a new public health agency, the Communicable Disease Center. In addition to mosquito control campaigns, the newly formed agency would handle all bug-borne illnesses and be responsible for a nationwide tracking system for outbreaks of infectious diseases.

It wasn't until the arrival of Alexander Langmuir, however, that the young agency began to take on the contours of the worldwide colossus it would become. The bespectacled physician had trained at Harvard and Cornell and left the Johns Hopkins faculty to become the CDC's chief epidemiologist in 1949, a position he held until 1970. A tall man with a deep voice and a razor-sharp intellect, he was a commanding presence with a will of iron who thrived on controversy. At the time, the CDC had plenty of engineers, entomologists,

and other scientists left over from wartime. But they lacked epidemiologists, the intrepid public health warriors in the John Snow and
Alice Hamilton mold who waded into the community to track down
real-time outbreaks and identify the miscreants causing all the trouble. There was a dearth of epidemiologists mainly because there were
few places for them to train.

Langmuir decided that the CDC would train their own and created the Epidemic Intelligence Service (EIS)—the shock troops of
public health. He cast the embryonic EIS as a crucial element of the
nation's frontline defense against biowarfare, a medical CIA comprised of highly trained disease detectives who could be instantly sent
out around the country when early warnings flagged possible dangers. As the government's chief disease detective, Langmuir advocated what he called "shoe leather epidemiology," which emphasized
boots on the ground and dispatching investigators into the field to
collect their own data and see problems firsthand.

In response to growing fears that germ warfare could be unleashed to deliberately contaminate reservoirs and the food supply,
Langmuir also pushed for the establishment of a nationwide disease
surveillance network—an innovative and unprecedented program.
This proposed nationwide system would track dozens of diseases and
analyze patterns to take steps to prevent clusters and outbreaks from
exploding into epidemics. A dedicated disciple of John Snow, Langmuir was adamant that public health, at its very taproot, must be
data-driven; that we need to know how many cases of a disease are
occurring, where the infections are occurring, when they're occurring, and who is getting sick. He set up a network that connected the
CDC with every single health department in the country, in big cities
like New York and Los Angeles and in rural outposts, and encouraged
them to voluntarily report their data to the CDC. The data were then
analyzed to see if there were patterns of illness. "Was there a blip of
measles in Illinois?" said Dr. Philip Landrigan, who was an EIS officer
in the early 1970s. "Or smallpox in South Florida? When we saw a
blip, our mission was to jump on an airplane the same day or the next

morning and get out to wherever the problem was happening, find out what was going on, and then do something about it."

The Cutter Incident

The first real test of this system came in 1955, with what came to be known as the "Cutter Incident," which occurred in the wake of the successful introduction of the polio vaccine—and which would firmly establish the CDC as the nation's flagship public health institution. On April 12, 1955, the tenth anniversary of the death of President Franklin Roosevelt, the world's most famous polio survivor, health officials gathered in an auditorium in Ann Arbor, Michigan. Just three years before, in 1952, the nation had experienced the worst polio outbreak in its history: About 57,000 people were infected, about 21,000 were paralyzed, and 3,145 died. Before a packed house filled with scientists, reporters, and television news crews, they announced the results of the field trial of the polio vaccine, which had been tested on more than 200,000 youngsters nationwide.

It worked.

The news grabbed headlines, church bells rang across the country, sirens blared, and Jonas Salk, the polio vaccine inventor, became a national hero. But in less than two weeks, the elation turned to doubt.

On April 25, the CDC received a report of a baby in Chicago with polio; the infant had been inoculated nine days earlier. An EIS officer arrived in Chicago early the next morning. An EIS officer in Napa, California, reported another case the following day. Before that day's end, a total of six cases were identified, and one of the children, seven-year-old Susan Pierce of Pocatello, Idaho, died. Within days, EIS officers had interviewed dozens of people who had contracted polio and found that they had two things in common: The paralysis first appeared in the inoculated arm, and the vaccines had all come from the Cutter Laboratories in California, in what became one of the worst pharmaceutical disasters in U.S. history.

On that critical day, on April 29, Langmuir was en route to Washington, D.C., for a scheduled meeting, but upon his arrival, he was ushered into an emergency summit convened by Dr. James Shannon, deputy director of the NIH, that included nearly a dozen high-level officials from several agencies and an EIS officer. It lasted for more than eight hours until it disbanded at four A.M. Time was of the essence: A massive polio vaccination clinic in Los Angeles using the Cutter vaccine was scheduled to begin in a few short hours. The surgeon general, Dr. Leonard Scheele, called Cutter and requested that all outstanding lots of their vaccine be recalled, while Dr. Malcolm Merrill, chief of California's department of health, canceled the Los Angeles vaccination program.

But the fate of the entire inoculation campaign hung in the balance—and along with it, the goodwill and trust of the American people. Instead of scuttling the polio vaccine effort, Langmuir proposed creating a nationwide polio surveillance network that could immediately spot whether vaccines made by other manufacturers were tainted, too. Everything "points that there is something about the Cutter vaccine . . . and nothing about any other vaccine yet that makes sense," he said at the top-secret meeting at the NIH on Friday, April 29, according to Elizabeth Etheridge in *Sentinel for Health: A History of the Centers for Disease Control*. As daily case reports came in over the next five weeks, it became abundantly clear that a bad batch of Cutter vaccines was to blame, and that the other vaccines were safe.

Subsequent investigations revealed that the Cutter Laboratories vaccines contained polio viruses that hadn't been completely deadened. More than 200,000 children had received these shots, which ultimately caused ten deaths and left 200 children with varying degrees of paralysis. In the ensuing lawsuits, Cutter was cleared of negligence—their lack of expertise and experience was cited as the main reason for the disaster, along with the fact that the inactivation procedure they used had unanticipated flaws. The Cutter incident was an inflection point in the history of the CDC, and the value of the EIS and the agency's surveillance program became obvious.

Nearly thirty years later, the CDC's vaunted surveillance network would rise to the occasion once again: The agency was the first to alert public health officials about the presence of a new and highly contagious pathogen that would soon claim millions of lives. In early May of 1981, Michael Gregg, editor of the *Morbidity and Mortality Weekly Report* (*MMWR*), a CDC bulletin distributed to health-care professionals that tallies illnesses and deaths, received a worrisome phone call from Wayne Shandera, an EIS officer assigned to the Los Angeles County Department of Health. Michael Gottlieb, a UCLA emergency room physician, had uncovered five cases of young homosexuals who were at an age when they should have been in perfect health, yet their immune systems were so severely damaged that they couldn't ward off even the most benign germs; their bodies were ravaged by normally innocuous infections—yeast infections and Pneumocystis pneumonia, a rare pneumonia that strikes cancer patients whose immune systems have been depleted by chemotherapy.

Publishing these findings in a medical journal would take several months, and Gregg, Shandera, and Gottlieb agreed that this information needed to get out right away. On June 5, 1981, the *MMWR* published the first reports about a new and deadly disease—and doctors across the country who had seen similar patients realized they were somehow connected to the Los Angeles cases. It became chillingly clear they were dealing with a looming public health crisis. Because it appeared out of nowhere simultaneously in three different cities, the disease, whatever it was, had a long incubation period. If the new pathogen had been a more recent arrival, the pattern of infection would follow a more traditional route, starting in one city, which would be the point of entry, and then spreading to other nearby locales—not appearing full-blown in three geographically diverse areas. Consequently, if it did have a long latency period, there was no telling how many people were already infected and spreading the disease, and how many time bombs were out there that could explode anytime.

The public health implications were staggering, and doctors were terrified. But unlike the heady days of the 1950s when Americans trusted science and people like Jonas Salk were revered icons, the emergence of what became a deadly pandemic couldn't have come at a worse time for the CDC—although there is never a good time for a disease outbreak to occur—because sensible public health measures based on science had become derailed by politics.

Still, in the decades during and after Langmuir's long tenure, EIS officers were in the forefront of dozens of campaigns, including to trace the effects of environmental toxins and to identify the culprits behind Legionnaires' disease and toxic shock syndrome, and they led the successful global crusade to eradicate smallpox, which is considered a triumphant landmark in the history of public health.

Boots on the Ground: The EIS Parachutes In

Like so many EIS investigations, the probe that would eventually force fossil-fuel companies to phase out lead in gasoline started with a phone call. In 1971, Bernard Rosenblum, director of the El Paso, Texas, health department, contacted the CDC because he was worried about the toxins being spewed into the atmosphere by a local smelter company, Asarco. Over the previous three years, the company had belched out more than 1,000 tons of lead, 12 tons of cadmium, 1.2 tons of arsenic, and 560 tons of zinc into the air, according to court documents from a lawsuit filed by local officials.

"It was an amount vastly greater than anybody in the health department had imagined," Dr. Philip Landrigan recalled. "While there weren't any obvious cases of lead poisoning, where kids were lethargic or had sustained blatant damage to the brain or other vital organs, Rosenblum wanted the EIS to determine whether there were any health effects from inhaling all these pollutants on kids living downwind from the smelter."

Landrigan had arrived at the CDC in 1970. He was a reluctant EIS recruit. After completing his pediatric residency at Boston Children's Hospital at the height of the Vietnam War, the Harvard-trained physician knew he'd be drafted and opted instead for the EIS. He

planned on a career in academic medicine and had a pediatric neurology fellowship lined up at Johns Hopkins after he finished his EIS
stint. But his time in El Paso changed the trajectory of his career.

Landrigan and another EIS officer were sent to Texas, where they
went door-to-door taking blood samples from about forty young
children. They found that kids living closest to the smelter suffered
the most damage, with blood lead levels that were "strongly elevated,"
he remembered. "In those days, an elevated blood lead level was anything greater than 40 micrograms. Today the limit is 3.5 micrograms,
but back then we didn't know as much. It was very clear that there
was a common source of the lead poisoning outbreak, and that nothing else could account for it except the smelter."

Around this time, Landrigan became friends with Dr. Herbert
Needleman, a pediatrician at Harvard who believed that even minuscule amounts of lead caused profound damage to health and mental
acuity, even in the absence of noticeable symptoms of lead poisoning.
To test this theory, Landrigan did a large study in 1972 (which was
published in 1975) that confirmed Needleman's research. Kids with
higher lead levels had significantly slower motor skills and an average
reduction of as many as seven IQ points. With this new information, Landrigan thought they had enough evidence to shut down the
smelter. But he soon discovered he was fighting entrenched vested
interests. "We were dealing with one of the largest employers in
El Paso, and they commissioned a counter-study conducted by a local
pediatrician and a psychologist," he recalled. "They found no difference, and this escalated into a major food fight at several national
[scientific] meetings."

The controversy was finally settled with the publication of Herbert Needleman's landmark study in 1979 in *The New England Journal of Medicine* that compared levels of blood lead in children with
their school performance and IQ. In examining more than 2,100
youngsters, he found that even small levels of lead had a dramatic
impact on intellectual development and behavior, a discovery that
helped propel the phaseout of lead in gasoline. The work done in El

Paso and Needleman's work in Boston helped establish the principle of what's called subclinical toxicity. In other words, lead could do irreparable harm even at levels that were too low to cause the grossly visible symptoms of lead poisoning. Kids seemed healthy, but real damage was being done. "This was a huge breakthrough finding and all new science," said Landrigan. "But it was also very powerful actionable information from a public health perspective. Because if you can show that this stuff is causing children to lose brain function, then you damn well better do something about it."

Ferreting Out the Invisible Killers

Over the decades, the CDC's responsibilities expanded almost exponentially, from mosquito-borne pathogens to environmental toxins, from HIV/AIDS to guns. Then and now, the agency has had to be ready to identify anything and everything that would bring harm to the public's health. At the same time, it has to find and implement ways to protect and promote health—which is not a small task.

Lead poisoning is just one example of the silent killers of human potential. That's why data collection across large populations is crucial. The data help us to distinguish these clear signals out of the noise of human life. One person getting ill doesn't tell you anything; it is only when you look at hundreds of people that trends in illness can become apparent. However, diverse voices provide an added dimension to the data, a wider aperture, if you will, that enhances perspective, and another lens through which data is analyzed and interpreted. Dr. Diane Rowley's experience underscores the importance of these diverse perspectives. Her groundbreaking research began the long process of upending many of the once widely accepted reasons for disparities in health.

THE WELLESLEY COLLEGE GRADUATE JOINED the CDC in 1980 after finishing medical school at Meharry Medical College in Nashville and her pediatric residency at the Medical College of Virginia. She later earned her Master of Public Health at Harvard. There were only a handful of women in her EIS class, and only one other Black woman, who came in the year before. "It was clearly an old boys' network," Rowley recalled. "Even though I was a double minority, as a Black woman, I shared their excitement around doing the work."

Initially, Rowley worked on environmental health and spent much of her time hopscotching around the country. It wasn't uncommon for her to be met at the airport when she was returning from one assignment with her marching orders for the next. One month she'd be investigating meningitis outbreaks, and the next she'd be on her way to Bangladesh looking for the root causes of child mortality in conditions that could be described as a toxic stew of social and environmental risk factors.

But she soon turned her focus on what would become her life's work: maternal and child health and documenting the racial disparities that made the United States, the wealthiest country in the world, such a perilous place for Black mothers and their newborn babies. It was around this time that the administration of President George H. W. Bush was looking for ways to reduce the nation's high infant mortality rates. The United States' international ranking had dropped from twelfth in the world in 1960 to nineteenth in 1989, with 9.7 deaths per thousand births, more than double the numbers of the world's leader, Japan, where 4.4 newborns out of every thousand died before their first birthday. Rowley served on the staff for Bush's Commission to Prevent Infant Mortality and launched a CDC-wide initiative that looked at racial disparities in infant mortality.

What she and her CDC colleagues uncovered was profoundly disturbing. They weren't surprised that Black infant mortality rates were more than double that of their white counterparts. However, the common perception was that this wide gap was driven by poverty, differences in education and income, and lack of access to health insurance and prenatal care. But in a revolutionary 1992 study published in *The New England Journal of Medicine,* they looked at infant mortality rates in children born to college-educated parents, which presumably eliminated the underlying social and economic variables that experts believed were largely responsible for the stark inequalities. Yet even in this affluent and educated segment of the population, which did have access to care, the differences stubbornly persisted: Black babies were twice as likely to die—10.2 deaths per 1,000 live births versus 5.4 white infants.

In subsequent research that dug more deeply into why these differences persist, Rowley pushed for more community involvement, returning to public health's roots in disease detection and prevention. In research in Harlem, Los Angeles, Chicago, and Atlanta, the universities conducting this research had to have regular meetings with community advisory boards to get feedback on data collection and how to interpret that data. "The community actually took over the research and insisted that nothing could be published without their consent, which really made a huge difference," said Rowley, "and what we found contradicted what was an emerging idea at the time, that disparities occurred because people are not empowered to do anything. But the reality was that these inequities occur *in spite of the fact* that people *do* make major efforts for their health and their communities." Clearly, something else was at play here beyond the accepted wisdom about the causes of racial disparities in health. This was among the first studies that showed that racism itself, and not just social and economic factors, undermines health across the lifespan, a finding that would later be confirmed by an avalanche of evidence.

The Politicization of the Public Health

But these triumphs were often overshadowed by the agency's weaknesses, especially when sensible public health measures based on science were derailed by politics and the CDC neglected vulnerable communities. The agency failed Vietnam veterans who complained of grave health issues after being drenched with Agent Orange, the toxic defoliant used to carpet-bomb the tropical Asian nation in order to flush out troops hidden in the thick, lush forests. Even an abortion study from the 1960s, before *Roe v. Wade,* that revealed how many women's lives were saved or dramatically improved when abortion was readily available, was suppressed.

In 1980, to cite another example, overwhelming evidence emerged from five different teams of medical researchers, including one led by Dr. Diane Rowley, that when children were recovering from chicken pox, taking aspirin could cause Reye's syndrome, an often deadly side effect. Big Pharma pushed back, insisting that the research was ambiguous and that they would produce rebuttal studies (which never materialized). It would take another five years of wrangling before warnings were added to aspirin bottle labels, and in the interim, 1,470 children died unnecessarily.

However, public health's most shameful episode began long before the CDC existed but continued for decades after the agency's founding: the infamous Public Health Service Syphilis Study at Tuskegee, which continues to fuel the Black community's mistrust of the medical establishment to this day. Many alarms had been raised over four decades about how the wildly unethical study was conducted, but the warnings went unheeded.

Until William Jenkins came along.

The Whistleblower

William Jenkins was no stranger to social justice advocacy. He had been swept up in the Civil Rights Movement of the 1960s while growing up in a middle-class suburb of Charleston, South Carolina, where his father owned a funeral home and a restaurant and his mother was a schoolteacher. In high school he helped register people to vote, which was a dangerous undertaking in the Jim Crow South, and in his college days at the historically Black Morehouse College, he was a foot soldier in the Student Nonviolent Coordinating Committee (SNCC). Dr. Martin Luther King Jr. was a frequent visitor to the Atlanta campus and had inspirational meetings with young student activists like Jenkins, who was arrested after protesting the whites-only policies of an Atlanta restaurant owned by Lester Maddox, who was later elected governor.

In 1967, Jenkins was hired as a statistician for the Public Health Service. In those days, Atlanta was still very much a segregated city. The agency reflected these almost invisible biases and was not friendly to African Americans. When Jenkins showed up for his employee physical, the receptionist at the front desk in the Atlanta office called security because she didn't believe a Black man could be a member of the Public Health Service's Commissioned Corps. He was forced to travel to Washington, D.C., to undergo his exam.

Even given his experiences, he was still shocked when a French-born Jewish physician at the agency alerted him about an ongoing experiment that echoed the horrors of Nazi atrocities. Jenkins did some digging that confirmed the doctor was right. He found at least a dozen articles in medical journals on the study, so it wasn't any big secret, but even the sketchy outlines of the research shook him to his core.

At the height of the Depression, in 1932, six hundred impoverished African American sharecroppers in Macon County, Alabama, were recruited for what turned into a forty-year federally sponsored observational study of a disease they knew colloquially as "bad blood." They later said they were motivated to join to protect their families. Of the original participants, 399 had latent syphilis and 201 uninfected men served as the control group. In exchange for being unwitting guinea pigs, the volunteers were offered free meals, burial stipends, medical exams, and so-called "treatments," which were actually placebo pills. The men were never told of their actual diagnosis, or that their potentially fatal disease could damage their heart and bones and eat away at their nervous systems, causing blindness, deafness, paralysis, and dementia. Or that they could inadvertently pass it on to their wives, who would then transmit it to their unborn children.

When penicillin became widely available in 1945, which effectively cured the disease, the men weren't informed and remained untreated, and the study continued even though their health was deteriorating.

Some died needlessly while others became blind or crippled, and they infected their families. What was equally unconscionable is that doctors thwarted the men at every turn when effective treatments were offered in other settings; they stopped authorities from giving them antibiotics when they were drafted into the service and prevented them from participating in government-sponsored disease-eradication clinics after the war. "Even when World War II started . . . they got the men exempted from the military so that they wouldn't be treated for syphilis," Dr. Jenkins said in a keynote address to the American Public Health Association in 2010. "After penicillin was established as the treatment for syphilis, the men were denied penicillin so that they could be followed to death."

They were simply being watched until they died.

Jenkins shared his deeply troubling discovery with his supervisor. "Don't worry about it," he responded. Jenkins couldn't believe that his boss would so casually dismiss this blatantly unethical and immoral research that callously disregarded the lives of Black Americans and their families. But he later learned that his supervisor's hands weren't clean—he was one of the statisticians helping to run the study.

Dropping things was not in Jenkins's DNA, however. He distributed the journal articles to other Black professionals employed at the Department of Health, Education, and Welfare (HEW), which became the Department of Health and Human Services (HHS) in 1979, and to his friend Peter Buxtun, who worked in the venereal disease branch of the CDC, which had taken over administration of the study. Their concerns were ignored until July of 1972, when Buxtun, in frustration, leaked the information to the Associated Press and investigative reporter Jean Heller's story was carried on the front page of *The New York Times*. Public outcry was fierce, Senator Ted Kennedy convened congressional hearings, and all the sordid details came tumbling out.

By the time the study was halted in November of 1972, the toll bordered on criminal negligence: 28 patients had died directly from syphilis, 100 had died from complications related to syphilis, 40 of the patients' wives were infected with syphilis, and 19 children were born with congenital syphilis. All of this was probably preventable, although all those years later it wasn't possible to prove that conclusively.

In the wake of these revelations, a class-action suit was filed on behalf of the men in the study, and a $9 million out-of-court settlement was reached in the case. Congress passed legislation that established strict rules mandating institutional review boards and informed consent to prevent the exploitation of human subjects in research studies. The Tuskegee Health Benefit Program was established to provide medical care for the study's survivors and the benefit was later extended to their wives, widows, and children. For nearly a decade, Jenkins was the program director, and he worked to expand benefits for survivors and their families. "What they deserve is the best medical care we can provide," Dr. Jenkins told *The New York Times* in 1997. "I try to give them the care that I would want to give to my mother."

Jenkins later earned a PhD in epidemiology because he felt this would give him the credentials and expertise to do the most good. He devoted much of his career to drawing attention to racial disparities in health and was in the forefront of campaigns to shine a light on the often-neglected health concerns of minority communities. When the AIDS epidemic began in the early 1980s, Jenkins, as a mathematician, was one of the first people who understood how AIDS would spread in the Black community, and he directed the CDC's first community-based funding program for HIV/AIDS.

Jenkins also encouraged and mentored dozens of young Black professionals to establish a thriving and supportive network of public health scientists who came from communities of color. He believed that increasing the numbers of minorities as scientists and in positions of leadership would amplify their voices and help counteract the institutionalized racism both inside and outside the agency. At one point, it was said that at least half of all Black epidemiologists could track their careers back to Jenkins.

I was certainly one of them. I met him in the mid-1980s, when I was in graduate school at Harvard while I was standing in line at one of the eateries that dotted the campus. He struck up a conversation with me, and after finding out I was studying epidemiology, he opened a cumbersome 1980s-era Radio Shack laptop and entered all of my particulars. From there on out, I was part of the team. "He did this almost alone," said Bryan Lindsey, a CDC epidemiologist and lifelong friend of Jenkins who was later the program director of the Tuskegee Health Benefit Program. "For every Black epidemiologist coming through the CDC, and other federal agencies and universities, if you said you didn't know Bill Jenkins, you would not be taken seriously. Mentoring was almost a religion for him, and he expected you to pay it forward."

Despite these inroads, however, the CDC hierarchy was still not sensitive to the plight of communities of color. Dr. Cheryl Blackmore Prince, who was a CDC epidemiologist for more than three decades, remembers attending a meeting of all the CDC division heads prior to chairing a conference on HIV and AIDS prevention among racial and ethnic minorities in August of 1988. There were about fifteen people arrayed around a conference table, and all of them were white men. Blackmore Prince was the only woman or person of color at the meeting, and the only reason she was there was to report on the status of the upcoming conference.

When she walked in, the men's eyes all turned to her expectantly, clearly hoping for some guidance. They told her they had approached Dr. Reed V. Tuckson, public health commissioner for Washington, D.C., about studying the prevalence of AIDS; it would involve dispatching contact tracers to ring doorbells, and recruiting volunteers to be interviewed about AIDS and to donate blood. Tuckson turned them down flat, telling them, "You can't come to my city and do that."

"They were wondering what they did wrong and how they could have approached Reed Tuckson to get him to buy in on this," she recalled.

I've worked with these men, and they are genuinely good people who did not consider themselves racist. But they did a very racist thing, and I was appalled that they couldn't see it. I had to call them on it. "You don't realize what it's like to wake up Black every day," I told them. "Race is always on our mind. You're going into a predominately Black community, 70 percent Black, and you're asking people to participate in a study to find out the incidence of HIV infections. You didn't try to do this is San Francisco, where cases among gay men are exploding, but in a Black community. And you wonder why people think this is like Tuskegee.

For this community, outsiders coming in to take blood samples was Tuskegee all over again, a manifestation of the original sin of Black oppression that is woven into the very fabric of our history. The way we overcome this handicap that our country is steeped in is to uphold the importance of diversity and inclusion. Cheryl Blackmore Prince is the perfect example of the importance of having that diverse voice in the room where a public health mistake was about to be made. It's not because her colleagues were inherently bad, but their tone-deafness was due to their insularity.

In 1997, while Satcher was still at the helm of the CDC, he was instrumental in bringing about some closure of this ghastly chapter in the history of public health that had taken place in his home state of Alabama. In a long-overdue reckoning, his boss, President Bill Clinton, issued an apology to the eight survivors of the Tuskegee study and their families. "What was done cannot be undone," Clinton said, calling the research deeply, morally wrong. "But we can end the silence. We can stop turning our heads away. We can look you in the eye and finally say on behalf of the American people, what the United States government did was shameful, and I am sorry."

Laudable sentiments to be sure but belated, at best.

More than two decades later, in April of 2021, CDC director Dr. Rochelle Walensky declared racism a public health problem, a victory in a long battle waged by people like William Jenkins. Unfortunately, the visionary epidemiologist did not live long enough to savor this triumph, dying in February of 2019 at age seventy-three in Charleston, South Carolina. But Bill Jenkins's legacy lives on. "We are making a difference," said Bryan Lindsey. "Is it enough? No. That's why we have to continue to do the work. We have to continue to bring along the next generation, because every generation has the work to do."

Still, the stench of the morally and scientifically flawed syphilis study lingers. For Black Americans, "Tuskegee" has "become shorthand for past medical betrayal, abuse, and exploitation at the highest levels," journalist Melba Newsome noted in *Scientific American*. Yet many are unfamiliar with the gruesome specifics. Many mistakenly think the study subjects were purposely injected with syphilis rather than given the lifesaving medicine that would heal them. This has played out in their resistance to receiving the coronavirus vaccines—"despite contracting, being made severely ill by, and dying from coronavirus at elevated rates," Newsome wrote—because of their "well-justified mistrust of public health initiatives . . . and a misreading of medical history [that allowed] the crisis to take an outsize toll on the Black community."

The syphilis study was one of the most disgraceful episodes in public health history, but the agency's most catastrophic failure was in battling the Covid pandemic. Despite our vast resources and technology, more than one million Americans died, more than anywhere else in the world. "Here we are, having to come to terms with the fact that during a global pandemic, the U.S. has led the world in the grimmest of distinctions," Isabel Wilkerson, a Pulitzer Prize–winning journalist wrote in an essay in *Time*. "Not only has the U.S. exceeded all other countries in the number of recorded Covid-19 deaths, it has led the world in the number of confirmed cases, millions more than the nation with the second-highest outbreak—India. The numbers in the U.S. are in line, not with our peer nations, but with the developing world."

We must do better.

CHAPTER SEVEN

The Burning Bed: Women Are Not Safe

Structural violence against women isn't just intimate partner violence—it's
embedded in our medical, social, political, legal, and economic systems
designed to deprive women of agency over their lives.

E VERYTHING WAS FALLING INTO PLACE FOR CHANIECE AND
Anthony Wallace. Chaniece had completed her fourth year
as a pediatric chief resident at the Indiana University School
of Medicine and had taken her specialty boards, Anthony was a special education teacher, and they had a baby on the way. Chaniece's
patients adored her, and her supervisors called the vibrant thirty-
year-old physician with the incandescent smile a "beloved" "warrior"
for her kids. The young Black couple, who met when they both attended Alabama A&M University and married in 2015, were considering job offers in their native Alabama because they wanted to be
close to family. Chaniece had gotten her medical degree from the
University of Alabama at Birmingham, and she was committed to
treating families and children in underserved communities. "We were
building our life together and this was the next step," said Anthony,

who is now a school counselor. "Everybody was excited and we were even talking with my mom about moving in with us to help out with the baby."

But their dreams were shattered in October of 2020. When Chaniece went in for her third-trimester checkup at thirty-five weeks, her doctor noticed that her blood pressure was dangerously high and there was protein in her urine, which are both symptoms of a potentially life-threatening complication known as preeclampsia. This is a serious blood-pressure condition that can cause stroke, blood clots, and seizures, and damage the kidneys, liver, and brain.

That afternoon, she was admitted to the hospital with "severe hypertension," according to the legal complaint filed by the Wallace family attorney. She called Anthony at work, who raced to the hospital, and four hours later, she had an emergency cesarean section. Baby Charlotte arrived on October 20 at 4:38 P.M., weighing four pounds and five ounces, and was quickly ushered into the neonatal intensive care unit (NICU).

Anthony hoped Chaniece would be able to come home, but doctors assured him she needed a few more days to recover. In the recovery room, however, Anthony began to have an unsettling feeling of dread. Her condition deteriorated over the next few days, but Anthony felt powerless to help her. He spent as much time in the hospital as he could, but because of Covid restrictions, he had to leave at six o'clock every evening.

Doctors were giving her magnesium injections to relieve her high blood pressure and Chaniece began exhibiting symptoms of magnesium toxicity—fogginess, lethargy, nausea, and severe drops in blood pressure and kidney function. Because of her malfunctioning kidneys, which were shutting down and failing to urinate and eliminate fluids properly, her sodium levels were quite low. This can trigger a severe life-threatening complication called tonsillar herniation, which is what happens when the brain swells to the point where it can't be contained inside the skull and the pressure forces the brain to push out of the bottom of the skull where the spinal cord connects to the brain.

Were there several checkpoints where Chaniece's life could have been saved if she had been treated differently? We will never know. But apparently the first doctor on her team to notice her low sodium levels was Dr. Arielle Russell, the only physician of color to treat Chaniece. This is not surprising: Studies consistently show that Black patients do better on virtually every metric—compliance, patient satisfaction, recovery, and even longevity—when they're treated by a Black physician.

In fact, one groundbreaking 2023 study conducted by a team of researchers from the U.S. Department of Health and Human Services and the Association of American Medical Colleges came to an astonishing conclusion: Black residents in counties with at least one Black physician lived longer. These counties had lower mortality rates and lower disparities in mortality rates between Black and white residents—*even if the Black residents never actually saw these doctors*. And the more Black doctors there were in a county, the longer Black residents lived. While the researchers didn't come to any definitive conclusions as to why the mere presence of Black doctors improved outcomes, they speculate that a county that supports Black doctors supports Black lives in general, and that these doctors are probably doing more to advocate for better care in their community.

Arielle Russell, a young African American anesthesiologist, had volunteered to do extra shifts during the period when hospital staffs were shorthanded during the first year of the pandemic. When Dr. Russell arrived at Chaniece's bedside in the early-morning hours of October 24, she quickly reviewed her lab work and realized that Chaniece's extremely low sodium levels were life-threatening. She ordered an IV of sodium chloride, but it was already too late. Her brain had tragically herniated out of the bottom of her skull.

That afternoon, the doctor called Anthony to tell him to come to the hospital right away. Chaniece was unconscious. "I was not expecting that phone call," recalled Anthony, overcome with emotion remembering the awful moment when his life was ripped apart. "I asked him how long is she going to be unconscious? When is she coming out of it? When is she coming home? I had all these questions running through my mind, but he wouldn't answer."

Shrouded in a cloud of confusion, and disbelief, Anthony sped to the hospital where doctors gave him the bad news. A scan done at five P.M. that day revealed that Chaniece was brain-dead.

Her colleagues and patients were devastated by her untimely death, and in 2021 the Indiana University School of Medicine established the Dr. Chaniece Wallace Health Care Disparity Research Award in her memory. But Anthony and their families remain grief-stricken over the loss of his soulmate and the fact that Charlotte, now an inquisitive, chatty youngster, will never know her mother. "The last words I ever said to her," he recalled, "were 'I love you. I'll see you in the morning.'"

Chaniece and Anthony had talked about the dangers of childbirth for Black women when they wanted to start their family. But they never imagined that Chaniece would become another statistic—one of about 1,200 women who die every year during pregnancy or in the year after giving birth, according to CDC statistics from 2021. Mortality rates are exceptionally high for Black women, who die at double the average rate of all other women, and nearly three times the rate of white women. Chaniece's education and her status didn't protect her: Maternal mortality rates of the highest-earning Black mothers were considerably higher than those of low-income white women. But while death rates are unacceptably high for Black women, there is a maternal health crisis in the U.S. for all women. Maternal death rates are dropping around the world, even in poorer, developing countries, but not here. Although we spend two to four times as much on health care as most other affluent nations, we have over three times the rate of maternal mortality of most other high-income countries. This is largely due to shockingly high pockets of poverty, lack of access to decent medical and prenatal care, and chronic ills like obesity-related disorders such as type 2 diabetes, hypertensions, and some cancers.

"But the deaths are the tip of the iceberg," said Dr. Jeffrey Gould, a professor of pediatrics at Stanford University and the principal investigator for the California Perinatal Quality Care Collaborative. These numbers are eclipsed by an even more serious problem, the staggeringly high rates of what's called "severe maternal morbidity." More than 50,000 women every year—which translates to 135 expectant or new mothers every single day—suffer grave and sometimes near-fatal complications that can result in emergency hysterectomies, sepsis that can damage vital organs, severe depression, and permanent disability, and leave them financially drained from months of unexpected medical care and unemployment. Yet up to four out of five pregnancy-related deaths are preventable.

When I first read Dr. Wallace's story, it was like a gut punch. The statistics are tragic: It's more dangerous for a woman to give birth in the United States—a country that spends nearly 20 percent of its GDP on health care and claims to be a world power—than in Saudi Arabia or Bahrain, countries where women are so severely constrained that they can only be seen as second-class citizens. But what's pernicious about what's happening in the United States is that we have a mythology that we have rights and privileges, but the reality is that for all the money we spend on health care, American women are even worse off than their counterparts in repressive regimes because of the historical way our health-care system was designed. These statistics are amplified by orders of magnitude for poor women and women of color. And underlying these depressing numbers are the stories of real women, like Chaniece Wallace—stories of heartbreaking, unimaginable, and possibly wholly preventable loss.

When I reflect on it, I can only conclude that this is nothing less than a national disgrace.

Why can't we do better?

We have inherited a world where half the population was considered less-than-human, and this is magnified when gender intersects with race and class. A thriving society has to lift the blinders that derive from these antiquated and persistent ideas of whose life actually matters. Removing those blinders requires diligent work, but it has to begin with the realization that women's health is more than just about women's health. It's a societal issue, because you can't leave half the population behind. We pay a huge price by not investing in women's health, and the framing of women's health as being solely a women's issue couldn't be more wrong. "Addressing the women's health gap could potentially boost the global economy by at least $1 trillion annually by 2040," according to an analysis by the World Economic Forum and McKinsey Health Institute. So we all should care. It's race, it's poverty, and it's gender that make us vulnerable as a population and as a nation.

The Pervasive Structural Violence Against Women

The reality is that these failures are part of a larger pattern of structural violence against women in the United States. Women simply are not safe in this country, and they never have been. Structural violence against women can be defined as the discrimination entrenched in our cultural, economic, and political systems that perpetuates physical, sexual, and psychological violence. It is so commonplace that it has become almost invisible; structural violence against women isn't just intimate partner violence—it's embedded in our medical, social, political, legal, and economic systems, which are designed to deprive women of agency over their lives.

Since colonial days, our laws have enshrined structural violence against women. English Common Law, which was adopted by the early settlers, sanctioned wife-beating, and even spousal murder wasn't considered a criminal offense. The Laws of Chastisement allowed men to discipline their wives with a rod. Our founding fathers didn't see women as equal—we didn't earn the right to vote for another 130 years—and we've been working ever since to correct that historical misalignment of the value of women in a society that still tolerates unequal pay for the same work.

WE'VE CERTAINLY COME A LONG way, but it's not nearly far enough. That overt violence long used to keep women "in their place" throughout history has been replaced by covert, implicit threats. Because in the United States, if you're poor, if you're a minority, and if you're a woman, things like the "Mississippi appendectomies" happen: poor women being sterilized without their consent. Even today, in our supposedly more enlightened times, a woman faces the barbaric prospect of bleeding to death in her car in a parking lot outside a hospital emergency room because of states' strict abortion bans. Why? Because these women have fewer choices, and they have fewer choices because of the societal obstacles that are stacked against them.

We think of violence as a physical force or intention to harm, but indifference is a form of violence, and neglect is a form of violence. Neglect, and indifference, especially aggressive indifference, is even more insidious than a slap in the face, because it is harder to pin neglect down, and harder to communicate its presence and impact, which makes it easier for us to blame the victim. While this structural violence takes many forms, it is principally a public health issue because our failures to protect women prevent them from meeting their basic needs and undermine their physical and mental health in a multiplicity of ways, leading to premature death, disability, and unnecessary suffering. Women may live longer than men, but they spend a quarter of their lives in poor health, sidelined in their most productive years not only from gynecological disorders but from higher rates of debilitating headaches, depression, and autoimmune disorders, according to the WEF analysis.

Our medical system is geared against women for many reasons:

• Because we still don't take their complaints seriously, which often leads to deadly delays in care—a problem that is even more pronounced for women of color like Dr. Wallace.

• Because up until quite recently, women were excluded from clinical trials of new medicines and treatments—and women of color are still woefully underrepresented—which means that we don't really know what treatments are truly most effective for women. We put more money into solving erectile dysfunction than we do into diagnosing and addressing endometriosis—and that indifference leads to the health gap that we are living with today.

• Because of economic inequality that denies women equal access to lifesaving care.

• Because of laws and policies that make women vulnerable to wage theft that erodes their financial and mental stability, and to violence at home, and to threats on the streets.

• Because of the cruelty of harsh abortion restrictions that sentence poor women and their children to a life of devastating poverty from which there is no escape. The majority of women seeking abortions already have low incomes, and when they are prevented from terminating an unwanted pregnancy, they are often held back from pursuing their educations or advancing their work prospects, which perpetuates their lifelong economic marginalization.

The structural violence against women filters down through generations, traumatizing our children. Childhood is the crucible that forms our character, and the scars from the wounds inflicted when we are young and vulnerable greatly influence the course of our lives. The children of the traumatized have always carried their mothers' suffering under their skin. We now know much more about the life-long impact of childhood trauma, known as ACEs (adverse childhood experiences). This concept emerged from a 1998 study that found that children exposed to abuse, neglect, and other negative experiences had increased risks of many common chronic health conditions, ranging from substance abuse, depression, and other mental health issues to heart disease, cancer, and emphysema.

The Burning Bed

Structural violence and the gendered society that we live in, where women find themselves facing significant obstacles at every turn, create the fertile soil for intimate partner violence to happen, that soul-crushing threat of physical violence that thousands of women face every day. It's the persistent gender norms that tolerate unequal pay for equal work. It's the wink and nod that male police officers might give each other when they're called for a domestic violence case. It's the inquisition of what the rape victim was wearing when the assault happened. It's the persistence of child marriage. All of these factors are at the root of gender-based violence. When these things are baked into our normal conduct in the criminal justice system, in the social fabric of how we define relationships, we end up putting women at risk.

Domestic violence and wife-beating has been a topic of discussion since the early days of the suffragettes in the 1900s, but it wasn't until 1977 that this violence against women finally came out of the shadows and was seen for what it is—felonious assault that trapped battered women in loveless marriages, exposed children to lifelong trauma, and perpetuated cycles of generational violence—and not some dirty family secret that should be hidden behind closed doors. It took a twenty-nine-year-old mother of four who was struggling to educate herself and better her family's lives to burn it all down and finally, at long last, get our collective attention.

In March of 1977, in a small town about twenty miles south of Lansing, Michigan, Francine Hughes had had enough.

For thirteen years, her ex-husband, Mickey, who had moved back in after a brief reprieve when they divorced, regularly beat her, smashed up the furniture, terrorized their four kids, and even killed their daughter's kitten. One night was especially awful, and that afternoon, when she returned from her secretarial classes, he demanded she quit school and burn her books. He dumped garbage on the floor, rubbed it into her hair, and savagely beat her. At her wits' end, she called the police, but they refused to arrest him because they hadn't witnessed the beatings, even though she was visibly bruised and bleeding.

Even more enraged because she called the cops, Mickey raped her before falling asleep in a drunken stupor. This final assault pushed Hughes over the edge. She was convinced that when he awakened, he'd make good on his constant threats to kill her. She told her frightened children to wait in the car. Then she poured gasoline on Mickey's bed, lit a match, and sped away as the house burned down. Hughes drove straight to the nearest police station and turned herself in.

What happened next was a watershed moment in a justice system that had consistently failed to recognize domestic violence as a crime. Instead of spending the rest of her life in prison, as so many other women did who had killed their abusers, Hughes was acquitted on a plea of temporary insanity. Battered wife syndrome, the defense that saved Hughes and has since been shown to be a form of PTSD that results from repeated intimate partner abuse, became part of the legal lexicon.

The incidence of domestic violence has plunged by about 67 percent in the past two decades because of recent reforms, such as the recognition by law enforcement that domestic violence is a crime, and women's growing economic independence. But nearly half a century after Hughes had had enough, domestic violence remains rampant, a virtually invisible epidemic that results in fifty women shot to death every month, killed by their partners after years of physical and psychological abuse. About one in three American women will experience intimate partner violence in their lifetimes, and more than 80 percent of women who are homeless with children are victims of domestic violence. It's pervasive, it crosses color lines, it's multigenerational, and it impacts a woman's social, economic, mental, and physical health. And this violence often spills over into the larger community: Many mass shootings had their roots in domestic-violence incidents that escalated out of control, and 80 percent of hostage situations are initiated by an abusive partner. Many of these perpetrators are damaged themselves and have been victims in an endless cycle of abuse that reverberates through generations.

Whereas it affects poor women and women of color much more sharply, it transcends race, class, and education. Even a 2006 survey conducted by University of Washington researchers in Seattle of upper-income white women revealed that one in ten said they were victims of domestic violence. And that was just the numbers of women willing to report it. That latter point was made abundantly clear in August of 2014, when police officers were called to a hotel room in Atlanta in response to a domestic-violence dispute. The woman who answered the door, Kelli Fuller, had "visible lacerations to her mouth and forehead," according to the police report. She and her husband, Mark, had an argument in which she accused him of infidelity. He "threw her to the ground and kicked her," the report noted. "Mrs. Fuller also stated she was dragged around the room and Mr. Fuller hit her in the mouth several times with his hands." What distinguished this otherwise unexceptional case, in an incident that is doubtless repeated countless times each year, is that Mark Fuller was a federal judge, on the U.S. District Court in Alabama, and had been on the bench since he was appointed by George W. Bush in 2002.

But there is a double standard for the powerful: Fuller was charged but let off with a slap on the wrist—under terms of a plea deal, he entered counseling, and the record of his arrest would be expunged. He finally did resign from the federal bench a year later, but only after he was consistently and roundly condemned by his Republican colleagues. Given the moral collapse of the current GOP, it's doubtful this would happen today.

The fact that violence often goes unpunished, especially for the affluent, and is not met with stiff prison sentences allows toxic relationships to spiral out of control. Francine Hughes had every reason to believe that Mickey would kill her, if not that day, eventually, because that cycle of violence can escalate so easily into a deadly fury: In America three women are murdered by a partner every day, and male partners are responsible for the deaths of more than half the women who are killed in the United States every year. Leaving is often not a viable option; evidence shows that's the time women are most vulnerable to being slain.

Unfortunately, these incidents still occur with almost metronomic frequency. On an otherwise quiet Wednesday evening in August of 2023, John Snowling, a retired twenty-five-year veteran of the Ventura Police Department in California, went to a bar and restaurant that he knew his estranged wife frequented in Trabuco Canyon, a sleepy hamlet in the foothills of the Santa Ana Mountains east of Los Angeles. Armed with multiple weapons, he found her having dinner with a female friend and instantly opened fire, in a murderous rampage that left three dead and wounded six others. Marie Snowling, who had filed for divorce a few months earlier, survived, but her husband was killed in a shootout with police outside the restaurant.

Although some women kill their abusers in sheer self-defense, acquittals like Hughes's remain rare. Most such women end up with lengthy prison sentences, and not surprisingly, Black women are imprisoned at higher rates than white women. To cite one particularly shameful example, in 2005, a Black woman in Ohio named Thomia Hunter was sentenced to life in prison for murdering her ex-boyfriend who had abused her for years and had trafficked her into prostitution. He was literally choking her when she stabbed him to death, but her plea of self-defense was ignored, and her history of abuse was hardly mentioned at the trial. Her sentence was finally commuted in 2019 after she had served fifteen years in prison.

When Domestic Violence and Maternal Mortality Intersect

Unfortunately, all too often domestic violence and maternal mortality intersect. Women are their most vulnerable to violence when they're pregnant or are new mothers. Study after study has shown that homicide is a leading cause of death among pregnant and postpartum women, who are twice as likely to die by homicide than by any other cause of maternal mortality. The statistics are stunning, but this is hardly a new story, and they reflect what I've seen in my own research over the past thirty years. In 1989, more than three decades ago, while I was working on my doctoral dissertation, I was sitting in the basement of Brigham and Women's Hospital in Boston, going through the medical records of women who were in various stages of pregnancy or had recently delivered a child. I read through one police report after another about the violence that was being inflicted on these women, and their stories still haunt me. Women in these kinds of situations are often trapped, particularly if they already have children, and they are usually stuck asking themselves, "Do I get out of this environment and put my children at the mercy of a system that, depending on the state, might split up the whole family, creating even more victims?" It's an ugly system that allows for intimate, interpersonal violence to persist.

The Abortions Wars and Right-Wing Misogyny

It all happened so fast. She was only twelve years old and playing outside her home in rural Mississippi when a man came down the street and grabbed her. The stranger covered her mouth, dragged her to the side of her home, and raped her, according to the report in *Time*. The shy sixth-grader was too ashamed to tell anyone what had happened. It was only three months later, when she began vomiting uncontrollably, that her mother took her to an emergency room and discovered that she was pregnant.

She was more than eleven weeks along, which meant it was too late to take pills to terminate her pregnancy, and a conventional medical abortion was a challenge, because she lived in the heart of the abortion-ban belt. The closest abortion provider was in Chicago, a nine-hour drive away that would necessitate paying for gas, food, and lodging for a couple of nights as well as for the procedure itself. Her family simply didn't have the money. So at age thirteen, she gave birth. None of her friends at school knew she was a mom, her mother was keeping the secret from nosy neighbors, and she was hoping to start seventh grade.

A stranger stole her innocence, but the government stole her future. Stories like this are becoming commonplace. The overturning of *Roe v. Wade* in June of 2022, and the institution of draconian restrictions on abortion access in nineteen states across the nation, criminalize abortion even in cases of rape and incest, subjecting pregnant people and abortion providers to heavy fines, suspension, and even imprisonment. Not only is this unspeakably cruel, but it accelerates a public health crisis already in the making because the people who will bear its consequences are poor women, who already face significant challenges.

Half the counties in rural Mississippi, where this adolescent was forced to give birth, are classified as maternity-care deserts, according to a 2023 report from the March of Dimes, which means there are no places within a thirty-minute drive to give birth or to see an obstetrician. There are just nine obstetrician-gynecologists to serve an area larger than Rhode Island, and each time one retires, there's no one to replace them. Younger doctors and medical students, even those in specialties other than obstetrics, don't want to practice in states with abortion restrictions, studies show. The inevitable consequence is that where abortion is banned, more babies are being born in places where there are already not enough doctors, and where it's almost impossible to recruit qualified physicians. While governors in states like Mississippi vow to "take every step necessary to support women and children," the reality is the opposite. States with abortion bans have the weakest social services and are racing to the bottom in every measure of health and well-being, with higher rates of death for infants and mothers, and double the rates of teen births and uninsured women and children, compared to states where abortion is legal.

In a nation that does not mandate paid family leave, a nation where it's acceptable for states to hoard billions in federal welfare money instead of giving it to needy families, a nation that does not guarantee universal health care and tolerates Black women dying in childbirth at the same rate as women in Uzbekistan, a developing nation that spends far less on health care, this is egregiously wrong. From a public health perspective, and from a humanitarian perspective, denying millions of women the right to control their own bodies and stripping pregnant people of access to fundamental health care exacerbate deep health and economic disparities, pushing women of color further and further behind, and perpetuating the dangerous history of structural violence against women.

If there was any question about the depth of the misogyny embedded in the decision, a quick read of Supreme Court Justice Samuel Alito's incendiary majority opinion in the *Dobbs v. Jackson Women's Health Organization* case that overturned *Roe v. Wade* should quell any doubts. In that decision, Alito cited a seventeenth-century English jurist who supported marital rape and who sentenced two elderly widows to be hanged from the gallows for the crime of witchcraft.

Any time women gain some autonomy and control over their reproductive lives, whether it's through the availability of contraception or abortion allows them to flourish and be independent, the backlash is ferocious. The legalization of abortion in the 1970s unleashed a wave of violence from religious zealots who turned abortion clinics into battle zones, and allowed right-wing politicians to use abortion as a wedge issue in the nation's divisive culture wars, revealing our patriarchal society's profound animosity toward the liberation of women. Since 1977, there have been thousands of criminal incidents, according to the National Abortion Federation, that include 11 murders of doctors, nurses, patients, and staffers, 42 bombings, 196 arsons, and 491 assaults.

One of those embattled doctors was LeRoy Carhart, perhaps the unlikeliest of defenders of progressive causes. A registered Republican who served for two decades in the air force, he married his high school sweetheart and moved to a large farm in rural Nebraska. The obstetrician had been performing abortions part-time when arsonists set fire to the farm in 1991, a blaze that killed his dog, his cat, and seventeen of his horses. The next day he received an anonymous letter letting him know precisely why he had been targeted.

But they clearly didn't know who they were dealing with.

The attack turned the Midwestern doctor into an activist. He started offering abortions full-time and renamed his medical facility the Abortion and Contraceptive Clinic of Nebraska just to make sure there were no doubts about what he was doing there. When his friend Dr. George Tiller, who performed late-term abortions at his clinic in Wichita, Kansas, was shot and killed, Carhart began offering them at his own facility and called abortion opponents the American Taliban, guilty of "religious terrorism." Undeterred, Carhart continued performing abortions until a few weeks before his death in April of 2023, when he was eighty-one. What drove him, he told *The New York Times,* was his memories of being a young doctor, when he regularly witnessed the side effects of self-induced abortions before abortion's legalization. "It was horrible," the air force veteran told the *Times,* "worse than watching people die in a war."

We may soon go back to the misery of these back-alley abortions.

But the landmark *Dobbs* decision, which upended nearly fifty years of legal precedent, was only the culmination of a thicket of legal battles that have been waged in our nation's courts since the right to abortion became the law of the land in 1973. "For me, the struggles for reproductive rights for women and civil rights for African-Americans are intertwined and at the same time parallel," wrote Dr. Kenneth Edelin, a prominent Black physician and former chair of the department of obstetrics and gynecology at the Boston University School of Medicine, in his autobiography, *Broken Justice: A True Story of Race, Sex and Revenge in a Boston Courtroom.* "The denial of these two rights is an attempt by some to control the bodies of others. Both are forms of slavery. We must never let slavery in any form return to America."

Edelin himself was at the center of one of the earliest and most controversial courtroom cases, in Boston in 1974, when he was indicted for manslaughter after performing a perfectly legal procedure. In what newspaper editorials called a "disgraceful" "witch hunt," he spent two traumatic years with the threat of losing his medical license and serving prison time hanging over his head. Edelin was inspired to devote his life to women's health after watching his mother die a slow, agonizing death from breast cancer when he was twelve. "Ken was very close to his mother, and he felt that because they were poor and because she was a Black woman, people didn't take her illness as seriously as they should have," said Barbara Edelin, Kenneth Edelin's widow. "He struggled after she died and felt that the way he could honor her death was by finding a path to help other women like his mother, who were poor and Black and did not have access to good care."

His own life experience convinced him of the importance of a women's right to choose. As a young man, he discovered that his grandmother had had an illegal abortion, which had been performed when she was hidden deep in the woods of Washington, D.C. She probably lay on the ground on a blanket, surrounded by the makeshift tools of illegal abortions—the construction tubing, plastic syringes, and mason jars filled with Lysol. Yes, Lysol, the strong, corrosive disinfectant, was often the chemical of choice injected into the uterus to induce the expulsion of an unwanted fetus. Early formulations contained cresol, a compound that induced abortion, and the household product was cheap and readily available.

Doctors estimate that, in those dark days, between 200,000 and 1.2 million illicit abortions were performed every year. Hospital wards were filled with young women who had undergone botched procedures. Mortality rates for those admitted to the hospital hovered around 20 percent—although who knows the numbers of women who died in agonizing pain in seedy hotels where illegal abortionists practiced, or in their own homes—but more than 60 percent of the desperate women whose uteruses were pumped with hot fluid containing Lysol died. In 1965, there were 235 abortion-related deaths nationwide, accounting for 20 percent of all pregnancy-related deaths, according to a never-released 1981 CDC report, and "it was not unusual for half of all beds in the gynecological units of large public hospitals to be occupied by women suffering complications" of illegal abortions.

In the spring of 1966, when Edelin was in his third year of medical school at Meharry Medical College working his ob-gyn rotation at Hubbard Hospital in Nashville, he personally witnessed the horrific effects of these illegal procedures. The young African American girl on the stretcher in the emergency room couldn't have been more than seventeen. Her face and body were swollen, and a severe infection had rampaged through her body. She had no family or friends to support her, nurses told him. Someone had abandoned her nearly lifeless body at the front entrance of the ER.

She was rushed into the operating room, where the surgeon heroically struggled to save her. But there was a gaping hole on the side of her uterus and floating inside her stomach was a red rubber catheter, a telltale sign that someone a couple of days earlier had stretched the catheter on a knitting needle or coat hanger and inserted it inside her womb to induce an abortion. But instead, they punctured the back wall of her uterus. The teenager was septic—the infection had invaded every organ. "With tubes and drains emerging from every opening of her body, she lay in bed, with [the surgeon] by her side, holding her hand," Edelin wrote. "It was the only thing left for him to do as life slipped away and she died."

Seven years later, in October of 1973, several months after the *Roe v. Wade* decision, when Edelin met another pregnant teenager in distress, he did not hesitate. By this time, Edelin was an experienced doctor. He had served as a medical officer in the air force, rising to the rank of captain, after which he moved to Boston in 1971 where he became the first Black person to be the chief resident of the ob-gyn service at Boston City Hospital.

The scared young girl's name was "Evonne," she was about seventeen, a high school senior with plans to attend college, and she was sixteen weeks pregnant. The abortion was a relatively simple procedure, Edelin explained to her and her mother. On the following Monday, he would inject saline into the teenager's uterus to expel the fetus. She would be home by Wednesday and could return to school on Thursday. "Dr. Edelin, do what you have to do," the grim-faced mother sighed. "I can't take her home pregnant."

But all did not go according to plan. The saline infusions didn't work, and Edelin was forced to perform a hysterotomy to terminate the pregnancy. This is a surgical procedure often used in second-trimester abortions in which the fetus and the placenta are removed from the uterine cavity. Mercifully, the surgery went well with no complications and when Edelin removed the fetus, it had already died in the womb. Evonne was discharged three days later, and presumably went on with her life.

But Edelin didn't. In April of 1974, a grand jury indicted him for manslaughter. Boston City Hospital did not stand behind him—they suspended him from his residency and the medical board considered revoking his license. "It was harrowing, and he was in disbelief because he knew he had not done anything wrong," said Barbara Edelin. "It's also important to remember that Ken was not advocating for abortion—he was just at work that day." He was simply doing his job.

Fortunately, the rest of the medical community realized he was being scapegoated. Dean Friedman of the Boston University School of Medicine looked into having the university's lawyers represent him, his fellow residents pressured the hospital to reinstate him so he could finish his residency, and other doctors, philanthropists, charitable foundations, and people in the community banded together to form the Kenneth Edelin Defense Fund (KEDF) to raise money for his legal fees. There were well-attended rallies on the hospital steps, and dozens of prominent physicians across the country would later take out full-page ads in *The New York Times* in support of Edelin because they all knew what was at stake.

"We knew the anti-abortionists were looking to bring a suit over the handling of fetuses because at that time there weren't any specific rules and they would come through the pathology departments [in the city] looking for specimens," recalled Dr. Vivian Pinn, a pathologist at the Tufts University School of Medicine at the time and one of the co-founders of Edelin's defense fund. "It was a horrible time for him and for all of us who were pro-abortion and who felt he was being unfairly prosecuted and being made a sacrificial lamb. The medical community as well as the community at large provided that nurturing and support that he needed to show he was not alone."

The indictment was based on flimsy evidence—that somehow the fetus had been alive outside of the womb, which was not true. But the prosecutor was gunning for the DA's job, the all-white jury was comprised of nine men and three women who were mostly working-class Irish Catholics, and this was the Boston of the 1970s that had been ripped apart by riots over forced busing to desegregate the schools, with angry white mobs overturning buses carrying frightened Black children, causing deep racial animosities. Add in a Black doctor and a Black teenager at a public hospital and it was the proverbial perfect storm for a gross miscarriage of justice.

Despite a parade of medical experts who all said that Edelin's actions fell completely within medical standards, he was convicted. "Boston was just a powder keg and there was that undercurrent of how angry white people in south Boston were about Black children bused for school," recalled Barbara Edelin. "At the same time, this Black doctor is on trial for manslaughter but really he was on trial for performing an abortion. The Irish Catholics in Boston felt there was no way they were going to allow this to be happening at their city hospital."

The judge sentenced him to only a year's probation, however. That evening after court, Edelin returned to work and did what he did best: He delivered a seven-pound, eight-ounce baby girl named Ayanna. His conviction was appealed, but Edelin was left in a tortuous limbo for nearly two years until the Massachusetts Supreme Judicial Court reversed the decision. Still, the court case had a chilling effect on abortion providers across the country, who were increasingly reluctant to perform second trimester abortions. Edelin went on to a distinguished career as a physician and activist as managing director of the Roxbury Comprehensive Community Health Center, which served Boston's Black community, associate dean at the Boston University School of Medicine, and chair of Planned Parenthood Federation of America. "After he was exonerated, he felt like it was his mission to continue to fight for women to have this right," said Barbara Edelin, "that women should be able to make this decision in the privacy of their relationship with their doctor, and not be scrutinized by the government, and to decide their own reproductive future."

Our Bodies, Ourselves: The End of Bikini Medicine

But women's bodies, especially Black women's bodies, were never treated equitably in the medical system and were subject to inferior care and humiliating treatment in ways large and small. Dr. David Satcher, who served as director of the CDC and as the nation's surgeon general (the first Black physician to hold both those positions), remembers a telling incident in his third year of medical school at Case Western Reserve University. He was on his first day of the obstetrical-gynecological rotation at the University Hospitals with nine other students. They were all led into a room to learn pelvic examination. Because Medicaid hadn't been fully implemented, patients who couldn't afford to pay were asked to be subjects for the teaching program.

That day, the four women waiting to be prodded and poked by medical students were all Black. "We were in line waiting to begin," Satcher wrote in his book *My Quest for Health Equity*. "I was immediately struck by the lack of privacy and dignity (there were no curtains) with which the women were treated. I refused to participate and walked out of the room."

The medical school dean requested a meeting with Satcher the next morning, and he fully expected to be expelled, with his future in shambles and all his hard work down the drain. But he was in for a welcome surprise. "Do you know what happened this morning?" the dean asked him. Satcher shook his head glumly. He told him the other students had walked out, too, because they thought he was right—this treatment of patients was callous and cruel.

But these victories are still far too few. Dr. Vivian Pinn believes that her mother died an agonizing death because of her race and gender. The 1910 Flexner Report had nearly shuttered the educational pipeline for Black physicians and led to the closure of all but two Black medical schools. Up until 1968, the American Medical Association had significant barriers to admitting Black physicians, which meant they didn't have admitting privileges to white-run hospitals, especially in the segregated South. Consequently, Pinn's mother, who lived in Lynchburg, Virginia, was forced to see a white orthopedic doctor when she complained of severe pain in her hip.

During her summer break from college, Pinn accompanied her mother to the specialist and was appalled by what she witnessed. He prescribed gold shots and orthopedic oxford shoes for her "arthritis," neither of which did anything to relieve her pain. But he ignored her complaints and instead lectured her about doing the exercises he had suggested. "He had such a dismissive attitude," Pinn recalled. "Later on, when my father massaged her hip, he felt a knot. But by the time she was correctly diagnosed, her bone cancer had eaten through the bone and spread throughout her body. This doctor was obviously not practicing good medicine. To miss the tumor completely meant he must never have done an X-ray, which could have revealed the tumor early on."

To compound his negligence, the bone biopsy was botched, and the wound never healed properly. The elder Pinn had an oozing incision on her hip for more than six months and was in constant pain until she died. "She did not get the care and attention initially that she should have had," said Pinn, who took a leave of absence from

Wellesley College for a couple of semesters to care for her ailing mother, who died when Pinn was nineteen. "I don't know if it would have saved her life if they found the tumor earlier, but she would not have gone through such a miserable and very painful prolonged death. It was a terrible thing, but it solidified my desire to go into medicine and to help women."

When she entered the University of Virginia School of Medicine in 1963, Pinn was the only woman and only person of color. At that time, women's health was limited to what one female physician called "bikini medicine." When treating women, medical professionals focused on the bikini-defined areas, the breasts and reproductive organs, and ignored the rest of a woman under the misconception that women were the same as men. That mistaken belief began to change in the wake of the second-wave feminist movement of the 1960s, when a group of women doctors in Boston produced a 193-page stapled pamphlet called "Women and Their Bodies."

It was the first practical manual that dealt honestly with a woman's anatomy and encouraged women to get to know their bodies. It included illustrations on how to use a mirror to inspect their vagina, and frank discussions of such taboos as abortion, the broad spectrum of female sexuality, the mechanics of sexual arousal and why masturbation and orgasm are natural and necessary for good health, subjects that had been stigmatized and shrouded in shameful secrecy. That makeshift booklet quickly expanded into a book that became a cultural phenomenon, *Our Bodies, Ourselves*, which sold millions of copies and became the bible of the women's health movement. "For my generation, the focus on women and their bodies really started with *Our Bodies, Ourselves*," said Pinn.

But it would be another two decades before women's health research began to get the financial backing needed to do rigorous studies. In 1991, a tough, no-nonsense, Harvard-trained cardiologist who had served as president of the American Heart Association and directed research at the Cleveland Clinic Foundation was appointed director of the National Institutes of Health by President George H. W.

Bush. Her name was Bernadine Healy, a Republican and an unapolo-getic feminist, and she took over a demoralized agency that had been without a director for two years and was rent by bureaucratic power struggles and turf wars. "I am willing to go out on a limb, shake the tree, and even take a few bruises," Healy, the first woman NIH director, told reporters. "I'm not particularly concerned about being popular."

Healy got her wish: She was not popular with the entrenched old guard. Still, she cleaned house, challenging the old boys' network and bringing recalcitrant underlings into line, hiring fresh faces, expand-ing the Human Genome Project, and stubbornly requiring that the NIH study women's health and reverse the standard practice of ex-cluding women from clinical trials. But her signature accomplishment was the Women's Health Initiative, a $625-million long-term study that involved more than 100,000 women and looked at the causes, prevention, and treatment of diseases that afflict middle-aged and older women, including cardiovascular diseases, osteoporosis, and cancer. The ongoing research effort ultimately yielded significant findings that saved thousands of women's lives. Among other revela-tions, the study uncovered key differences in heart disease between men and women, and the dangers of hormone replacement therapy in post-menopausal women, which was an untested treatment that women had taken for decades but that closer scrutiny revealed could increase risks of breast cancer, stroke, and heart attacks. Other re-search uncovered the link between the BRCA genes and aggressive breast cancers, saving even more lives.

Healy recruited Pinn, whom she knew from the early 1970s, when she was a medical student at Harvard and Pinn was a patholo-gist at Tufts, to be the first director of the newly created Office of Research on Women's Health at the NIH. "When Dr. Healy offered me the job, it was out of the blue but I initially said 'I can't take this job—I'll get fired because I like to say what I think and I won't last in government,'" recalled Pinn, who was then chair of the department of pathology at Howard University College of Medicine in Washing-ton, D.C. "She said, 'Well, I do, too, but come try it anyway.' Driving home from that meeting with her I thought, Why not? Maybe I can make a difference."

Pinn stayed for twenty years. During her lengthy tenure, she pushed for greater awareness of women's health issues, especially for women in underserved communities; ensured that federally funded research included women; and urged and inspired women to enter the medical and scientific professions. "I realized when I got into this position that no one has ever done this before and we needed to make sure that everything we did was based on science and underwent the same reviews as every other grant that came through the NIH," she recalled. "In essence, we set the first national research agenda for women's health research."

Still, in the early years, they faced raging institutional headwinds from fellow scientists, both men and women, who thought what they were doing was "politically correct" junk science that was a waste of money and time. To counteract this perception, Pinn and her team formulated strategic plans based on dozens of public hearings both in Washington and nationwide. "I wanted to make sure we were representing women across the country," she said.

> The people who participated were your average next-door neighbor, a woman or a husband of a woman or a father, or those who were involved in research, or health-care advocates, or simply someone who had a personal gripe. But we really wanted to get beyond the Washington, D.C., Beltway and make people feel their voices were being heard. And I think that helped with our office being accepted in the community and it got people in Congress to pay attention to what we were doing.

Despite these considerable strides, women remain second-class citizens when it comes to medical research. This lack of data on what works and what doesn't—the unnecessary deaths and illnesses from hormone replacement therapy are just one example—translates to consistently inferior care. Only 4 percent of Big Pharma's research and development monies are earmarked for female-specific conditions. In 2022, the FDA approved thirty-seven prescription drugs, yet only two were for female-specific conditions. When the Covid vaccines were approved, pregnant women were given little guidance about whether the shots were safe for them and their unborn children because they were last in line for clinical trials.

There has been a growing recognition of the physical factors that contribute to our rising maternal death rates, to cite yet another example, but little research has focused on the mental side of the equation, which is even more important. The conventional wisdom is that pregnancy and childbirth are a time of emotional well-being when women are awash in feel-good hormones. But the studies that are available show that quite the opposite is often the case. Mental health conditions are the underlying cause of more than 30 percent of pregnancy-related deaths, according to recent research, and suicide deaths among pregnant and postpartum women were higher than the most common causes of maternal mortality, such as severe bleeding or hypertensive disorders like preeclampsia. The incidence of depression during hospital deliveries has skyrocketed, exploding from 4.1 diagnoses per 1,000 hospitalizations in 2000 to 28.7 in 2015—a 700 percent increase. Yet mental health conditions are underdiagnosed and underreported, and most women don't get adequate care.

With abortion bans now in effect in large swaths of the country, the situation will become even more dire. Given that almost half of pregnancies in the U.S. are unplanned, research consistently demonstrates that lack of access to legal methods of terminating a pregnancy are associated with a nearly 6 percent increase in suicide, which is a leading cause of maternal death. With ultra-right-wing judges trying to ban one of the pills used in medication abortions, which would cut off the one lifeline that women in the abortion ban belt still have, we'll see more teen pregnancies, more women whose lives are derailed, and more deaths from despair.

Unfortunately, the ongoing war on women is imperiling the lives of millions. We need to get back to the basic principles of public health. We need data to understand who we're leaving behind and how to correct that. In California, for example, public health experts used data to find out precisely why women were dying in childbirth. They found that the main causes were hemorrhages, infections, and pulmonary embolisms (the deadly clots in the lungs that almost killed the tennis champion Serena Williams when she had her first child). They've used this information to institute systems—such as crash carts when a mother starts bleeding out—to cut death rates in half. Title IX had bipartisan support and helped give girls an opportunity in sports, which helped develop their leadership skills. These are a couple of examples, but we have hard work ahead of us. We need to push for equal pay, for childcare, for reproductive justice and affordable housing, and for the kind of social justice for women and girls that has been lacking for too long.

CHAPTER EIGHT

Ending the Killing Fields: Public Health Confronts the Epidemic of Gun Violence

"Violence is the leading cause of lost life in this country today. If it's not a public health problem, why are all these people dying from it?"

—DR. DAVID SATCHER, former director of the Centers for Disease Control

JEVON STANDBACK PANICKED. WHEN HE GOT PULLED OVER FOR a routine traffic stop in the early-morning hours of October 25, 2019, he hit one of the police officers with his car and bolted. He raced his Chevy Impala at speeds of up to 100 miles an hour through the deserted streets of the South Side of Chicago before the cops caught up with him. He was charged with a series of felonies, including aggravated battery of a police officer, illegal possession of a firearm by a convicted felon, and fleeing the scene, and was released with an electronic monitoring device on his ankle after posting bail.

While he sat at home under house arrest, his brother and his aunt died, and two of his friends were murdered. Then thirty-one, Jevon had a lot of time to think about what to do with the rest of his life. Growing up as a lonely child who lived with a mother and grandmother who were gone at work most of the time, he had found companionship on the streets. And the streets—for Jevon—meant a world, in large part, defined by guns: He bought his first gun as a teenager for $100, nearly a dozen of his friends and family have been victims of gun violence, and his long rap sheet included numerous gun charges, several stints in jail, and a shoot-out that left him hospitalized with a bullet in his back that couldn't be removed. At this point, he knew his opportunities were severely limited because of his criminal history. "Once you have a felony, and you apply for all these city jobs, who's going to take a chance on you?" Standback recalled. "And all these barriers undermined my self-confidence. The only situation I felt confident in was on the streets. There's no room for a regular life."

In 2019, he got thrown a lifeline when he enrolled in Chicago CRED, one of the numerous "violence interrupter" programs across the country that use basic public health approaches to reduce the toll of gun violence. Standback was able to alter the trajectory of his life. He earned a BA in social and criminal justice, and he now works as a CRED life coach with young men who are in the same predicament that he was in, helping them learn the skills to navigate the real world and get a decent job. After going through the program himself—he was initially a reluctant, belligerent recruit, but counseling helped him control his anger—he serves as a role model to prove that it is possible to escape from the intense gravitational pull of the streets. "I'm trying to get these guys to understand and look a few years down the road," says Standback. "If you utilize these tools, and follow this plan we give you, you do have a future."

Jevon Standback could so easily have been just another casualty of our nation's perilous, mean streets, ending up dead after that police chase, or forced to scratch out a life at society's margins with no chance of redemption. He reminds me of a kid who grew up across the street from me, who has spent most of his life on Rikers Island, New York City's jail. I grew up with so many people who aren't here or are locked away, trapped forever in the criminal justice system. It's far too easy to lock them up and throw away the key without looking at the root causes and the circumstances that led them into situations that could cost them their future and even their lives. Society has failed these young men, who've been left behind. But it doesn't have to be that way. By providing basic public health interventions when they need them the most, these lives are salvageable, and they can become productive members of society. People are better than their worst mistakes. Jevon Standback is a living example of that.

In 2022, more than 48,000 Americans lost their lives because of a firearm. While mass shootings garner the headlines, the reality is that fatalities from these incidents account for a tiny fraction of all gun murders that occur nationwide each year. More than half of firearm deaths are from suicides, while the remainder are the result of homicides and the street violence that plagues poor urban communities. But public health experts believe that the epidemic of gun violence—whether it's mass shootings, suicides, or the carnage in impoverished neighborhoods—is largely preventable by employing the same disease-control methods that are used to stop the spread of infections. Urban violence prevention programs like Chicago CRED are modeled on the three basic public health tenets used to control contagious outbreaks: Interrupt transmission, contain the contagion—in this case, by recruiting the soldiers on the street like Jevon Standback—and change community norms, which here means giving young men an attractive alternative to gang life instead of railroading them into prison.

It would be nice to report that over the years, we've applied the basic methodology of public health to curtail the epidemic of gun violence. That in mounting the same kind of research juggernaut that identified other threats to public health, like contaminated water and the spread of cholera, or cigarette smoking and cancer, we have moved forward and become a safer society. But that is not the case. Any meaningful studies about the root causes of gun violence—whether it's on the street, in the home, or in the mass-shooting incidents that have become an inescapable fact of American life—and how to prevent it were derailed for decades by the National Rifle Association and the powerful gun lobby. Political interference in science has resulted in perhaps hundreds of thousands of needless deaths.

In 1996, Congress passed the Dickey Amendment, an initiative pushed by the National Rifle Association that banned the use of federal funds to do research that would "advocate or promote gun control." The NRA told gun owners and sympathetic politicians that you can either have research into preventing gun violence, or you can have a right to own guns; there was no middle ground. This created an unbridgeable and highly polarized division between gun owners and anti-gun factions—and we've been shouting at each other across this breach ever since. In other words, this state of paralysis and mistrust is by design. The intentional lack of investment in gun-related injury-prevention research creates an ecosystem where misinformation, disinformation, mistrust, and policy paralysis thwart the work of public health professionals. The net result is that almost 50,000 Americans die from gun violence every year.

How Gun Violence Metastasized

The thinking that gun violence could be diminished by public health measures is relatively new. Throughout history, the two major causes of early or premature death have been infectious diseases and violence. Beginning with the first vaccines for smallpox in the late 1700s, vaccinations, antibiotics, and pesticides, along with better housing, sanitation, and improved nutrition, have enabled us to control infectious diseases. But violence has defied efforts by the health profession and was largely relegated to the criminal justice system, the police, the courts, and the penal system.

As far back as the 1960s, however, the CDC's own data were pointing to the importance of social factors, including gun violence and tobacco use, as the root causes of premature mortality among Americans. Public health scientists led in-depth studies that conclusively showed how dangerous cigarette smoking was to our health.

Despite enormous efforts by the tobacco industry to discredit this research, the number of American adults who smoked cigarettes regularly declined from 42 percent in 1965 to 11 percent in 2022, a seismic shift in personal habits that saved millions of lives.

Then in 1979, Dr. Julius Richmond, the nation's surgeon general, issued the landmark public health report *Healthy People,* which outlined what was killing most Americans and strategies to prevent those deaths. He reported that of the five leading causes of premature death, three—injuries, homicide, and suicide—are related to violence. In the early 1980s, public health researchers began to view violence through a public health lens. "We thought the gun violence problem was solvable, and we could approach it using an evidence-based scientific set of questions and answers about the causes, and especially the questions about what works," said Dr. Mark Rosenberg, who helped found and was the director of the National Center for Injury Prevention and Control, which was established at the CDC in 1992.

Researchers at the CDC were inspired by how studies into the causes of car crashes, which was one of the biggest sources of injury and death, eventually saved more than 600,000 lives over fifty years. In the 1950s, Swedish engineers at Volvo focused their efforts on safety and invented the three-point safety seat belt in 1959, which they refused to patent in order to make this lifesaving innovation widely available. Americans turned up their noses, calling Volvo an "old man's car," while they snapped up record numbers of snazzy high-performance sports cars—the Corvettes, the Thunderbirds, and the Mustangs—that were more suitable for the racetrack than residential streets.

But lawmakers couldn't ignore the growing carnage on the road. More than 53,000 Americans were killed in traffic accidents in 1969, and that was when the U.S. population was 200 million. Starting in 1970, Congress earmarked $200 million per year to study the problem, and what they uncovered led to a redesign of cars and roads, and campaigns to reduce drunk driving. Automobiles are now equipped with a suite of safety features: seat belts, harnesses, airbags, collapsible steering columns, padded dashboards, and rollover impact protection. And instead of long straightaways, which encourage speeding, highways and roadways are curved so drivers slow down, among numerous other innovations. These simple, research-based interventions on how to make cars and driving safer have saved hundreds of thousands of lives. Why couldn't the same evidence-based approaches be applied to our epidemic of gun violence?

With the 1991 publication of "Violence in America: A Public Health Approach," CDC scientists persuasively outlined how the tools of public health can be used to prevent gun violence in its various forms, whether it was suicide, urban bloodshed, or domestic violence. When Dr. David Satcher took over the CDC in 1993, he encouraged these efforts.

Momentum was clearly building for a large-scale research effort into the causes of all forms of gun violence—suicide, intimate partner violence, street violence, and mass shootings—and possible methods of prevention. A long list of questions needed exploring: Should we focus on mental health? Should schools install metal detectors or arm teachers? Does raising the legal age to purchase weapons from eighteen to twenty-one curb violence? Will banning semi-automatic weapons solve the (then-growing) problem of mass shootings? Do red-flag laws identify would-be shooters? Can waiting periods to buy a gun prevent people from killing themselves? All of these questions are too complicated to simply work out in our heads because there are so many variables involved, said Rosenberg. "But it's possible a well-designed study could and would in turn build public trust in any resulting legislation," in much the same way that safety studies finally convinced reluctant Americans to wear seat belts.

But that never happened. The National Rifle Association fought back hard against these research initiatives. The Dickey legislation had a "chilling effect" and essentially halted any real research into gun violence. Thirty-plus years after Dickey, after literally depriving public health investigators of the resources needed to build an evidence base that could drive population-based interventions and public policies that curb gun violence, the United States tops the list of industrialized countries of per capita lives lost to gun violence.

As a consequence, what research is available is sketchy, undermining efforts at constructive and effective reforms, and strategies are frozen in the 1990s. That's unfortunate, because it was the scientific rigor of well-designed studies that definitively demonstrated that seat belts save lives, that wearing helmets can greatly diminish the chances of sustaining a severe brain injury after a motorcycle or bicycle accident, that tobacco use can cause cancer and heart disease, or that exercise and better nutrition can stave off heart disease. Think how far along we'd be in containing the gun violence epidemic if public health scientists had spent the past thirty years investigating the causes and truly effective methods of prevention.

Instead, gun violence has metastasized. From 2004 to 2021, deaths by firearms soared by 45.5 percent, according to a 2022 JAMA study, and in the first year of the pandemic, homicides grew by 30 percent. The nation convulses each time there is another mass shooting, which is happening with such regularity that we've become accustomed to the bloodshed. Each incident predictably renews calls for banning assault weapons, a strategy that is only one in a long list of remedies that could help bring this monstrous scourge under control if there was any political will. But there isn't, and it remains easier for a malevolent gunman to buy an arsenal of weapons, even from licensed dealers, than it is for chronic sinus sufferers to stock up on decongestants.

Since 1999, we have had Columbine, Parkland, Virginia Tech, and Sandy Hook. And more recently, the horror of the Uvalde massacre in May of 2022, when a suicidal teenager killed nineteen children and two teachers at Robb Elementary School in Texas. Most of the postmortems in the anguished aftermath centered on the catastrophic failure of law enforcement to intervene for nearly an hour. (Officers were rightfully scared out of their wits to face the firepower of an AR-15 machine gun, which hopefully put to rest once and for all the wrong-headed idea that a good guy with a gun can stop a bad guy with a gun.) But a crucial part of this tragedy hasn't been talked about: the fact that it might have been prevented from happening at all if threat-assessment procedures and red-flag laws had been enforced or even in place.

Before he opened fire that fateful day, the gunman, Salvador Ramos, a former student at Robb Elementary, took numerous actions that loudly telegraphed his intentions, according to an investigation conducted by a committee from the Texas House of Representatives in July of 2022. But no one heeded the flashing warning signs. A year before the massacre, he had descended into a deep well of despair, making such frightful, rage-fueled threats that people who played online games with him nicknamed him "school shooter." He terrorized women on social media and stalked a girlfriend after she broke up with him in 2021.

The day he turned eighteen, Ramos ordered 1,740 rounds of 5.56mm 75-grain boat-tail hollow-point bullets that an online retailer delivered to his home, according to the report. He also ordered an AR-15–style rifle and had it shipped to a gun store in Uvalde, and purchased another AR-15 type of weapon, along with 375 rounds of ammunition. When the rifle arrived at the gun store on May 20, he had the staff install a holographic sight on it. One can only imagine what that gun-store clerk was thinking when he attached a gun sight meant for only one thing—killing humans—to an automatic weapon that can fire forty-five rounds per minute, which he just sold to a teenager in a nation that has mass shootings on a weekly basis.

When authorities have previously done profiles of shooters, they have found certain common characteristics: a history of misogyny, mental deterioration, threatening communications, and methodical preparation. Ramos fit the profile: He was a mentally unstable eighteen-year-old with a history of harassing women who spent $5,000 over a handful of days amassing a deadly arsenal that was suitable for mass killings in a war zone. Yet not one person thought to sound an alarm?

Could this slaughter have been avoided if gun-violence research had been allowed to continue? If we had red-flag laws or a nationwide computerized system that could identify when someone is stockpiling weapons of war? We'll never know.

Made in America Carnage

Yet these tragic deaths, in supermarkets, synagogues, churches, shopping malls, outdoor concerts, and classrooms, are only the tip of the iceberg in an enormous epidemic. The real carnage is largely invisible, in impoverished neighborhoods and in the quiet, lonely rooms where desperate people take their own lives. Despite the disinformation campaign of the gun lobby—and the partisan lawmakers on their payroll—that attempts to divert attention from the real issue by talking only about mental illness, the reality is that the root of the problem is the guns.

The statistics are almost beyond comprehension in what is supposed to be a civilized society. Americans own nearly 400 million guns, which translates to 67 million more firearms than people, a difference larger than the entire population of the United Kingdom. The U.S. has the highest death rates from firearms of any developed country, with nearly five times the mortality rates of France, the nation with the second-highest rate. Firearms are the leading cause of death for children, guns are the weapon of choice in cases of domestic violence, and American women are twenty-one times more likely to be killed by firearms than in any other peer country. *Twenty-one times.*

Then there is the financial toll: the health-care costs of gun violence, which leads to 30,000 hospital stays and 50,000 ER visits, at an intial cost of $1 billion annually. The Deep South, where gun-owning has been part of the cultural landscape for literally centuries, accounts for nearly half of inpatient hospital stays and the attendant costs. In the aftermath, victims are left with sizable medical bills, averaging nearly $2,500 a month, and survivors are often disabled and unable to resume their normal lives, and suffering from PTSD and substance-abuse disorders. The overall financial costs of gun violence to our nation are astonishing: more than $557 billion annually, a figure that includes medical costs, lost productivity, police and criminal justice expenditures, and the loss of quality of life of the victims and their families, according to a 2022 report by Everytown for Gun Safety.

More than half of the people admitted to hospitals for gunshot wounds are Black. Young Black men between the ages of twenty and twenty-four are, by far, the principal victims of gun violence, and they die from firearm homicides at a rate that is 22.5 times higher than any other group of Americans. Overall, Black people account for 60 percent of firearm homicides every year, even though they comprise only 14 percent of the population. In poor communities, every child grows up with the trauma of knowing an aunt, uncle, cousin, brother, mother, father, or friend who was killed by gun violence. Some have even witnessed these murders at tender ages, leaving them with permanent psychological scars, which are exacerbated by the everyday adversities of growing up in impoverished neighborhoods where substance abuse, domestic violence, homelessness, and even hunger are rampant.

Those who aren't lured into a life of petty gang crime—and more than a few join simply because they fear for their lives—find themselves virtual prisoners in their own homes after school, unable to play basketball or stickball with their pals because they are afraid of being caught by a stray bullet in the crossfire of a drive-by shooting. And the statistics do not tell the whole story. There are myriad other adverse outcomes that stem from this epidemic, including the sedentary lifestyles—and all the attendant clinical implications of obesity and related illnesses—among adults and children feeling unsafe and at a risk of neighborhood violence. There are also the lack of social cohesion, lingering mental health issues from trauma and social isolation, and finally, lost income. These kinds of routine, everyday bloodshed and lost opportunities for health and wellness are facts of life in these neighborhoods.

"This is a made-in-America problem—it doesn't exist in any other industrialized country," says Arne Duncan of Chicago CRED, who was previously Obama's secretary of education.

> Every other country has mental illness. Every other country has violent video games. Every other country has angry white men. They just don't have this access to guns and access to weapons of war. This is not intellectually difficult. We just lack the courage to do what every other country's done to keep their children safe, to keep their citizens safe. And the amount of fear and trauma that our kids grow up with in Chicago and other places is mind-boggling. And we just allow that to happen and act like that's normal and we continue to sacrifice our kids.

Can Public Health Stop Urban Violence?

Violence-interruption programs like Chicago CRED (Create Real Economic Destiny) are based on a basic principle of public health: Contain the contagion. In the case of street shootings, studies consistently show that a small fraction of the population is responsible for most of the violence. It's often the result of turf wars that erupt between small groups of people who know one another. Intervening directly with those at highest risk for perpetrating a shooting—or of being shot themselves—may interrupt transmission and contain the risks by stopping the endless cycle of retaliation and mobilizing the community to establish norms to prevent violence, in much the same way as designated-driver campaigns have reduced traffic-accident deaths from drunk drivers. These programs often employ people who have criminal records and a long history of violence to use their street cred, experience, and contacts to build relationships with those who are most likely to engage in violence, and to mediate disputes, defuse volatile situations, and thwart the dynamic of constant reprisals. They also encourage gang members to participate in programs and social services to give them other, better choices, and help young men like Jevon Standback avoid becoming another casualty.

In the past few decades, community violence intervention programs have been adopted across the country. Dr. Deborah Prothrow-Stith, dean of the college of medicine at Charles R. Drew University of Medicine and Science, was a pioneer in this movement, and her educational strategies for preventing gun violence are now taught in schools in all fifty states. In the late 1970s, she saw firsthand the destruction of gun violence when she was a resident in the ER at Boston City Hospital, an inner-city facility that treated gang members coming in with gunshot wounds. "We were stitching people up and sending them out," the Harvard-trained physician recalled. "One night, one young man said, 'Hey, I'm going to go out and get the guy who cut me.' It was almost as if there was nothing we could do, and this was just inevitable. It started me thinking about what we should do."

She realized that this demanded a public health response, not a criminal justice one. The toll it takes is, of course, on health and life. And because a lot of violence is directed at friends and family members, it is not easily amenable to law enforcement and criminal justice. Prothrow-Stith's *Violence Prevention: Curriculum for Adolescents*, which outlines strategies for families, schools, and communities to reduce gun violence, is similar to the kind of public awareness educational campaigns that have been so successful in reducing smoking, drunk driving, and teen pregnancy.

In the 1990s, during her tenure as commissioner of the Department of Public Health for Massachusetts, Prothrow-Stith also worked with a broad-based coalition of leaders in government, law enforcement, education, and health. They developed a comprehensive violence-prevention blueprint that became known as the "Boston Model," which emphasized dealing with the factors that provoke youth violence, like poverty and domestic abuse, and methods of prevention, such as conflict resolution. The program proved so successful that in a three-year period, the youth homicide rate dropped by nearly two-thirds, from an average of around forty annually to the low teens in 1996. But like so many similar programs, it withered because funding dried up and cities failed to continue to implement the strategies that had been shown to work.

Other violence-prevention initiatives are modeled on a program developed by Gary Slutkin, a veteran epidemiologist who was horrified by the killings in his hometown of Chicago. Among a population of 2.7 million, there were more than 3,500 shootings, including some 800 homicides, in 2021 alone. This is nearly as many shootings and deaths as in New York and Los Angeles combined, even though the city has one-fifth of their combined populations.

Slutkin had spent the late 1980s and early 1990s in Central and East Africa with the World Health Organization as a public health foot soldier in the drive to contain the AIDS epidemic. When he returned to where he grew up in Chicago, he was struck by the fact that the gun violence that gripped the city had all the properties of the epidemics he had spent his career combating. "It qualifies as a contagious disease, as it has characteristic signs and symptoms causing morbidity and mortality, and it's contagious, as one event leads to another," he told *The New Yorker.*

Slutkin saw early on that the core methodological pillars of public health investigation and response can be applied universally. When we talk about domestic violence or climate change being a public health crisis, the underlying message is that we need a public health approach for understanding the problem and then solving it or mitigating its impact on humans and our planet. Under the auspices of the University of Illinois in Chicago, Slutkin devised a program that employed essentially the same strategies used to combat AIDS and other outbreaks, and that deploys public health workers to reach the people who were most vulnerable to infection. In 2000, he launched what eventually came to be called Cure Violence, which used a team of so-called "trusted messengers," people like Jevon Standback who grew up on the streets, to work with the shot callers—the people most likely to incite violence—and ease tensions in the city's most high-risk communities.

Research shows that more than half of the shootings on Chicago's South Side take place in less than 8 percent of the blocks, according to the University of Chicago Crime Lab. Shootings dropped by 68 percent in one of the more violent neighborhoods where Cure Violence had a strong presence, and street violence declined by an average of 30 percent in six other hot spots where they had outreach workers. Cities that have applied these methods have seen as much as 73 percent drops in shootings and killings.

These kinds of successes inspired similar initiatives across the country, like Chicago CRED, which was founded in 2016 by Arne Duncan, the former U.S. secretary of education. Before serving in the Obama administration, Duncan spent seven years as superintendent of the Chicago school system. Once every two weeks on average, one of their students was killed by gun violence. "It was a staggering rate of loss, and having to meet with parents after they had just lost their son or daughter was, by far, the hardest part of my job," he said. "I kept a picture above my desk that a young middle school boy had drawn for me, of him climbing up a ladder outside a burning building. And his caption was 'If I grow up, I want to be a fireman.' *If I grow up*, not when," Duncan emphasized. "That's the reality of so many kids here in Chicago."

When Duncan returned to Chicago after Obama left office, the situation on the street had gotten worse, prompting the launch of Chicago CRED, which has focused on the communities where it could do the most good. The presence of these programs in vulnerable communities does seem to save lives. Another violence-prevention program in Chicago called FLIP (Flatlining Violence Inspires Peace) dispatches unarmed men and women who have trusted relationships with street gangs to hot spots in the most violence-prone blocks in fourteen communities during summer evenings and weekends, when most shootings occur. In the summer of 2021, FLIP outreach workers settled 639 disputes that could have erupted into violence and helped hammer out 47 nonaggression pacts between rival gangs, according to research from Northwestern University, which also found that when FLIP workers are patrolling vulnerable pieces of real estate, shootings drop to near zero. In a similar vein, on Memorial Day weekend of 2022, there were more than fifty shootings that included nine fatalities. But in the two neighborhoods where Chicago CRED has concentrated its efforts, North Lawndale and Roseland, there were none. "It is hard to measure shootings that don't happen and even harder to link them directly to our efforts," Duncan has readily admitted, but he does think the absence of violence is "reassuring."

Since its inception, about one thousand people have gone through Chicago CRED's comprehensive program, a number that includes participants from two partner organizations that CRED funds. Typically, the program takes about eighteen months to complete at a cost of about $30,000 per participant. While $30,000 may seem like a lot of money to help someone turn their life around, if this gives them the leg up they need to become law-abiding members of society, then that price tag is a bargain. After all, it costs $37,000 a year to house someone in prison in Illinois, and $52,000 for a yearlong stay in the Cook County jail. An analysis conducted by Bain Consulting estimated that the financial return on investment for scaling up violence prevention efforts is 19–1. When the costs of health care, policing, and prosecution are factored in, each prevented shooting can save as much as $1 million. And these figures don't include the incalculable social benefits: saving lives, reducing trauma, transforming communities, and restoring hope and dignity.

Hundreds of their graduates are now gainfully employed in more than forty different companies, and some of them, like Standback, now work for the organization. "Jevon may have been part of the problem at some point, but he is invaluable to the solution," said Duncan. "We have trained psychologists, and a team of lawyers and people with PhDs, and then we have people like Jevon who have PhDs in the streets. He's a remarkably gifted leader, but he is not unique. There are lots of others who just need a chance to lead and do something else with their lives. Those closest to the problem always have the best answers."

Still, it is difficult and painstaking work, and it can be dangerous. To cite just one of several examples, in 2021–22, over a period of thirteen months, three outreach workers with Baltimore's highly lauded Safe Streets initiative, including the organization's charismatic leader, Dante Barksdale, were shot and killed. Unfortunately, many of these programs withered in places like Philadelphia, where one pilot program after another disappeared because funding dried up. In part, that's because there was resistance on many sides: from city officials leery of hiring serious offenders, police departments reluctant to work with men whom they had arrested, and the interrupters themselves being just as wary of the cops—and many of them falling back into crime. According to Arne Duncan and other experts, the truth is that we need hundreds of outreach workers patrolling the streets, not just a few dozen people in targeted neighborhoods, to make a real, lasting impact and genuinely rein in a prodigious problem that hemorrhaged out of control long ago. As well-intentioned as these programs are—and intuitively, they do seem to make a difference—evidence, which is largely derived from small-scale studies, is unclear as to whether they actually work. As Duncan says, it's hard to measure crimes that don't happen, and, in some cities, where homicides dropped, the overall crime rate declined, too, which may have contributed to the reduced gun deaths. Part of the problem is that we have failed to invest in the kinds of studies that would rigorously assess multiple urban violence prevention programs' impact and scalability across diverse urban communities.

Is the violence interruption model, which relies heavily on trusted messengers in the community, most effective? Or does the "focused deterrence" intervention program developed by Harvard researchers, which involves police, gang members, the clergy, and other community leaders, deliver the most consistent anti-violence effects? The available research is inconclusive because there hasn't been enough funding or political will to do the large-scale studies that would clearly demonstrate efficacy. Was the program directly responsible for the reduction in deaths, or were other factors in play, too? The results are mixed at best. And more to the point, can we really curtail street violence without addressing the tinderbox of underlying issues—poverty, lack of opportunity, police brutality, the school-to-prison pipeline—that provoke simmering tensions to boil over into rage-fueled violence? Or the inescapable fact that the political deadlock about gun control and our lax gun laws make it easy for a teenager—like Jevon Standback once was—to buy a gun?

More Guns = More Suicides

More guns translate inevitably to more suicides. In scientific circles, this is not open to debate. That's because most suicides are not methodically planned, according to decades of research. The impulse to kill oneself is usually a fleeting one—often an impetuous response to a temporary crisis, especially in the case of teenagers, who may have gotten a bad grade, had a run-in with a teacher, or been bullied by classmates. If it's deflected, most people don't go through with it, and they find a way forward. It is the ready accessibility of guns that can make a bad decision in the heat of the moment turn deadly. A 2009 study by a team of Austrian psychiatrists found that the time from when someone has suicidal thoughts to the time they actually attempt to take their own life was less than an hour. In another study of people with near-fatal self-inflicted gun injuries, in which, for instance, they missed their heart by a quarter of an inch or miraculously hit a non-essential part of their brain, they were asked how long they had been considering suicide. About a quarter of them had deliberated for less than five minutes.

"The majority of people who experience a suicidal crisis wind up alive and totally fine," said Brett Bass, a program coordinator for Safer Homes, Suicide Aware, a suicide prevention program at the University of Washington.

Only a small minority of people actually attempt it. Suicide only happens if you have both capability and the desire. If you're missing one of the two, there's not going to be a death. If we can delay somebody from accessing something highly fatal for five to fifteen minutes, it is potentially the case that we could save half of these people. More than 90 percent of people who survive attempts do not go on to kill themselves. One of the big myths is that if somebody wants to die they're going to do it, it's inevitable. But that's simply not true.

An unlocked and loaded gun in a home is the number-one predictor of suicide, and increases the risk by 300 percent, according to numerous studies. Our children have ten times the gun-suicide rate as kids in France, Australia, and other developed countries. We have the highest rate of firearm suicide of all twenty-seven developed countries, and half of all suicides here in the U.S. are by firearms. The toll is staggering. Nearly half a million Americans took their own lives between 2010 to 2020, and the suicide death rate increased in that period by 12 percent. As of 2009, suicide has surpassed motor vehicles as the leading cause of death for Americans. Here again, the argument can be made that at least part of the reason we've failed to confront this problem is the same reason we haven't stopped mass shootings—because liberal access to guns plays such a significant role.

What happened to Matthew Adler is a tragic cautionary tale. In 2010, he had become deeply depressed and slowly descended into a suffocating cocoon of despair despite the best efforts of his family and trained professionals. A successful attorney in Seattle, he was suddenly unable to sleep and gripped with such anxiety that he took a leave of absence from the job he loved. Therapy and medication didn't provide much relief, and even his wife, Jennifer Stuber, a social work professor at the University of Washington, didn't realize how dire his circumstances were.

On February 18, 2011, he saw only one way to finally relieve his crippling anguish. That afternoon, this clinically depressed man walked into a gun store and purchased a revolver, and on that dark winter day, he shot himself. He was forty years old and left behind a grief-stricken family that included his wife, a five-year-old son, and a one-year-old daughter. The mental health system failed him because he felt stigmatized and filled with shame, and because a series of psychiatrists had little experience dealing with someone in the throes of suicidal despondency. "It's a myth that, when someone wants to die, there's nothing you can do to prevent it," Jennifer Stuber, Adler's widow, said in a recent interview. "My husband died because no one knew what to do. If he had had a different set of interventions, he would be very much alive."

But our lenient gun laws, which allowed someone in Adler's mental state to buy a firearm, no questions asked, failed him, too, even in a state like Washington that has greater restrictions than average. In states with fewer rules, there are twice as many suicides by firearm than in states with more laws. Even in Washington, nearly two-thirds of firearm-related fatalities are suicides (317 homicides versus 696 suicides by firearms, according to 2023 CDC data). In nearby Utah, a mostly rural state with permissive laws where nearly half the residents own guns, 85 percent of gun deaths are suicides, while 12 percent are the result of homicides. (Nationwide, those figures are 58 percent of gun deaths from suicide and 38 percent from homicides.)

Two years after Adler's death, Jennifer Stuber co-founded the University of Washington's Forefront Suicide Prevention to help counteract the erroneous information and lack of firearm-suicide prevention skills among public health professionals and gun owners. The group is part of the Safer Homes task force, which is an unlikely coalition of public health experts, suicide-prevention advocates, gun-rights enthusiasts, and Second Amendment groups. "It's not always easy," Stuber told *The Oregonian*. "But having everyone at the table is exactly what needs to happen. The conversation has not been focused on firearm suicide."

Brett Bass, who was a sharpshooter in the marines and is a handgun expert, now works full-time for Safer Homes, Suicide Aware

doing community outreach programs that focus on suicide prevention and gun-safety techniques at gun shows and community events,
and to Second Amendment groups. But he fell into the job quite by
accident. He was working as a gun-range manager at the Bellevue
Gun Club in a suburb of Seattle when his boss asked him to attend a
forum on suicide prevention and gun violence. Bass listened politely
to the presentations at the daylong event but quickly came to the realization that he was the only firearms expert in the room. When he
finally got up to speak, he asked the audience for a show of hands of
gun owners. In a roomful of about two hundred health professionals,
only two hands went up—and that's in a state where one-third of the
residents own at least one firearm.

"This shouldn't be a partisan issue," he admonished them. "This
whole 'Red Team, Blue Team' nonsense is a distraction. This is a serious issue that affects people and people die. We ought to be able to
find some common ground here."

Much to his surprise, he received a standing ovation. Afterward,
as he colorfully recalled, "I'm nervously spooning hors d'oeuvres
onto a paper plate, coming down off of the adrenaline rush of making
public comments to a room full of folks from public health that I've
never met before, when Jennifer Stuber corners me and says, 'Oh my
god, that was perfect, I need you on my task force.' And I'm thinking,
'There's a task force?'"

Today, Bass, who now manages a three-person team, drives
around Washington State in his Dodge Durango full of gun-storage
safes. He does trainings for firearms-safety instructors and gun-shop
retailers, distributes suicide-awareness videos, gives away free locking
devices for firearms, and talks about how to keep a gun safely stored
but able to be quickly accessed in the event of a break-in. "The challenge is that two-thirds of people purchasing firearms in the United
States are doing so explicitly for the purpose of personal safety," said
Bass, citing a 2017 study by the Pew Research Center. "So we tested
a variety of gun safes to figure out which one opened the fastest and
was the most reliable when the lights are low and your adrenaline is

spiking. Turns out the safes with a drum lock, where the key fits correctly only one way, is the quickest of the things we tested in that environment."

Similar programs have been launched across the country, and it's not unusual to see people like Brett Bass staffing suicide-prevention booths at gun shows. The National Shooting Sports Foundation, a trade association for the firearms industry, carries suicide-prevention information on its website. Gun-shop owners and gun-range operators are now trained to look for possible signs of depression when new customers come in, and they give out postcards with suicide-prevention hotline numbers. Do these strategies work? Here again, there is some evidence that making guns less accessible can lower suicide risks. In Israel, it had been common practice within the Israeli Defense Forces to send soldiers home on leave on weekends. It's a small country, and you can drive across it in about an hour. Soldiers would travel home in uniform, and they'd take their service rifles with them. As part of a comprehensive suicide-prevention program, the IDF changed the policy in some units and soldiers would go home in civilian attire and leave their rifles locked up in an armory. Without the easy access to a gun, suicide rates in the IDF dropped by 40 percent. If those kinds of numbers were the case in the U.S., as many as 10,000 lives could be saved every year, and 10,000 families would be spared the lifelong guilt, grief, and trauma of losing a loved one to suicide.

Still, many of these groups, like the NRA, and the Second Amendment Foundation, don't support the measures that public health experts believe can help stop senseless deaths, including universal background checks, mandatory waiting periods, and red-flag laws. They argue that these policy changes only apply to legally purchased guns and do little to stop the flow of illegal weapons or guns bought through straw purchases or other unlicensed methods that are used in violent criminal activity. However, the statistics that track domestic trafficking patterns show that red-flag laws are a deterrent. States that have robust gun-sale regulations have found them effective in reducing the rates of illegally trafficked guns. In New Jersey, which has strict gun-safety laws, over 80 percent of guns used in the commission of crimes were purchased in another state. And the majority of crime-gun recoveries in major cities with strong firearms rules, such as New York City, Chicago, Baltimore, and Los Angeles, were bought in states with weaker gun-safety laws.

Even though Bass is optimistic that we're moving in the right direction, until we change the cultural norms around guns, especially in the parts of the country where gun ownership is highly concentrated, we may not make any real progress.

Can Science Stop the Carnage?

"Science is the only thing that can break this stalemate," says Dr. Mark Rosenberg. The depressing fact is that early research funded by the CDC was promising and could have been the catalyst for building a scientific foundation for sensible gun laws. In 1993, the CDC researchers published a landmark study that showed that while many people keep firearms in their homes for personal protection, those guns pose a terrible danger to the families. Keeping a gun in the home increased the risk of a family member dying by gun violence by 300 percent, and the risks of suicide went up by 500 percent. What's more, the researchers found that even when there was a break-in and a struggle with an assailant, guns not only offered no protection but made the situation even more deadly because the intruder often used the gun against the homeowner.

"This first study looked at the question of whether having a gun in your home protects you," said Rosenberg.

The answer was very clear: Not only does it not make you safer, but it increases the risk that someone in your family will be shot and become a homicide victim with a gun. These are huge increases in risk. To put that in perspective, when the FDA approves a new drug, if the risk of side effects with the new drug is 20 percent greater than with existing drugs, you won't get it approved, because a 20 percent increase in risk is deemed excessive. Here we're talking about a 300 percent increase in the risks of homicide and a 500 percent increase in the risks of suicide. The NRA, which had been pushing gun ownership as a way of protecting families, didn't like it and told their members that if you let this go on, every civilian is going to lose all their guns. The NRA saw these results and they really scaled up the attacks that had been going on for years.

It all came to a head in 1996 during a Congressional hearing on funding for the CDC. The NRA recruited Jay Dickey, a congressman who was a born-again Christian from rural Arkansas and a lifelong member of the NRA, to lead the effort and sponsor an amendment to the bill that would curtail research. "We got ambushed by the NRA and it set off a big fight in Congress," said Rosenberg. "They wanted to abolish the whole injury center and put us out of business. It was an awful attack, and I couldn't understand how they could want to stop a research effort that could save lives."

Despite the best efforts of CDC director Dr. David Satcher to protect them, the NRA ultimately succeeded. Funding was frozen, the National Center for Injury Prevention and Control was dismantled, and Rosenberg was fired. But then something surprising happened. Jay Dickey and Mark Rosenberg became friends.

In the wake of the passage of the Dickey Amendment, Dickey had asked Rosenberg to come to his office and brief his staffers on gun-violence research. While Rosenberg was there, he noticed that Dickey had photos of his family prominently displayed. He struck up a conversation with him about his own kids, and it turned out that they had children who shared some common problems. Dickey then invited Rosenberg's son and his classmates for a tour of the Capitol. Afterward, Rosenberg's six-year-old, Ben, in his childish scrawl, wrote Dickey a thank-you note, which the congressman posted on his wall, where it remained until he left office in 2000. That initial discussion led to more talks, Dickey came to regret how his amendment had been used, and the two men became an unlikely team, writing op-eds and pushing lawmakers to fund gun-violence research.

When Dickey died in 2017, more than five hundred people came to his memorial, including the governor of Arkansas and the state's entire congressional delegation. His family asked Rosenberg to deliver the eulogy.

What the two men came to believe is that the way out of this deadlock is to formulate policies that satisfy camps on both sides of the equation: that prevent gun-violence deaths and that also protect the rights of law-abiding gun owners. Assault rifles are a good example of how good science can help us formulate policies that work for everyone. When they were banned, shootings went down. But that doesn't prove cause and effect—this is merely a correlation, and other factors could have contributed to the decline. That's why we need to do big studies that involve multiple states and have the support of the police, the judiciary, public health departments, and hospitals. And only the federal government is equipped to conduct research on this scale and to deploy teams of epidemiologists who can design these studies and decipher patterns in the reams of data that can point to solutions.

But there is finally some hope. After the country had been handcuffed by the Dickey Amendment for decades, the Biden White House recognized that gun violence is a public health crisis. In April of 2021, the administration unveiled a comprehensive strategy to combat gun violence and to close many of the loopholes that give criminals easy access to firearms because of our loose gun laws, and that allow the illegal flow of guns across state lines. But the centerpiece of this package is a $5.2 billion investment in funding for community violence intervention programs, and for research. Said Rosenberg:

> I think the biggest enemy we have is not the violence, or the gangs, or drugs and alcohol. It's fatalism—it's the sense that there are 400 million guns in this country, and we can't do

anything about them. But if we systematically go through and do the research, if we can get the data, we can get people to support things that make sense and find things that are acceptable in both red states and blue states, to Republicans and Democrats, and to gun owners and gun-control advocates.

CHAPTER NINE

Wasted Lives: Environmental Toxins Doom Poor Communities

Communities of color are forced to live in the least desirable hellscapes, sacrifice zones downwind from industrial facilities and highways where residents can't escape.

WHEN FREDDIE GRAY DIED OF A SEVERE SPINAL INJURY in the early-morning hours of April 19, 2015, the twenty-five-year-old West Baltimore man had been a victim of horrific, almost unspeakable police brutality. A week earlier, he had been arrested by police after a foot race in his neighborhood, although it remains unclear to this day why he was pursued.

He didn't resist arrest, but he was dragged into a police van after he was handcuffed, witnesses said. A citizen's video of his arrest showed Gray screaming in pain. Other witnesses reported that he was thrown face down, headfirst, and so hard into the metal van compartment that they could hear a loud thump and Gray's agonized cries. He was shuttled around the city without a seat belt, but his hands and feet were shackled.

By the time he arrived at the police station less than forty-five minutes later, he was unconscious and not breathing, his spinal cord nearly severed. Paramedics were summoned and Gray was rushed to R Adams Cowley Shock Trauma Center, where he was swiftly wheeled into surgery. He remained in a coma and never regained consciousness.

What happened in that police van to an otherwise healthy young man is still a matter of intense dispute. But his family said he was treated for three fractured vertebrae and a crushed voice box, the kind of grave injuries doctors see in serious car accidents. Medical experts later compared the physical damage to what happens when someone dives headfirst into too-shallow water.

Yet the circumstances of Freddie Gray's entire life sealed his fate, perhaps even before he was born. His life and tragic death embody a much larger issue: the pernicious and cumulative effects of centuries-old practices and policies that have created conditions that are inhospitable to human development and thriving. Poverty and racism intensify this vulnerability, and even when we have the scientific knowledge to mitigate these risks, social safety nets fail the most vulnerable. All these factors converged in the life of Freddie Gray: He was born prematurely to a drug-addicted mother, he was poisoned as a toddler by the lead-based paints in his family's dilapidated home, and his constant exposure to lead left him so physically damaged that he was virtually incapable of leading a functional life. At every conceivable checkpoint, the system had failed him.

Like so many other young men who grew up in the same bleak circumstances, Freddie Gray's life ended in a deadly confrontation with police.

The conditions faced by people like Freddie did not appear overnight. Historical practices, like Jim Crow and systemic racial segregation, forced Black Americans and people in poor communities of color to live and work in some of the nation's dirtiest environments, victimized by what activists call "environmental apartheid." The tragic fate of the Freddie Grays of this world underscores the fundamental connection between place and health. The places of our lives—our homes, workplaces, schools—and the built environment surrounding us—the buildings, roads, green spaces, sewage systems, and access to clean water, nutritious foods, and fresh air—exert powerful influences on our health, our vulnerability to disease, and our overall well-being. The toxic stew of unrelenting environmental threats that Gray faced, from contaminated housing and exposure to toxins to police violence and despair, were almost impossible to overcome.

When people hear of public health, they think of medicine, medical care, vaccinations, or restaurant inspections. But everything—our history, our regulatory ecosystem, our indifference or unwillingness to act on scientific evidence, how we vote, how we govern, how we regulate corporate impulses, how we police communities—all collectively contribute to the conditions that determine the health of individuals and populations. This is why I believe all policies are, at their root, health policies.

Freddie Gray's story, and that of millions of people who faced the same thicket of virtually insurmountable environmental and societal threats, illuminate the lasting, multigenerational impacts that seemingly unrelated policies and practices can have on our health. Reversing these long-standing environmental injustices will require a strong political will and the perseverance and commitment of multiple stakeholders working together to determine the best solutions.

Environmental Apartheid Is Deliberate

The convenient narrative is that these segregated communities are the result of decades of de facto segregation, notes economist Richard Rothstein in his excellent book *The Color of Law:* that it *just happened* and was purely an unfortunate result of generations of private practices, such as "white flight," when Blacks moved into urban neighborhoods after World War II and white families escaped to the growing suburbs. Or social norms that prompted real estate agents to steer middle-class Blacks away from white communities, a racist custom that would sometimes be spelled out in restrictive racial covenants that forbade white residents from selling their homes to people of color. This was compounded by banks refusing to offer mortgages to Black families, a practice called redlining, forcing them to remain concentrated in overcrowded neighborhoods and urban ghettos.

But the reality is that the housing segregation we see is, in legal parlance, *de jure;* in other words, it wasn't some awful coincidence but was usually rooted in government policy, and a deliberate and inevitable consequence of more than 150 years of laws and racist policies of federal, state, and local governments that left Black Americans and other communities of color with no alternative but to live in the most toxic neighborhoods. "The invisible arm of public policy works to create these underlying inequities," said DeMarcus Jenkins, an assistant professor in the School of Social Policy and Practice at the University of Pennsylvania. "Land use in this country has always been about race—racial exploitation, capital accumulation, colonialism, imperialism, and violence. We would be myopic to believe that those things are not inextricably linked and orchestrated."

Like a death by a thousand cuts, a cascade of inflection points—racist lending practices, prohibitive zoning laws that are still on the books, urban renewal and highway construction projects that tore up established neighborhoods—coalesced to create these intractable divisions. Even in the supposedly superior suburbs, which boast cleaner air, newer housing stock, and presumably better services, the same problems remain, driven by the same racist policies. Black towns have far higher rates of disease and death than their white counterparts in adjoining municipalities.

"Today's residential segregation in the North, South, Midwest, and West is not the unintended consequence of individual choices and of otherwise well-meaning laws or regulation, but of unhidden public policy that explicitly segregated every metropolitan area in the United States," noted Rothstein. "We have created a caste system in this country, with African Americans kept exploited and geographically separate by racially explicit government policies. Although most of these policies are now off the books, they have never been remedied and their severe effects endure."

Life in these bleak landscapes compounds the preexisting vulnerabilities across generations—the chronic stress of unrelenting financial insecurities, the unresolved traumas and profound wounds that never heal, the constant specter of police violence that kills unarmed Black Americans at nearly three times the rate of white Americans. These deeply ingrained inequities continue to sicken and kill Black Americans and other members of communities of color as well—and to rob us as a nation of what they might have contributed if they had been able to lead healthy, productive lives.

Like Freddie Gray.

Drowning in Environmental Dangers

Freddie Gray grew up in Sandtown, which got its name from the spillage that left a coat of fine grit on the streets from the horse-drawn wagons that once carted sand from a nearby quarry. The impoverished West Baltimore neighborhood, with its decrepit homes, abandoned buildings, boarded-up storefronts, and rutted roads, so reminiscent of the desolate environments in Philadelphia that W.E.B. Du Bois described a century before, was light-years away from the tony shops and upscale eateries of the affluent Inner Harbor, a scant three miles to the south. A child born in Sandtown isn't expected to live much past their sixty-fifth birthday—a full six years less than if they were raised anywhere else in Baltimore.

The neighborhood had roughly double the city's rate of unemployment, poverty, and shootings, according to a 2011 report. Lead-paint violations were nearly four times the city average, as was the percentage of vacant buildings. Sandtown and the adjacent Harlem Park had more residents in jails and prisons than any other neighborhood in the city, according to a study by the Justice Policy Institute, at a cost of more than $17 million to keep them locked up. These statistics paint a striking picture of the vast disparities that exist in these forgotten communities, places largely hidden in plain sight, where all of our society's inequities come together in a witches' brew that creates a populace suffocated by addiction, poor health, violence, poisonous chemicals, contaminated water, filthy air, and desperation.

Freddie Gray was a product of this environment. From the moment he was born, the deck was heavily stacked against him. His mother, Gloria Darden, was disabled and struggled with heroin addiction. She was in her early twenties when she gave birth to twins, a boy and a girl, two months prematurely. Freddie and his sister, Fredericka, were so tiny and underweight that they spent the first few months of their lives tethered to machines in the neonatal intensive care unit before Gloria was able to bring them home to the Gilmore Homes, a dreary, low-rise public housing project. Because he was premature, Gray's lungs never fully developed, and he was plagued by asthma all of his short life.

But what happened when Freddie was a toddler, barely two years of age, is what permanently derailed his life. He and his family moved into a home on North Carey Street in West Baltimore, a two-bedroom brick row house built in 1900, where they lived for four years. For decades, lead was everywhere—in paints, water pipes, food cans, toys, and even as an additive in gasoline. But it was especially problematic in older homes like the one where Freddie's family lived, which were covered in chipped-off layers of lead-based paints, with every available surface coated with toxic dust. Worse, the metal tasted sweet, making it irresistible to children, who ate the paint dust. When ingested or inhaled, a sugar-sized packet of lead dust in a house is enough to do permanent, irreversible neurological damage.

Before his second birthday, Freddie had already been severely poisoned, his life short-circuited before it even began. Even as little as two micrograms of lead in a deciliter of blood is considered unsafe, the point at which exposure to this neurotoxin can cause permanent brain damage and trigger serious learning disabilities and a propensity for aggression. Freddie's blood levels were more than thirty-seven micrograms per deciliter, more than fifteen times the levels that are deemed dangerous today. Every few months throughout Gray's childhood, nurses took blood tests to monitor his levels of lead, court records show. Over the course of four years, the hazardous blood levels persisted—yet nothing was done to remove him or his family from this dangerous environment, in chilling echoes of the criminal negligence of the infamous public health syphilis study at Tuskegee.

At the time of Freddie's exposure, however, so many houses in Baltimore were loaded with lead that health officials rarely enforced anything below 45 micrograms per deciliter, which even then was nearly twice the federal limit. "This was a child who had repetitive lead blood tests and whose family moved four times, fleeing bad conditions, but there was no redress, no laws to protect him or his siblings," said Ruth Ann Norton, head of the Green & Healthy Homes Initiative and a founding member of the Maryland Lead Poisoning Prevention Commission. Parents desperate to find a safe place for their kids were faced with a nightmarish catch-22. "In the nineties, if they told their landlords there were high levels of lead and their kids were getting poisoned, they knew they'd get evicted no matter what, and their stuff was thrown on the street," said Norton, who has witnessed generations of residents—grandmothers, fathers, daughters, and sons—crippled by lead poisoning. "And if they told prospective landlords their kid had elevated blood levels, they wouldn't rent to them."

What's truly unconscionable about all of this is that by the time lead was detected in Freddie's bloodstream, in 1991, there had been more than a decade of ample evidence that inhaling even faint traces of the toxic metal could do irreparable harm. This was the result of research done by Dr. Herbert Needleman, a child psychiatrist and pediatrician who is considered one of public health's true heroes. Needleman, a strapping six-footer built like a linebacker, with broad features and thick Coke-bottle glasses, spent the early part of his career in the 1950s practicing medicine in one of Philadelphia's poorest neighborhoods.

Still, he was shocked the first time he saw a case of lead poisoning because he had no idea it could do so much damage. The child's desperate mother had brought the sickly toddler to the emergency room when she was barely breathing. The comatose three-year-old was rushed to the infant ward where she was seen by Needleman, who towered over his tiny patient and her anxious mother.

Blood tests revealed that the child's lead levels were off the charts. Therapy cleansed the child's body of the toxic metal and brought her back to life. "It was a gratifying experience and I felt very smug," Needleman recalled. "I told the mother she had to move out of the house. 'You cannot go back to that house, because if she has a second episode she's going to be retarded.'"

"Where am I going to move to?" the single mother retorted. "All the houses I can afford are the same age." A stunned Needleman realized that lead poisoning wasn't just a health issue but a by-product of poverty, too. At the time, though, scientists thought the body could withstand a fair amount of exposure to lead and that recovery after exposure was possible. However, an incident that happened one night, when he spoke at a Black church to a group of adolescents, changed his mind—and the course of his career.

"At the end of the talk, a kid came up to me and started telling me about his ambitions," Needleman remembered in a later interview. "He was a very nice kid, but he was obviously brain damaged . . . I thought, how many of these kids who are coming to the clinic are, in fact, a missed case of lead poisoning?"

Needleman realized that many of these seemingly healthy children had sustained irreparable harm. This observation prompted the pediatrician, who later moved to Boston and joined the Harvard faculty, to embark on a series of studies that transformed thinking about the effect of lead on children's health. His initial findings, published in 1972 in *Nature,* revealed that lead poisoning was an undetected epidemic in poor urban neighborhoods. Children in the central city had more than five times the amount of lead in their bodies than their suburban counterparts. Later, in a landmark 1979 study published in *The New England Journal of Medicine,* he showed that even exposure to low levels of lead could have a dramatic impact on intellectual development and behavior. Children who tested for high levels of lead but had never been identified as having any problems with lead had lower IQ scores, poorer language functioning, problems with impulse control, and serious learning deficits.

In another groundbreaking study in 1996, Needleman measured lead levels in young men who were incarcerated. They had higher lead levels than their peers who were not in prison. This finding linked lead poisoning to criminality, to the epidemic of violence in inner cities and to the inescapable fact that many ended up imprisoned, in part because of brain damage that walled them off from legitimate pathways of economic mobility and robbed them of a productive future.

Like Freddie Gray.

In 2008, Gray's family joined with 480 others in a lawsuit because of their children's exposure to unsafe levels of lead, which they believed had caused permanent injury. Freddie had behavior problems in school and had been tracked into special education classes, forced out of a regular classroom by his intellectual disability, according to the lawsuit. By fifth grade, he was four grade levels behind in reading, and his attendance in elementary school was spotty. He played football in middle school and made the junior varsity team at Carver Vocational-Technical High during his freshman and sophomore years, but he never graduated.

Ironically, a report by two Harvard economists, Raj Chetty and Nathaniel Hendren, that was released shortly before Gray's death, identified the best and worst places for children born into poverty. And Baltimore had the dubious distinction of coming out on top—the absolute worst city in the United States in which to be born poor. Generations of discriminatory practices cut off any pathway that residents of the West Baltimore neighborhood where Gray grew up might have had for improving their lot in life. They ranged from redlining and predatory banking practices that prevented people from moving into better neighborhoods or stopped them from even owning homes, to inferior and underfunded schools. The institutions they relied upon to protect them or prepare them for a productive future—

the police, the schools, social services, even the public health and medical systems—fell disastrously short, wrecking their chances for a better, longer, healthful, and more rewarding life.

Freddie Gray had hopes and dreams, too. He often talked with his girlfriend about getting married, and he doted on her young daughter, by all accounts. He yearned to have a family, a real family, and a home that was cozy, warm, and inviting. But Freddie Gray never stood a chance.

He drowned before he reached the far shore.

"In April of 2015, when Freddie Gray was on that corner, that should have been no surprise to anyone because we ensured this pathway," said Ruth Norton. "He missed school frequently, could barely read, and dropped out of high school, he grew up in chaotic housing situations and experienced that disruption and trauma, he suffered from asthma that was exacerbated by his living conditions, and he was poisoned.

"But if he wasn't poisoned, if he had been in stable housing," Norton poignantly wondered, "would he have been on that corner?"

Forced to Live in Hellscapes

Freddie Gray's life is a microcosm of what happens to millions of Americans who are forced to live in these toxic environments with no way of escape, often traumatized by violence, and disabled by chronic diseases and grave cognitive impairments that deprive them of any opportunity for a meaningful, satisfying life. In Flint, Michigan, in another predominately Black community, the water crisis rages on. In April of 2014, in order to save money, city officials switched the city's drinking water from Detroit's system to the Flint River. But it turned out that the river's water supply was heavily contaminated with lead—a situation that has yet to be resolved and has caused terrible damage. Poor neighborhoods in cities like New York continue to grapple with the severe health consequences of too much lead in their drinking water. The city has spent billions replacing lead pipes in New York's aged housing stock, which is among the oldest in the nation, but serious problems persist. About 21 percent of New Yorkers may be drinking water transported through lead service lines, according to a 2023 report, and city officials are struggling to replace all these contaminated lines.

But it's not just lead. Communities of color are forced to live in the least desirable hellscapes, downwind from industrial facilities and highways where residents can't escape the fumes from diesel truck emissions, chemical plants, and refineries, and that contaminate the water and shroud playgrounds in noxious clouds. Even noise pollution, the incessant sounds of traffic, factories, wailing sirens, and construction, is intensified in segregated urban neighborhoods, studies show, and can contribute to a host of health problems. These range from high blood pressure and heart disease to sleep disturbances, stress, and hearing loss. For children, exposure to the constant drumbeat of loud noises, especially if they live near airports or busy streets, is linked to deficits in memory, attention level, and reading skill.

Research has also shown that neighborhoods with higher numbers of Black, Hispanic, and Asian residents or renter-occupied housing have more exposure to ambient light at night. Too much artificial light at night increases the incidence of sleep disorders. The disruption of circadian rhythms, our natural sleep cycle, plays a role in depression, obesity, diabetes, heart disease, and cancer.

The toxicity of these neighborhoods is compounded by the deplorable conditions of the housing stock. More than 30 million Americans live in older and badly weatherized housing that is literally making them sick. These dilapidated dwellings are poorly ventilated, with cancer-causing asbestos insulation, and tar roofs that trap heat in the summer and leak during the rain, causing infestations of mildew and mold. These poor housing conditions played a key role in the higher incidences of mortality during the pandemic, which ravaged communities of color who were trapped in these harmful environments.

Some communities even lack basic sanitation. It is hard to believe that in twenty-first-century America there are places in the rural South, in Appalachia, and even in the suburbs of St. Louis and New York City that have sewage backing up into residents' living rooms because of our failures to invest in infrastructure. In Lowndes County, Alabama, an impoverished region situated between Selma and Montgomery, as many as 90 percent of households have deteriorating or inadequate systems for flushing out wastewater. Cesspools and septic systems have failed, and gravity pushes the wastewater back into residents' gardens and homes, gushing out of bathtubs, and flooding their houses with stinking raw waste. Such conditions are so deplorable that according to a 2017 Baylor College of Medicine study, at least one-third of residents were infected with intestinal parasites, most notably hookworm, a tropical disease that was thought to be eradicated here in the early 1900s, which can cause anemia and developmental delays in children. The consequences of what environmental activist Catherine Coleman Flowers called "America's dirty secret" in her influential book *Waste* can be life-threatening.

But again, all of this didn't "just happen." Numerous factors and forces led to the creation and persistence of these harmful environments, in which a myriad of old and new threats—from lead and inferior housing to unsanitary conditions and extreme heat—combine to threaten our health, particularly those of us in poor communities. A century of racist policies and practices contributed to the aggregations of risks in Black and poor communities.

What happened to the Freddie Grays of this world is a public health system's failure. Even with lead screening and the documentation of risk, without a prompt implementation of remediation protocols, those cleanup procedures that are proven to eliminate the presence of lead, we failed Freddie Gray in the most painful way. The voices of public health heroes like Catherine Coleman Flowers and Dr. Herbert Needleman need to be heeded, not sidelined. These problems are complex and require multifaceted solutions and the social and political will to curb or even outright eliminate these threats by acting on the scientific evidence generated from public health research like that conducted by Needleman.

Fenceline Communities

For decades, Black and poor communities with little political clout became convenient dumping grounds for the toxic runoff of our industrial society. Corporate polluters were rarely reined in because they were big political donors. This is precisely what happened in the so-called "fenceline" communities in Louisiana's Cancer Alley, the eighty-five-mile industrial corridor on the Mississippi River between Baton Rouge and New Orleans that is overrun with more than 150 oil refineries, plastics plants, and chemical facilities. These historic towns are separated only by chain-link fences from the fossil fuel companies belching foul chemicals into the air. They are mainly populated by the descendants of enslaved people who faced unimaginable hardships on the plantations there, in some of the most brutal conditions of all the states of the Confederacy.

Numerous studies show that these residents suffer and die more from cancer, diabetes, and respiratory illnesses than people do anywhere else in the nation. The rates are even markedly higher than in other parts of Louisiana, a state that ranks dead last in most measures of health. Air pollution in the corridor is so poisonous that cancer risks are 95 percent higher than in the rest of the nation, and during the pandemic, death rates skyrocketed. Children at one mostly Black elementary school were exposed to a hazardous cancer-causing chemical at levels that were eleven times what is considered acceptable, according to the EPA. And an investigation by ProPublica revealed that parts of Cancer Alley had up to forty-seven times the lifetime cancer risks that the EPA considers normal.

Not surprisingly, every family along the River Parishes has lost droves of loved ones—mothers, fathers, siblings, cousins, friends—to cancer and other pollution-related ailments. Many families live in an-cestral homes that were passed down through generations. Local res-ident Mary Hampton recalled that her father scrimped and struggled to buy a parcel of land he could give to his nine children. "He thought he was leaving us a legacy," Hampton, eighty-four, told NBC News. "Actually, he left us a death sentence."

At least three rural towns on the industrial corridor have been wiped off the map by decades of environmental racism. Places like the River Parishes are "sacrifice zones," forgotten corners where Ameri-cans are trapped in toxic environments while the corporations that cause the destruction escape penalty. This lack of any real regulation is especially true in big oil-producing states like Texas and Louisiana, whose economies are dependent on the fossil fuel industry. As one EPA official bitterly said, "They do what they please because they know we can't come after them."

Climate Change Amplifies Adverse Health Effects

The costs of these failures are not inconsequential, and these threats are permitted to escalate because of the failures of civic leaders to stand up to corporate polluters. It is now increasingly clear that the lethal conditions that characterize fenceline communities will only worsen because of climate change, which is a threat multiplier that amplifies these adverse health effects and intensifies existing threats. As the weather becomes more extreme, we'll see higher summer tem-peratures that turn urban neighborhoods into sizzling heat islands, more frigid winters, gale-force winds that cause lengthy power out-ages because grids weren't built to withstand superstorms, and drenching rains that engulf neighborhoods whose antiquated drain-age systems fail and wash away homes built on flood plains.

But some areas will be hit harder than others. Neighborhoods that swelter under the hottest temperatures, with the bleakest land-scapes marked by block after block of heat-trapping concrete unrelieved by any canopy of trees or grass field or park, and that remain underwater after floods because of inadequate drainage systems, with the highest air pollution and record numbers of kids with asthma, all have one thing in common. These are the communities that were redlined—the racist housing policy dating back to the New Deal that remains a chief contributor to the housing segregation we see today.

Studies show that in dozens of urban neighborhoods across the country, in nearly every city, the neighborhoods that had been redlined were up to 13 degrees hotter than other communities. These poorer neighborhoods lack the trees and green spaces that can ease temperatures, in an urban heat-island effect that can add up to 8 degrees in major cities like New York, Houston, and Los Angeles. In 2023, as we were writing this book, we experienced the hottest summer in recorded history, with nearly half the world's population, more than 3.8 billion people, exposed to extreme heat from June through August, according to an analysis by the nonprofit group Climate Central. And it's only going to get worse, with longer, more intense, and more frequent heat waves that have deadly consequences.

Around the world, extreme drought and heat will push millions toward starvation, and beginning in 2030, more than 250,000 people will die annually from the direct impact of climate change, according to estimates by the World Health Organization. Farmworkers in hot, humid regions, in Sri Lanka, India, Egypt, and Sudan, are dying of end-stage kidney failure from extreme dehydration, hospitals in Nepal are overflowing with construction workers on dialysis who had helped build the towering skyscrapers in Dubai, and kidney failure is now a leading cause of death in El Salvador.

Here in the U.S., we're already seeing the toll that extreme heat will have on vulnerable populations, including the very young, the elderly, people who work outdoors, and the poor, who often have no way to escape blistering heat. Heat waves claim about 800 lives in the U.S. in an average year—although that number could escalate into the thousands during extreme weather, which is what happened in

Europe's 2003 heat wave, when more than 70,000 people died. On July 6, 2023, Efraín López García, a twenty-nine-year-old farmworker in south Florida, died on the job on one of the hottest days recorded on Earth in nearly half a century. Agricultural workers are thirty-five times more likely to die from heat stroke than people employed in any other occupation, and these deaths will continue to climb as temperatures rise.

And it's not just heat. When Hurricane Katrina hit New Orleans, it was the Lower Ninth Ward, a mostly Black neighborhood along the Mississippi River, that was the hardest hit. Once an orderly, thriving community of more than twenty thousand people with comfortable single-family homes and well-tended lawns, only one quarter remained in the aftermath of the storm. The two-mile-square district became a jungle of weeds and twelve-foot-tall grasses, a dumping ground for the city's debris and home to roaming packs of abandoned dogs. The people who were permanently displaced by the floods, many of them from Black families who had lived in New Orleans for generations, were the nation's first wave of climate refugees, with numbers rivaling the Midwesterners fleeing the 1930s Dust Bowl.

These disparities are the direct result of more than a hundred years of exclusionary city-planning decisions, on both the local and national levels. The vast differences that we see in the health and well-being of a child growing up in West Baltimore, like Freddie Gray, and a kid raised in Baltimore's affluent Roland Park, one of the very first suburbs to enact racial covenants in the early 1900s, can be traced back to these roots. "Racial residential segregation is a fundamental cause of health disparities across the board," said Martine Hackett, a professor and director of public health programs at Hofstra University in Hempstead, New York. "In New York City, there are neighborhoods that will have the highest rates of infant mortality, hypertension, infectious diseases, and even Covid. The thing they have in common is place. And that's not just true in the city, it's also true in the suburbs, that there is obviously a relationship between where you live and your health." In other words, place is a potent driver of health.

The New Deal and Segregation

Ironically, like so many other well-meaning initiatives that had disastrous unintended consequences, redlining originated in efforts to revive the struggling economy when the nation was mired in the depths of the Great Depression. In 1933, many homeowners lost or were in danger of losing their homes to foreclosure, only a handful of Americans could afford a home at all, and the construction industry was at a complete standstill. Under the New Deal, the federal government created the Home Owners' Loan Corporation, or HOLC, a state-sponsored lending program that purchased mortgages on the verge of default and reissued new ones with repayment schedules of up to fifteen years to lower monthly costs.

The government, however, wanted to ensure that the loans would be paid back, and gauged the risks based on racial composition. The HOLC generated color-coded maps of two hundred metropolitan areas of the country: green neighborhoods were considered the safest, yellow was marginal and declining, and red was hazardous. Neighborhoods of Black people, even if they were solidly middle-class with single-family homes, were redlined; racial segregation was thus codified into law. The Federal Housing Administration was created in 1934 to insure up to 80 percent of bank mortgages so that average middle- and working-class American families could purchase homes, but the FHA discouraged lenders from making loans to people of color.

After World War II, the restrictive lending practices of the FHA further divided and hardened housing segregation. Huge housing tracts like Levittown on New York's Long Island sprouted up virtually overnight thanks to government guarantees for the full cost of these developments. The FHA had congressional authority to back bank loans for dozens of mass-produced subdivisions like Levittown across the country. Banks were willing to finance the construction and land-acquisition costs because of these federal protections. Developers could never have raised the kind of capital needed to build these vast projects on their own. But the FHA financing, along with that of the newly established VA, which was backing mortgages for veterans, was contingent on a commitment not to sell to Blacks.

Municipal zoning ordinances added another restrictive layer and were weaponized to perpetuate segregation. The most desirable areas were reserved for the elite—the neighborhoods that had the best housing and schools, and that were free of environmental hazards. These same zoning laws shunted people of color to communities that often lacked basic amenities, like sewer lines and paved roads. Some of these neighborhoods were even rezoned to permit industrial plants, toxic-waste disposal incinerators, and other environmental hazards that turned these areas into slums.

By the time of the postwar building boom, more than 70 percent of housing developments had these restrictive rules. Even affluent Blacks were forced to live in areas that were questionable. Baldwin Hills, the swank suburb known as the Black Beverly Hills that was home to luminaries like Ray Charles, Ike and Tina Turner, Lenny Kravitz, Debbie Allen, Art Tatum, and John Singleton, boasts breathtaking jetliner views of Los Angeles's celebrated coastline. But the area is perched directly above the Inglewood Oil Field, which is still dotted with the towering drilling cranes used to extract crude oil from deep beneath the ground. Plans to build a power plant in those hills were scuttled only after residents banded together to stop what they called a clear case of environmental racism.

Redlining and Health Disparities

The health-care challenges in the inner cities—industrial pollution, lack of access to care, and a scarcity of social services—have spilled over into the suburbs. A 2015 Brookings Institution study of the nation's most populous metropolitan areas revealed that more people lived in poverty in the suburbs—more than sixteen million—than in nearby major cities, which accounted for thirteen million impoverished residents.

Two towns that sit next to each other on the South Shore of Long Island, Roosevelt and Merrick, exemplify this inequality and are a microcosm of how racial segregation has led to wildly divergent health outcomes even though they share a border. Nearly 90 percent of Merrick residents are white, and the median household income is about $147,000. In Roosevelt, about 98 percent of residents are Hispanic or Black, and about half of the public school students receive free or reduced-price lunches.

Roosevelt started off as a white enclave. But in the early 1960s, forced busing was used to integrate the school district which, in turn, triggered "white flight." Unscrupulous real estate speculators took advantage and "blockbusted" the community, buying houses at bargain-basement prices from terrified white residents who thought their property values would plummet because of Blacks moving in, and then sold them at a profit to middle-class Blacks. In the 1970s, social-service agencies began encouraging families on welfare or who were receiving housing subsidies to settle in Roosevelt—a practice called "welfare dumping"—and the community was trapped in a downward spiral. Middle-class Black families fled, too, taking their tax base and resources with them, and slumlords converted abandoned homes into multifamily dwellings with poorer people of color moving in. An industrial laundry, which washed linens and uniforms for institutional facilities, was abandoned and never remediated, leaving behind a toxic "brownfield," a previously developed industrial site. Today, there isn't much access to green spaces or social services, and the tiny hamlet is a food desert, with only one supermarket but at least three dozen mini markets, one on practically every corner, according to Dr. Martine Hackett.

Given this, it's no surprise that infant mortality rates for Roosevelt are 8.8 infant deaths for every 1,000 births. In Merrick, the infant mortality rate is 1 per 1,000 births. Infant mortality rates are one of those benchmarks that reveal a lot about health-care access and quality, because they are tied to the socioeconomic status of the parents. After all, babies can't take care of themselves and are influenced by the stressors in their environment. When there are such stark differences in survival between children born within a few miles of each other, said Hackett, "that tells us that something is happening in one place that is not happening in another. In a place like Merrick, you have the protection of the environment, a shield around you that does not expose you to the same level of stress."

In the same vein, residents of Roosevelt experience higher rates of diabetes, liver disease, and premature death, and kids with asthma end up in the hospital *ten times* more often than children in neighboring communities. "Why does a kid get hospitalized for asthma?" Hackett asked.

> Because you're not able to control what is a chronic disease—no quick access to doctors or medications—and you live in a place that has triggers for your asthma—dust, and the high levels of particulate matter in the air from industrial run off. This has to do with the highways and the way the roads are constructed, the placement of homes, and environmental hazards like brownfields and superfund sites that are present in Roosevelt. But in general, these problems are invisible in the suburbs, not just in Nassau County but across the country, because we've been sold on the idea that suburbs don't have city problems, that there's more space, and that it's safer, with cleaner air and better schools. Part of the reason that it's deliberately not addressed is to maintain property values. Otherwise, why live here?

Can We Fix This?

Over the past century, numerous court decisions challenged housing segregation practices, dating back to the Supreme Court's 1917 decision in *Buchanan v. Warley*, which struck down ordinances that were used to deny housing to minority groups in white-zoned neighborhoods. Later court rulings determined that "racially restrictive covenants" were unenforceable, and that federal law prohibits racial discrimination in the sale or rental of property. In 1968, Congress passed the Fair Housing Act, which outlawed racial covenants and made racial discrimination in the sale and rental of housing illegal.

But most of these rulings were not enforced, and by the 1960s, it was too late to undo the collateral damage of decades of segregation. Housing patterns were set in stone and virtually impossible to reverse. In 1973, the U.S. Commission on Civil Rights grimly observed that the "housing industry, aided and abetted by Government, must bear the primary responsibility for the legacy of segregated housing . . . Government and private industry came together to create a system of residential segregation."

The bigger problem by the late 1960s was affordability. Many Black Americans didn't have the wealth to tap into to pay for skyrocketing housing costs, because they were never given a chance to participate in the postwar housing boom that generated so much equity for white families—and with no-money-down mortgages. "By the time the federal government decided finally to allow African Americans into the suburbs, the window of opportunity for an integrated nation had mostly closed," noted Richard Rothstein in *The Color of Law*. "The advantage that FHA and VA loans gave the white lower-middle class in the 1940s and '50s has become permanent."

The environmental justice movement has made some inroads in rectifying some of these injustices. However, any victory is the result of decades-long, uphill battles against entrenched corporate interests that have much deeper pockets than grassroots groups. That's what ultimately happened in the place where the environmental justice movement started more than forty years ago, in Warren County, North Carolina, and it underscores how difficult it is to reverse these injustices, especially when a community's interest collides with that of corporations.

In September of 1982, dump trucks first arrived in Warren County carrying hazardous waste laced with toxic PCBs. They were headed for a landfill in the town of Afton, a poor rural community that was over-whelmingly Black. Many locals—in a crusade that eventually united college-educated environmentalists with civil rights leaders and be-came the nucleus of the environmental justice movement—were in-furiated that authorities had ignored their concerns about poisonous chemicals seeping into their drinking water. They stopped the trucks by lying down on the roadways leading to the waste dump, which ignited six weeks of protests. More than five hundred people were arrested, which generated national media attention—and launched a potent and enduring grassroots movement.

Despite the intense news coverage, however, that story didn't have a triumphant ending. Then-governor Jim Hunt made deals with the polluters to turn Warren County into a gigantic depository for hazardous materials from all over the region. More than 60,000 tons of toxic PCBs were eventually dumped in the county, which later saw higher rates of cancers and immune-system disorders among the residents.

However, the Warren County protests did generate a raft of re-search that documented the relationship between race and these haz-ardous waste sites. In 1983, a Government Accounting Office analysis revealed that three out of four toxic landfills in the southern U.S. were situated in poor communities with below average per capita in-comes, and that Blacks comprised at least 26 percent of the residents. A 1987 analysis by the United Church of Christ's Commission for Racial Justice found that 60 percent of Black and Hispanic Americans lived in communities that housed "uncontrolled toxic waste sites," which were either closed or abandoned dumps that were leaking tox-ins harmful to residents' health. What was especially chilling is that researchers found that the single strongest predicter of the location of toxic waste facilities was race.

Four decades and $25 million later, the hazardous wastes still haven't been cleaned up adequately in Warren County, despite the efforts of federal regulators. The soil remains toxic and the runoff continues to pollute nearby rivers, poisoning local wildlife. "All the companies just bury this stuff in holes, but these landfills leak and there are no regulations," Deborah Ferruccio, one of the leaders of the Warren County movement, said in a recent interview. "It's not safe, people are sick, and it's a mess."

Build Back Better?

Numerous healthy-homes programs across the country are improving the abysmal housing conditions that many Americans are forced to live in, but we've made little progress in closing the widespread racial gaps in health and life expectancy that are tied to residential segregation, even twenty years after the publication of the landmark report *Unequal Treatment,* by the Institute of Medicine of the National Academies, which identified racism as a major contributor to racial health disparities. However, some initiatives across the country demonstrate that it is possible to clean up some of the culprits behind this persistent imbalance.

Ironically, Baltimore, of all places, which once exemplified the toxic legacy of lead contamination, has made remarkable strides in reducing the incidence of lead poisoning in children. Rates have dropped by an astonishing 97 percent since Freddie Gray was a toddler. However, the deep, transformative changes that overhauled the decaying housing stock took decades and required dogged persistence from activists, aggressive civic enforcement, and a steely political will to get it done—and the job still isn't finished.

Baltimore banned the use of leaded paints as far back as 1951. The real changes began in 1994, however, when the Maryland legislature passed a sweeping law that required intensive lead remediation, which included removing lead-based paints on walls and replacing lead-lined plumbing and pipes in rental units that were built before 1950. The mandate was strictly enforced, the state issued stiff fines for property owners who weren't in compliance, and a squad of state inspectors were dispatched when landlords balked. In the years between 2003 and 2006, then-mayor Martin O'Malley, who later became governor, began enforcing city lead violations. Within those three years, the incidence of lead poisoning in Baltimore dropped by 45 percent.

But that was just the beginning. Over the past two decades, state regulations were passed that formed a comprehensive lead-eradication package of programs, policies, and laws that has been copied by several other states. They included early-prevention efforts with home visits to evaluate lead hazards, mandatory lead testing and registering of all children starting at twelve months, tests for the presence of lead in drinking-water outlets in public and private schools, education for families, case management follow-up by local health departments for children with elevated blood levels, and legal tools for families to withhold rent if landlords failed to comply with the rules. "We kept going back to find the holes and we added to it every year to fix them," said Ruth Ann Norton. "But the heart of this was the tough enforcement."

These initiatives were done in concert with campaigns to weatherize homes, which included upgrading the old leaded windows, repairing leaky roofs, making dwellings more energy-efficient, and taking housing that was effectively toxic and obsolete and bringing it back to life. Improving these aging homes was salutary, reducing hospitalizations and emergency room visits for asthma by two-thirds. That translated to a 62 percent increase in school attendance and an 85 percent rise in work attendance because of fewer absences due to sickness or doctor visits.

But even after these massive initiatives, more work remains, which underscores just how difficult it is to do truly adequate and comprehensive remediation and to repair decades of neglect. There are an estimated 85,087 homes in Baltimore where families live that still contain "dangerous lead hazards," according to a 2022 report by the Abell Foundation, a Maryland-based public policy think tank; their research estimates that fixing the problem would require a herculean effort from federal, state, and local governments at a cost that could exceed $4 billion. And on a national level, the situation is even worse.

"Maryland is the gold standard because we have good, thoughtful, comprehensive laws and we enforce them," said Norton. "But we still have half a million children a year being poisoned in the United States. That's how insidious this is."

CHAPTER TEN

The Fire Next Time

Our security and continued health hinges upon developing global strategies to prevent the next pandemic. But we must end the epidemic of early death here at home.

WHEN PATRICK SAWYER WAS RUSHED BY AMBULANCE TO a hospital in Lagos, Nigeria, in July of 2014, Dr. Ameyo Stella Adadevoh could see he was deathly ill—and what she did next saved thousands of lives. Sawyer was a forty-year-old Liberian diplomat who had just flown in from Monrovia. He had collapsed at the airport, but he insisted his headache and fever were symptoms of acute malaria or hepatitis. Adadevoh suspected he was stricken with something far worse—Ebola, the highly contagious and deadly pathogen that kills half its victims, and which had rampaged across Sierra Leone, Guinea, Mali, and Liberia throughout that winter and spring, eventually claiming more than 11,000 lives.

He should never have been allowed on that plane, Adadevoh thought. She immediately quarantined Sawyer and barricaded him behind a wooden wall. Sawyer had been en route to a diplomatic conference in southern Nigeria. Even though Liberian authorities knew he had been exposed to Ebola, which had claimed his sister's life, he was still permitted to travel. Throughout the ensuing days, pressure mounted on Adadevoh from Liberian authorities to discharge him. It seemed like anytime the physician's cellphone rang, it was the Liberian ambassador making increasingly dire threats about the future of her career if she continued to refuse to release him. But the endocrinologist was steadfast, and her colleagues at the hospital backed her up. Sawyer himself was so angry about being detained, despite his rapidly deteriorating condition, that he became very aggressive, and even pulled out his intravenous tubes, which spilled blood everywhere.

If he did have Ebola, Adadevoh worried that he could have exposed hundreds of people on the airplane, in the airport, and then in the hospital. Nigeria is the largest country in Africa, with 227 million people, and Lagos itself is incredibly dense, with more than 20 million residents, a hub of commerce and international travel on the northwestern end of the vast continent. If the virus got a foothold there, an exponential outbreak could spread like an uncontrollable wildfire throughout Africa and even globally. Adadevoh shared her suspicions with health authorities and the hospital staff was provided with full protective gear. Four days later, Sawyer was found unresponsive in his room and later that afternoon, Adadevoh was vindicated: His Ebola test results came back positive.

When AIDS swept across Africa in the 1980s, the continent was completely unprepared for the deadly epidemic. There were few doctors, no medications to treat victims, and hardly any public health infrastructure to track and identify people who were infected to prevent further spread of the disease. The death toll was staggering: AIDS killed tens of millions and left millions of children orphaned. But the tide began to turn in the late 1990s, with better medications, and boots on the ground from international public health scientists, who buckled down to the arduous task of building a public health infrastructure that could respond to a massive outbreak.

Nigeria became a model. Funded with a $25 million grant from the Gates Foundation, public health scientists trained chemists, built a testing and disease surveillance infrastructure at twenty-two teaching hospitals across the country, set up computerized record-keeping systems, and educated thousands of public health staffers on how to fan out into the community in the event of an outbreak and track down anyone who had encountered a contagious victim. More than a decade later, when Ebola arrived, Nigeria was ready. The lessons that were learned from AIDS were used by Nigeria to stop Ebola in its tracks. Still, I was stricken with dread that we would repeat the same mistakes we had made with AIDS, which was allowed to spread out of control and claim millions of lives because we ignored an escalating threat that was unfolding in the Global South. AIDS had been present on the African continent since the 1930s, when it jumped from monkeys to hunters eating bush meat, and there were periodic outbreaks in the ensuing decades in remote regions. But until it emerged on our doorstep in the early 1980s, when young men in San Francisco and New York became sickened and swiftly died when their immune systems collapsed, we didn't pay any attention. We failed to recognize that an outbreak anywhere is an outbreak everywhere, and with increased travel within and across borders, everyone is at risk.

Our failure to contain AIDS was due, in part, to what I call othering: seeing people beyond our immediate, insulated world as something different, not like us, and able to be left behind. The act of othering is our Achilles' heel, making us profoundly vulnerable to contagions, and is costly for all of us. Othering is what allowed AIDS, which could have been contained or maybe even wiped out when viral risks emerged, to propagate and spread. For too long, AIDS was a scientific curiosity, studied by a few dedicated, underfunded scientists. It was only when the infection was no longer limited to isolated areas that we mobilized and invested in prevention.

But I was greatly relieved to see that the Obama administration took the Ebola threat seriously: They dispatched a team of medical support personnel and earmarked more than $100 million in funding to aid the containment effort. And what Nigerian health officials did next underscores the critical importance of a functional public health infrastructure. They immediately activated their Emergency Operation Center, and they met daily to monitor the outbreak. Disease surveillance experts were dispatched to hospitals, urban areas, and remote villages to catch the culprit before it claimed more victims, and to do the tedious work of contact tracing by backtracking through the infected person's recent life to identify anyone who they might have encountered. In the process, these Ebola hunters made approximately 18,500 face-to-face visits. Laboratories were put on alert, and a public relations campaign was launched to warn locals of the dangers.

Because they had swiftly identified and isolated the index patient (or "patient zero," that first case that is the tip of the spear of a fast-spreading contagion), Ebola was stopped in its tracks. "Because there were hundreds of people who were exposed on the airplane, potentially hundreds that would have been exposed at the airport and then the hospital, to Nigeria's credit, the minute they had the diagnosis, the country activated this emergency operations center," said Dr. Phyllis Kanki, an immunologist at the Harvard T.H. Chan School of Public Health, who created and directed the Gates Foundation's AIDS Prevention Initiative in Nigeria (APIN) in 2000. "They had that infrastructure that was in place—that's what saved Nigeria."

By September, Nigeria declared victory—the country was free of Ebola even as neighboring countries were gripped by an outbreak that killed thousands—thanks to a well-trained staff that was nimble enough to adapt to the threats. Dr. Ameyo Stella Adadevoh's bravery came at a terrible price, however. Like thousands of other frontline health professionals, she went into battle knowing full well that she might perish. Adadevoh, along with three of her colleagues who were also infected by Sawyer, died of Ebola in August.

The nation mourned her passing and she remains a revered icon.

Whereas Nigeria's public health infrastructure is lacking in many areas, their fast action in this crisis offers many lessons about how to contain an outbreak. Their timely response and their success in stopping Ebola motivated authorities to move forward with creating the Africa Centres for Disease Control and Prevention, which was on the front lines battling Covid-19. The Africa Centres for Disease Control and Prevention is now building a disease surveillance, prevention, and treatment network throughout the continent to be ready for the fire next time.

My own thinking was radicalized watching the carnage of the Black doctors, nurses, and community health workers during the Ebola crisis in West Africa; the bravery of that incredible workforce, who were in harm's way but ran toward the unknown in the service of others. It fueled my desire to avoid a repeat of Ebola when we were faced with the global crisis of the Covid-19 pandemic. I had hoped we'd learned our lessons.

But we failed miserably.

In the early stages of the pandemic, everyone everywhere was flying blind with few treatments and no vaccines. There was a reluctance, however, to listen to those who were ringing alarm bells, especially in the Global South, and there was only a minimal commitment to global health diplomacy and collaboration. Once vaccines became available, we hoarded them. *Hoarded them.* It wasn't until June of 2021, a full six months after vaccines were available domestically, that President Joe Biden committed to buying and distributing 500 million doses of the Covid-19 vaccine around the globe. This unconscionable behavior is the legacy of colonization of the Global South and left poor countries engulfed in needless misery and death. Experts estimate that by the end of 2021, more than a million people died in the Global South because of the lack of vaccines.

Many believe that the stubbornly high infection rates in these countries led to the emergence of the variants that prolonged the pandemic in rich nations, too (although a couple of variants emerged in first world countries, such as the U.S. and the U.K.). As the pandemic made abundantly clear, we are all in this together. Beyond the fancy rhetoric, we saw and are still seeing that a threat anywhere can have ripple effects that destabilize the global economy, global security, and civil society. This latter point is absolutely key. We ignore the Global South at our peril. The harsh reality is that our own safety and security hinge on fortifying public health structures internationally. We needn't be extending a helping hand merely out of a sense of moral obligation—it's in our direct interests to do so.

We must rethink the paradigm for global scientific cooperation. The scientific and political elite have long assumed that the Global North is the best place to develop solutions for challenges in Africa, South Asia, and Latin America. But we can no longer afford this arrogance and continue to ignore, marginalize, and patronize the Global South. Our top-down biases have blinded us to the enormous reserves of talent and ideas in nations that we should both learn from and engage with as thought partners. Pioneers in the Global South have made crucial scientific discoveries that include breakthrough research on Burkitt lymphoma and HIV treatment and prevention.

Ironically, the travel restrictions during the global health emergency allowed many African scientists to lead their own research studies. For the first time, crucial research about the pandemic's evolution and spread was done by African-led teams, which sparked a wave of investment in Africa's molecular biology capacity. There is perhaps no better recent example of that capacity building in the Global South than the Botswana–Harvard AIDS Institute Partnership. Established in 1996, the lab pivoted to genomic surveillance when the Covid-19 pandemic struck. It was this lab that first spotted the Omicron variant and alerted the world, giving us all precious time to prepare for the next stage in the pandemic.

Building manufacturing capabilities in the Global South, in countries like Brazil, Senegal, and South Africa, and creating networks to speed vaccine and drug distribution, can save lives. Fortunately, there is movement in this direction. The African Union and the Africa Centres for Disease Control and Prevention recently launched the Partnerships for African Vaccine Manufacturing, an initiative that aims to turn African universities into research and development hubs and ensure that at least 60 percent of vaccines needed in Africa are made on the continent by 2040.

But the real work in disease prevention and in halting outbreaks before they begin is upstream. Climate change will accelerate the transmission of infectious diseases, and our increasing intrusions into wildlife areas will amplify the incidence of zoonotic illnesses, which jump from animals to humans. And these outbreaks can escalate quickly because of international travel. We saw that with Covid-19. Within a month after China reported the first cases, it had spread to at least nineteen countries. With the increased mobility of air travel, the speed of spread is fast—an infected traveler can fly to virtually any other point on the planet within two days. That's why global partnerships to create early-warning surveillance systems, like the ones being set up in West Africa, are crucial. We must invest in building these international networks, which give us the tools to identify threats, and the infrastructure to stop them before they explode into a worldwide pandemic.

Such scientific excellence is not isolated, and targeted investments over the decades have improved infrastructure in nations across the region and saved millions of lives. AIDS is a case in point. In the early 2000s, at the height of the African HIV epidemic, 28 million people were living with the virus in sub-Saharan Africa, and more than two million Africans died of AIDS each year. In 2003, President George W. Bush announced the establishment of what became known by the acronym PEPFAR—the President's Emergency Plan for AIDS Relief—which became a massive relief effort to fight HIV and AIDS. In the two decades since, the program has provided about $120 billion in funding and delivered lifesaving treatment to more than 20 million people in 54 countries. Administered through the U.S. State Department's Global AIDS Coordinator, the agency has helped build a huge infrastructure that provides support to more than 10,000 labs and testing sites around the world, trained health-care workers, and increased surveillance to quickly pinpoint outbreaks.

The return on investment has been extraordinary, and even Bush's harshest critics, like Nicholas Kristof of *The New York Times,* have called it "the most important humanitarian program in American history." So far, more than 25 million lives have been saved. That's a staggering number that Kristof calculates is more than all the Jews killed in the Holocaust, in the genocides of Armenians, Cambodians, Rwandans, Bosnians, Darfurians, and Rohingya, all the global deaths from Covid-19, all the military deaths in all the wars in U.S. history, and all the auto and gun deaths in the last half-century—combined. Evidence of the initiative's success is everywhere—in the empty beds in hospitals in sub-Saharan Africa that previously overflowed with dying AIDS patients, in the thriving communities filled with middle-aged people who had once been decimated by the epidemic, and in the sharp uptick in longevity, which rose from the low point of fifty-three years in 2004 to sixty-six in 2022. "I knew it was going to be big, but I think it turned out to be even bigger and better than we thought," said Dr. Anthony Fauci, former director of the National Institute of Allergy and Infectious Diseases who helped design the program. "It should serve as a model of what can be done when you make a major commitment."

Why the CDC Failed During the Pandemic

On the domestic front, we must honestly confront our mistakes during the pandemic and understand why the CDC failed when we needed the agency most. Many experts believe that this crisis was largely inevitable because public health has been underfunded or outright ignored for too long, with antiquated equipment, anemic budgets, overworked staffers, and a sore lack of cohesive national leadership, all of which left the entire system unequipped to handle a global outbreak of this magnitude. The pandemic was unprecedented in some ways, but now that we've explored this history of public health and epidemics of various kinds, it's clear that we should have employed the basic principles that we do know work, much as Nigeria implemented the lessons of AIDS for Ebola. Protecting ourselves, however, all comes back to the foundation built by public health pioneers like W.E.B. Du Bois: Know the population that's affected; understand the risks; collect and use the data to promote change; and don't leave anybody behind.

FIRST PRINCIPLE: GET CLOSE: BOOTS ON THE GROUND

Alexander Langmuir understood the crucial importance of timely data collection and of having a well-trained army of public health epidemiologists who can parachute into a community—like the legions of other EIS officers—to determine what's actually happening on the ground. These two elements are the backbone of any effort at disease prevention and controlling outbreaks, and they were both inadequate during the pandemic, creating the nightmare perfect storm that contributed to the deaths of more than a million Americans.

Boots on the ground are public health's eyes and ears, and these frontline workers give us access to the communities affected. This enables us to gather and collect the data so we understand the magnitude of the problem and can then interpret that data in a humane and thoughtful way to develop an action plan. But good, solid data is only one crucial starting point. We need the data evidence to inform the design of interventions, to set priorities, to streamline coordination, and to build the scaffolding for collective action. That's when you're taking what you know and doing what you can with it at the moment.

During the pandemic, better coverage of what was happening on the ground would have enabled us to realize sooner that places where people were stuck in confined spaces from which they could not escape—nursing homes, prisons, mental institutions—were death traps, veritable incubators for the spread of disease. Employees who toiled in close quarters, those "essential" frontline workers who kept the engines of the economy running during the height of the pandemic, needed far better protections. This was especially true for the nearly two million people who worked in farm and food production, in dairy operations, agriculture, and meatpacking. They are primarily Black, Latino, and Indigenous; many of them are easily exploited undocumented immigrants who toil for meager pay and are often victims of wage theft.

What transpired in meatpacking plants is a national disgrace. An executive order by the Trump administration kept the plants open—they were deemed crucial to the nation's food supply. That forced the workers to remain on the job despite the health risks, which are reminiscent of the conditions that Dr. Alice Hamilton witnessed more than a century ago, and it stymied the attempts by horrified local public health officials to shutter the plants to stop the spread of disease. This really underscores that the successes and gains achieved by people like Hamilton are not etched in stone and must be fought for again and again, requiring a steadfast persistence to promote reforms and policies to protect human health.

However, the meat industry ignored even the most basic safety precautions, such as stockpiling masks and spacing out workers on assembly lines, according to a 2022 investigation by ProPublica. The results were as predictable as they were catastrophic. Up to 8 percent of all Covid-19 cases were connected to packing plant outbreaks by July 2020, researchers found, with workers transmitting the virus throughout their communities. As subsequent analysis revealed four months later, in October of 2020, community spread associated with meat-packing plants was responsible for 334,000 illnesses and some 18,000 Covid-19–related deaths.

While the pandemic raged, the public health experts who should have been leading containment efforts in factories, farms, food processing plants, nursing homes, and everywhere else there were outbreaks were sidelined or vilified. At the same time, it was nearly impossible to get timely data on the community spread of disease. Information systems were woefully outdated, unable to handle the avalanche of numbers from millions of test results and case reports. Some states' information systems even relied on archaic and agonizingly slow 1980s technology like fax machines to transmit crucial outbreak information, which created severe data-sharing bottlenecks.

SECOND PRINCIPLE: COLLECT AND SHARE DATA

"The CDC has very little ability to innovate new tools for surveillance and data collection in the time of a crisis," said Dr. Julie Gerberding, a CDC director during the George W. Bush administration, who is currently CEO of the Foundation for the National Institutes of Health. "The integration between the public health system and the health-care delivery system is very tenuous. We have information we need sitting in electronic health records and in public health databases, but putting these things together at a patient level or even a zip code level is very difficult."

Unfortunately, this problem didn't begin with the pandemic. The CDC's data collection system has long been broken, which is why many health-care experts don't think the agency is a credible source of information. It was only when the country was in a national emergency that its grave deficiencies became too blindingly obvious to continue to ignore. "The U.S. public health infrastructure has an anemic surveillance system that relies on stale data that is sometimes years out of date," said Dr. Karen DeSalvo, chief health officer for Google.

DeSalvo should know. She was the national coordinator for health information technology in the Department of Health and Human Services during the Obama administration. She remembers her first meeting with the CDC in 2015, when they presented the HHS secretary with the state of the nation's health report. "The data was more than two years old," she recalled. "I thought 'You've got to be kidding me? This is what the secretary of HHS has to work with? This rear-view data information? There's no weekly dashboard of what we're seeing in terms of trends in suicide or in substance abuse disorders?' No wonder we're always playing catch-up when it comes to treating big public health threats."

Unfortunately, the CDC and the public health community were squeezed out when Congress was doling out big bucks to upgrade our health-care data collection system. In 2009, the HITECH Act (Health Information Technology for Economic and Clinical Health) was passed. "Nearly 40 billion was earmarked to digitize health care in America," DeSalvo said. "But instead of supporting a broader infrastructure, all that money essentially went instead to buying electronic health records for doctors and teaching them how to use it. Public health monies were siphoned off, and it was a really significant challenge for public health because they wanted to have a pipeline for case reporting but they had no digital infrastructure."

Once again, public health got hijacked by the medical establishment. When the pandemic happened, the CDC didn't have the information they needed to figure out where best to deploy their resources. To use a familiar analogy, it wasn't a case of trying to build an airplane while it was already in the air, said DeSalvo. "They were building it while the plane was going down. Researchers at Johns Hopkins and other people in the private sector and in scrappy start-ups had to step in to do the surveillance for the entire country because our public health infrastructure at the national and local level couldn't step up at the beginning. And then, we were forever behind the eight ball."

THIRD PRINCIPLE: STREAMLINE COORDINATION
BETWEEN AGENCIES

Our public health system is a disjointed network of agencies, separate fiefdoms without any national coordination, which compounds all of the other existing problems. The Centers for Disease Control and Prevention has no real authority and relies instead on the good-faith cooperation of state and local health officials. We have nearly three thousand state, local, tribal, and territorial health departments. However, there is no individual or office at the Department of Health and Human Services to lead and coordinate their work.

Our current patchwork of federal institutions—namely the CDC, the Food and Drug Administration, and the National Institutes of Health—was simply not designed for a crisis like this one. Lack of coordination among them manifested in dangerous ways, from conflicting public guidelines to direct interagency conflicts. Early in the pandemic, tests were in short supply partly because the FDA was slow to approve them, and the CDC failed to communicate the imperative for these tests as a public health tool to monitor the spread of the infection at a population level. From new and reemerging infectious diseases to the myriad impacts of climate change, we know the next crisis isn't a matter of if, but when, and we must redesign our public health apparatus to meet the many global threats we will face in the coming decades.

Fortunately, we do have a model of what we can do. For decades, the U.S. military was mired in the same rivalries, infighting, and poorly delineated chains of command that we're now facing in public health. The Goldwater–Nichols Act of 1986 fundamentally transformed our defense establishment for the better by streamlining the chain of command and fostering cooperation at strategic and operational levels. It is time to do the same for public health and establish clear lines of authority within public health institutions at both the state and national levels, and bridge communication and execution gaps across agencies.

FOURTH PRINCIPLE: LEVERAGE THE SCIENCE

Operation Warp Speed, the Trump administration's push to accelerate the development of Covid-19 vaccines, shows what we're capable of when everyone puts aside their differences to work together for the common good. Vaccine development usually takes years, but that timeline was condensed into months for several reasons. We were able to leverage new vaccine technology, such as the breakthrough mRNA vaccines that had been germinating in private, academic, and government labs for years. Billions of dollars were earmarked not only for development but to help companies gear up their manufacturing capabilities so they could begin churning out vaccines the minute the FDA gave them the emergency green light. The government helped secure raw materials, convinced vendors to dramatically whittle down production times from months to just days, and collaborated with companies at every step of the supply chain, from syringes to glass vials to packaging, to speed the rollout.

It's literally miraculous that effective shots were devised within a year of the first outbreak. Then they had to translate that miracle into action—a robust, effective, and equitable vaccination program needed to be implemented, and on an unprecedented scale. The vaccine roll-out was initially plagued with production shortages and computer glitches—we can all attest to the frustrating hours spent on appointment sites trying to arrange for a shot—but the reality is that in six months, half the population got vaccinated—more than 166 million Americans. We dodged a massive bullet, and doctors saw the effects right away: Fewer and fewer severely ill patients were coming into emergency rooms.

By November of 2021, less than a year into the vaccination campaign, there would have been about 1.1 million more deaths and 10 million more Covid-19 hospitalizations in the absence of the shots, according to a December 2021 analysis by the Commonwealth Fund. Without vaccines, deaths would have tripled, and jumped as high as 21,000 per day, which is five times the level of the record peak of more than 4,000 in January of 2021 before vaccines were introduced. The coordinated effort among federal, state, and local public health agencies that got vaccines into the arms of tens of millions of Americans, noted Dr. Craig Spencer, a physician at Brown University, "serves as a blueprint for how to mobilize mass-vaccination campaigns in the future."

FIFTH PRINCIPLE: RESTORE BROKEN TRUST

Unfortunately, that sense of collegiality and shared mission among public health people at the federal, state, and local levels was missing throughout most of the pandemic. That goodwill was poisoned by the divisive political environment and attacks on public health experts who've dedicated their lives to public safety. "The CDC has never had national authority over what states do in public health, and yet we haven't had the problems we're having right now," said former CDC director William Foege, in a recent seminar. In the past, "if there was even an outbreak investigation, the CDC had to be asked by the state or a county or a city or a tribe to do that investigation. . . . Yet the system worked so well that it was never actually a problem. We didn't need more authority." But now Foege worries that the trust has been lost, and it is trust that cements that coalition.

It's a daunting task to rebuild that broken trust, which was deliberately undermined during the early stages of the pandemic. The national leadership and the sense of national sacrifice for the common good, which got the so-called Greatest Generation through the Great Depression and a world war, was crucial to controlling the pandemic. It was that shared ethos of commitment to the common good that catalyzed the successful public health campaigns to curb drunk driving and stop smoking, encouraged people to wear seat belts and cycling helmets, and vaccinate youngsters against the childhood diseases that killed millions in previous generations.

But during the pandemic this was lacking in many instances. In the lengthy post-mortems on what went wrong, we can't forget how basic public health efforts and sensible science became politicized. Conservative officeholders and TV pundits portrayed the refusal to adhere to basic lifesaving public-health initiatives, like lockdowns, wearing masks, and social distancing, as acts of heroic political defiance. During the pandemic, twenty-six states enacted laws curbing basic public health measures, such as mask and vaccine mandates, quarantines, and business closures, and there were more than one thousand lawsuits challenging Covid-19 measures put in place by health officials. Early in the pandemic, retail clerks and security guards were threatened with violence, and one was killed enforcing mask mandates on recalcitrant shoppers.

"Social media has created a world where people are drowning in information and they're starving for the ability to discern what's real and what's fake," said former CDC director Dr. Julie Gerberding. "They end up trusting people they know best who aren't public health experts, so we had a perfect storm for people to take matters into their own hands. The other thing that was drastically different was the intense politicization. Instead of trying to work collaboratively, we had leaders who used it as an opportunity to make political points to the detriment of their constituents. This disinformation was deadly and we're still seeing the consequences of that as we've got outbreaks of vaccine-preventable infectious diseases on the rise."

During those early dark days, public health officials were demonized while overcrowded and overwhelmed hospitals were erecting tents in parking lots, makeshift morgues filled with bodies lined the streets, and thousands of Americans perished every day in isolated wards, utterly alone and away from loved ones in their final hours. In an unprecedented exodus, hundreds of high-profile public health officials across the country resigned, retired, or were fired after suffering from burnout and enduring public hostility and even death threats.

Muzzling public health experts sabotaged our efforts at containment. During February of 2020, to cite just one example, evidence was mounting that the virus was being spread by people who were not yet visibly ill, which meant that simply quarantining people with symptoms was not going to be enough to stop the spread. Despite repeated attempts by public health experts to warn the public, it wasn't until nearly six weeks later, on March 30, that Dr. Robert Redfield, the CDC director, alerted the public about asymptomatic transmission. The delay had catastrophic consequences: A May 2020 report estimated that if social distancing measures had been deployed just a week earlier, 36,000 lives would have been saved.

In August of 2020, Michael R. Caputo, assistant secretary of public affairs at HHS, characterized CDC scientists—many of whom had been working sixteen-hour days, seven days a week—"as lazy and as traitors engaging in sedition," according to *The New York Times*. Morale at the agency plummeted, and there was a pervasive feeling of deep despair among the silenced staffers. "All of us knew tens of thousands were going to die, and we were helpless to stop it," Dr. Daniel Wozniczka, an EIS trainee, told *The New York Times*. "It was really heartbreaking and difficult on a psychological level not to be able to do anything."

Years later, we're still dealing with the aftermath. A 2023 study in *Health Affairs,* conducted by researchers at the University of Minnesota School of Public Health, the de Beaumont Foundation, the Association of State and Territorial Health Officials, and the Harvard T.H. Chan School of Public Health, revealed the depths of the toll this took on the demoralized public health workforce. Nearly half of employees at state and local public health agencies left their jobs between 2017 and 2021, researchers wrote, "a mass exodus accelerated by the pandemic." Even worse, the rates of defections among people who had recently come on board—who are the future—rose to three-quarters.

If these trends continue, we will have lost as much as half of the nation's public health workforce by 2025. We were already seriously shorthanded in dealing with Covid-19, and because there is no concerted effort to replace these scientists and practitioners, we will be feeling the effects of these losses for years to come. When the next pandemic occurs, as it surely will, the consequences of having a hollowed-out public health workforce could be severe, jeopardizing our centuries-long march toward social justice, improved health, safety, and economic prosperity. Unless these challenges find their way to the top of our agenda—Covid-19 was merely the opening volley—this century could be a disaster movie without a happy ending.

CHAPTER ELEVEN

Missing Americans: Our Nation's Epidemic of Early Death

"With a public health system underfunded, and understaffed,
keeping America healthy is almost impossible to do."

—GREGG GONSALVES, epidemiologist at the Yale School of Public Health

O UR FAILURES DURING THE PANDEMIC DIDN'T JUST HAPPEN. They were the inevitable consequence of decades of poor policy decisions and a tattered social safety net. As a consequence, we must strive to confront the deeper, structural inequities that kill millions of Americans. Otherwise, simply making the prescriptive changes to the CDC that many have advocated for, like improving data collection, boosting morale and recruitment, and expediting cooperation and communication throughout all the layers of government, is tantamount to rearranging furniture on the *Titanic*. We feed billions of dollars into a medical system that emphasizes rescue care—exorbitantly expensive high-tech acute care once we're already sick—but we starve the public health initiatives that keep us healthy, prevent disease, help us get better if we do fall ill, and genuinely save lives.

"For all the money we spend on healthcare, we spend a fraction of that on public health," Gregg Gonsalves, an epidemiologist at the Yale School of Public Health, wrote in a recent essay. "People have been frustrated by the public health response to Covid-19, but with these facts in mind, perhaps we can agree that the expectations here have been like asking a thirty-year-old used car to perform like a Ferrari just out of the showroom. With a public health system underfunded [and] understaffed, keeping America healthy is almost impossible to do."

Public health is the foundation of our modern world and is the story of our lives: How long we will live, and how well. Public health is what made it possible for my mother, Angelita Reynolds, to celebrate her first birthday, and for all the Jamaican babies born after her to get their birth certificates right when they're born, because of the expectation that they're not only going to survive but thrive. Public health providers, even in a poor country like Jamaica in the early 1960s, knew just what to do when a low-birth-weight infant was born with jaundice. I was that child, and in the absence of incubators, I was placed outside, to be bathed by the healing powers of sunlight. When my mother told me this story, she remembers being agitated when they took me from her and put me outside. But that's the right thing to do when you don't have an incubator, and the sunlight worked just fine.

But somehow, we've forgotten all these lessons, all the wisdom handed down through generations, and all the sacrifices that public health heroes have made throughout our history, from John Snow and W.E.B. Du Bois to Alice Hamilton and Frances Perkins, and the thousands of warriors who selflessly devoted their lives to making people better and to help all of us fulfill our human potential. Like Drs. Kenneth Edelin, Herb Needleman, Julius Richmond, David Satcher, Bernadine Healy, and Vivian Pinn, and even my two sisters, nurses who were on the front lines during the pandemic. I remember warning them about the carnage Ebola caused for health-care workers in West Africa. But they went to work every day anyway, because they were fighting for something bigger than themselves, even though the system failed them and they didn't have protective gear to let them work safely and were forced to take unnecessary risks. My younger sister, Jacqueline Thornton, who was then an ICU nurse, became gravely ill and was hospitalized for fourteen days, with much of that time spent on a ventilator. She recovered, but tens of thousands of medical professionals who put their lives on the line for the greater good didn't.

My good friend Gregg Gonsalves is right. We are losing precious ground because we've put public health last. All of the issues we've talked about throughout this book—gun violence, the structural violence against women, racial segregation, toxic living conditions and work environments, deep-seated racial disparities in health-care access, suicide, unconscionably high maternal and infant mortality, and the underinvestment in social determinants of health—converge into one frightening statistic: Longevity in the United States is lagging far behind that of other industrialized nations, and we continue to lose ground.

We rank forty-ninth, according to the World Bank, behind Cuba, Estonia, and Saudi Arabia, and we've lost more than 2.5 years of life expectancy in the past decade. In 2015, life expectancy dropped in the U.S. for the first time in decades. Then it dropped again in 2016 and 2017, which is unprecedented in highly developed countries, where life expectancy has been consistently rising for nearly a century. Longevity ticked upward slightly after the pandemic, but we still haven't reached pre-Covid levels. The only comparable situation in modern times is the decline in longevity after the 1991 collapse of the Soviet Union. In the three years afterward, men's life expectancy plummeted by six years, driven by the sudden massive increase in poverty and inequality after the breakup, and compounded by a spike in alcoholism.

This ominous trend began long before the pandemic, dating back to the 1980s, but it has since accelerated into a breakneck gallop, and we're falling disastrously behind other wealthy nations in virtually every metric of health and well-being. The chief culprits behind this death spiral are also the main reasons why the United States far outpaced other developed nations in the rate of Covid-19 deaths and why we had the worst outbreak in the industrialized world.

A 2023 study illuminated the profound depths of our failures. Jacob Bor, an epidemiologist at Boston University School of Public Health, and his colleagues looked at statistics from international mortality databases and the CDC, for every year from 1933 to 2021. Then they compared America's mortality rates with the averages of Canada, Japan, and nineteen Western European nations. What they found, says Bor, "was shocking." If the United States had the same mortality rates as other wealthy nations, one million deaths in 2020 and 1.1 million deaths in 2021 would have been prevented. Even worse is that about half of what the researchers call "missing Americans" died before age sixty-five, in what should be the prime of their lives. "The number of excess U.S. deaths relative to peers," they noted, "is unprecedented in modern times, at least since the 1930s."

What's more, Bor and his colleagues estimate that this is 26.4 million years of lost life in 2021 alone, and that doesn't include the years preceding the people's deaths, when they were hobbled by disabilities, illness, and despair that stopped them from fulfilling their potential, and robbed us as a society of what they might have contributed. And there is a ripple effect across communities and generations—the effects these early deaths have on children who grow up without a parent or in a family that becomes mired in poverty after the untimely death of their primary breadwinner.

Researchers looked at breakdowns by race and ethnicity to see if these trends were an artifact of systemic racism and—no surprise here—Black and Native Americans bore a disproportionate share of these excess deaths. The surprise was how poorly white Americans are doing, too: In 2021, they comprised 70 percent of those missing Americans. Over the past forty years, we're talking about millions of preventable deaths, and tens of millions of missed soccer games, high school graduations, camping trips, and anniversary celebrations, all the unrealized milestones of fully lived lives. It's all the preventable deaths of people who aren't here but should have been. We're talking about Dr. Chaniece Wallace and all the babies she didn't get to deliver, and of her own baby, who will grow up never knowing her mother. How could we have missed this? And why are other wealthy nations doing so much better at keeping their citizens alive?

There's been a huge amount of excellent research into racial disparities in health over the past two decades. But because of the way the studies were constructed, we failed to see the much bigger picture; namely, how bad off most Americans are compared to their counterparts in other wealthy nations. That's because virtually all of the population studies of racial disparities use white U.S. residents as the baseline or benchmark as a comparator. Perhaps it's the willful blindness bred by the pervasive myth of American exceptionalism, but we rarely looked beyond our borders to see how other countries were doing. Said Bor:

> Using the experiences of white Americans as a benchmark in studies renders the trends in the white population invisible, and these are important in and of themselves. In addition, it woefully underestimates the grim circumstances of Americans of color, in terms of their mortality shortfalls, their survival shortfalls and their health shortfalls because the baseline you're using is already sub-standard. We're wearing blinders if we only look at factors that are different between Blacks and whites, rather than looking at factors that are common across Blacks and whites.

This excess mortality is driven mainly by the usual suspects: structural racism, structural violence against women, economic inequality, lack of access to quality health care, a bloated and broken national health-care system, and underinvestment in public health and social-safety-net programs. People die because of gun violence, traffic accidents, heart disease and other metabolic disorders like diabetes, and from suicide, substance abuse, and drug overdoses.

The inescapable fact is that millions of white Americans are dying too young, their lives cut short because of the same policies and institutions that are killing Black, Latino, and Indigenous populations. The analogy that Bor uses is that we're all frogs boiling in that pot of water. It's just that white people are boiling a little slower. Yet somehow, they are led to believe they're better off, and we continue to simply muddle through this metastasizing crisis without doing anything about it. Policy experts like Heather McGhee, in her excellent book *The Sum of Us,* point out that the racial resentments of the white working class have been exploited by right-wing politicians as a wedge to dilute support for policies that benefit everyone, like universal health care.

The stubborn refusal of red states—Wyoming, Kansas, Texas, Wisconsin, Tennessee, Mississippi, Alabama, Georgia, South Carolina, and Florida are still holdouts—to take the Medicaid expansion funds as part of the Obama administration's Affordable Care Act is just one example of this incomprehensible self-sabotage. This translated into a loss of tens of millions of dollars in federal health-care subsidies that left more than two million Americans without health insurance and led to the closing of dozens of rural and urban hospitals. Local residents—Black as well as white—were stuck driving up to a hundred miles in an emergency, often on treacherous backwoods roads, which contributed to the epidemic of early deaths from heart attacks, pregnancy complications, drug overdoses, diabetic comas, and a host of other ills that could have been prevented with adequate and timely medical interventions.

In the years since, Republican governors have doubled down on their drive to cut health insurance for the poor. When the federal government declared the end of the pandemic emergency in May of 2023, the restrictions that protected Medicaid enrollees from losing their coverage ended. Nearly 16 million people were dropped from Medicaid, according to the Congressional Budget Office (although the KFF estimates that up to 24 million will eventually lose coverage), and that figure includes 6.7 million children.

Red state governors like Greg Abbott of Texas—which quickly

dropped 82 percent of recipients from its Medicaid rolls—and Arkansas's Sarah Huckabee Sanders moved swiftly to cut families' health insurance coverage. "This is the fastest pace in the nation . . . I'm proud Arkansas is leading the nation in getting back to normal," Huckabee Sanders wrote in an op-ed for *The Wall Street Journal.* A staunch right-to-lifer, she maintained that the people being dropped were ineligible and the state government wanted to "reserve resources for those who need them and follow the law." However, the reality is that of the 171,000 people Arkansas threw off of Medicaid, only about 35,000 were deemed ineligible. More than one-third of Arkansas residents who lost their coverage were children, including 11,000 newborns.

Yet studies consistently show that residents of these states continue to reliably vote for these same legislators who are putting them and their families into early graves. "There's the direct impact of racism on oppressed groups," said Bor. "But these public policies, both of commission and omission, hamstring us from responding to a public health crisis or from providing a robust social safety net." That safety net would benefit countless white, Black, Latino, and Indigenous Americans.

When the pandemic happened, the elderly were hit the hardest. But Bor and his colleagues looked more closely at these mortality statistics, and their research revealed why our death toll was markedly higher here than in any other wealthy nation. Half of our nation's excess deaths during the pandemic were of people under the age of sixty-five. From 2019 to 2021, deaths among working-age Americans increased by at least 233,000. Nine out of ten of these people would have survived if they had lived in any other peer nation. *Nine out of ten; more than 200,000 lives.* That's a staggering number. In 2021, young white Americans died at three times the rate of their counterparts in wealthy nations, and the death rates for young Black and Indigenous Americans were five times and eight times higher, respectively.

"Covid simply did more of what life in America has excelled at for decades," science journalist Ed Yong wrote in *The Atlantic,* "killing Americans in unusually large numbers, and at unusually young ages."

This crisis of early deaths began more than forty years ago, when America's peer countries recovered from the devastation of World War II and began to surpass us in building a social safety net, providing universal health care, and enacting policies that protected its most vulnerable citizens. We went in the opposite direction, and our mortality numbers began to diverge sharply from those of other wealthy countries, in a downward slide that coincides with the dismantling of the social safety net that began in the 1980s and continued throughout the 1990s and the aughts. This meant that poorer Americans had scant resources to rely on if they became sick or faced job, food, or housing insecurity. In fact, 66.5 percent of all bankruptcies are tied to medical issues, according to a 2019 study, and every year, about 530,000 Americans file for bankruptcy due to medical bills. These stresses were compounded by the wave of deregulation that began in the 1980s that left working-class Americans vulnerable to unhealthy foods, more workplace dangers, environmental toxins, and the unchecked spread of guns and opioids. The escalating numbers of Americans who died "deaths of despair," from substance abuse, suicide, and drug overdoses, contributed to this decline and mirror what happened after the dissolution of the Soviet Union. Two Princeton economists, Anne Case and Angus Deaton, first identified this trend in a 2015 paper, which revealed that working-age white men and women without four-year college degrees were dying at astonishing rates. Between 1999 and 2017, there were more than 600,000 excess deaths of Americans between the ages of forty-five and fifty-four.

But Case and Deaton dug deeper into the numbers and discovered that the chief causes of these early deaths weren't solely because of the easy availability and oversupply of opioids, or the epidemic of obesity that contributes to many chronic ills, or even poverty. Sifting through reams of data revealed an undeniable pattern of mortality: Death rates from suicide, drug overdoses, and alcohol-related illnesses were directly correlated with chronic joblessness in regions that were hit hardest by globalization, communities that had been set adrift by the export of once-stable jobs, in mining, manufacturing, and heavy industry, that had sustained blue-collar workers. Labor unions declined, and the federal minimum wage remains stuck at a mind-bogglingly low $7.25 per hour.

European countries were better at weathering the shock waves of globalization. Their workforces were buffered by a much stronger safety net and a national health-care system that was conducive to longer, healthier lives, and there were no sharp declines in real wages, because their employers weren't on the hook for insuring their medical care. In contrast, the U.S. did little to cushion the blow of this long-term economic stagnation. This steady drip of broken promises and unfulfilled expectations put the American dream out of reach, breeding the deterioration in social capital and hopelessness that has enveloped once-thriving regions.

The jobs that are now available are poorly paid, the hours are irregular, the duration is shorter, and they usually don't offer benefits like health insurance. Case and Deaton's research revealed that skyrocketing health-care costs and our reliance on employer-provided insurance is a prime contributor to this precipitous decline. The average family health-care policy costs around $20,000, according to a 2019 Kaiser Family Foundation analysis, which essentially discourages employers from hiring and retaining workers without a college degree because it adds so much to their overall compensation package. The net result is that in the U.S., employers are practically compelled to outsource or automate low-wage positions, especially in industries with thin profit margins. The next time you're shopping at your local pharmacy, home improvement store, or chain supermarket, and only one checkout counter is staffed by a human being and has such a long line that you're forced to use the self-service checkout, this is why.

"The grip of financial self-interest in U.S. health care is becoming a stranglehold, with dangerous and pervasive consequences," warned Dr. Donald Berwick, president emeritus and senior fellow for the Institute for Healthcare Improvement, in a scathing 2023 opinion piece in the *Journal of the American Medical Association*.

> Greed harms the cultures of compassion and profes-
> sionalism that are bedrock to healing care. . . . U.S.
> health care costs nearly twice as much as care in any
> other developed nation, whereas U.S. health status,
> equity, and longevity lag far behind. Unchecked greed
> is not the only driver of that failure, but it is a major
> one. Few, if any, other developed nations tolerate the
> levels of avarice, manipulation, and profiteering in
> health care that the U.S. does.

When Public Health Comes First

We are in a public health and health-care crisis that began long before Covid-19. Much of this deterioration is the unfortunate consequence of the uncoupling of our increasingly expensive for-profit medical care system from public health, in a process that began nearly a century ago. The pandemic was a reckoning that made our institutional failings impossible to ignore, and our shocking excess death rate is only one metric of the cost of that neglect. Costa Rica, however, a Central American nation of five million with a per capita income that is one-sixth of that of the United States, is a living laboratory of what can be accomplished when public health comes first, instead of dead last.

Despite their relative poverty, Costa Ricans live longer than their wealthier counterparts elsewhere, with a life expectancy that now approaches eighty-one years. Men who survive to age sixty have the longest life expectancy of any people in the world, surpassing even the long-lived Japanese. How did they do it? The key seems to be in the nation's familiar catchphrase: *pura vida,* or the pure life. Costa Rica is a centuries-old democracy with universal health care, no standing army, and the highest literacy rate in Central America, and it has been relatively insulated from the corruption, narco-terrorism, and civil wars that have plagued neighbors like Panama, Nicaragua, and Guatemala.

Researchers believe that their leisurely pace of life, network of family and friends, regular exercise, and purposeful lives seem to be their recipe for longevity. But the cornerstone of Costa Rica's blueprint for a long life is that individual health and public health are inextricably linked. As a nation, they consistently employ the basic tools of public health to keep residents healthy. They ensure that all their citizens are vaccinated, that they live in sanitary environments with clean running water, and that they have ready access to proper nutrition and health care through more than a thousand community-based clinics, even in remote rural regions in the mountains that can only be accessed by horseback.

This was not always the case. In 1950, one in ten Costa Rican infants died before their first birthdays, succumbing to the diarrheal illnesses, respiratory infections, and birth complications that the U.S. had brought under control decades before. Many children and adolescents didn't survive into adulthood. Life expectancy hovered around fifty-five years, which was about thirteen years shorter than here in America. In about half the homes, there was no running water or adequate sanitation, resulting in high rates of polio, parasites, and diarrheal diseases. Malnutrition was rampant, and children went hungry and their growth was often stunted.

All that began to change in the 1950s and '60s, when fundamental public health efforts began to transform the society. Water was piped into homes, national power generation electrified the country, and the government provided outhouses made of cement and embarked on vaccination campaigns against polio, diphtheria, and rubella. Each community had a public health staff that was dedicated to guarding against disease outbreaks and combating malnutrition and other hazards. These teams worked in tandem with the health-care system, which was still in its nascent stages.

The truly revolutionary reforms began in the 1970s, when the nation adopted a national health plan and set up clinics in rural areas that provided the same medical care as in the cities. But instead of treating patients on a scattershot, individual basis the way we do here, Costa Rica used its scant health-care dollars to identify the diseases that were killing most residents and then implemented strategies to prevent them. Maternal and child mortality were the first targets. Pregnant women were given prenatal care, and rural residents were transported to cities weeks before their due date to ensure a safe delivery in hospitals. Nutrition programs helped reduce malnutrition, sanitation and vaccination campaigns effectively lowered the incidence of cholera and diphtheria, and a nationwide network of clinics provided better treatments when kids did get sick. The results were astonishing: By 1980, infant mortality had dropped to 2 percent.

In the four decades since, Costa Rica has continued on this path, integrating public health services with their network of hospitals and clinics, and allowing public health officials to set the national health-care agenda—not Big Pharma, not health-care executives beholden to their shareholders, and not the lawmakers who rely on what my friend and public policy expert David W. Johnson calls the "healthcare-industrial complex" to bankroll their election campaigns. By 2006, nearly the entire country enjoyed universal primary care, and the lack of access to care that plagues many Americans is a foreign concept to Costa Ricans; at birth, they are assigned a local primary-care health team that includes a doctor, a nurse, and a community health worker, who will follow them throughout their lives.

There are now more than a thousand neighborhood teams that visit each household at least once a year, and the outreach workers are well versed in the health status of all the residents and deliver care that emphasizes prevention and public health. The system is not perfect—because of the nation's limited budgets, there can be months-long waits for advanced imaging and procedures, and specialists are in short supply. But the wide health-care disparities that are endemic in the U.S. are virtually nonexistent in Costa Rica, where such things as differences in infant mortality based on a family's income or where they live have been erased.

We can do better.

Navigating an Uncertain Future

We need to take several actions to fully realize the benefits of translating the science of public health into action. The pandemic was not a one-off—this is our new normal, and we must modernize our public health system to face the twenty-first-century threats of fast-spreading disease outbreaks and the consequences of climate change, which become more evident and more catastrophic with each passing day. "The leadership of our country at every level needs to recognize that health security is national security," said Dr. Julie Gerberding, the former CDC director. "We need to approach our public health system with the same investment, strategic intent, and discipline that we approach our national defense in other ways. That's the kind of mindset we need to move forward in public health and get out of this crisis-to-complacency cycle we've been trapped in for decades."

Close the gap between what we know and what we do. For far too long, there has been little connection or communication between public health researchers in academia and people in the field. Whereas curiosity-driven and goal-oriented research advances science, knowledge generation is only one part of our mission in public health. Acting on that knowledge matters, too.

When I finished graduate school, I was disheartened to realize that academic colleagues, particularly those in the most elite institutions, who were on the fast track were largely technocrats, not hands-on community organizers. Salaries and promotions were based on publishing papers in scientific journals rather than doing the arduous community work that feeds our souls. Training grants and research monies poured into exploring biomedically related determinants of health, such as identifying risk factors that made individuals more vulnerable to disease, rather than looking at the big picture, namely the systemic inequities that we now know play key roles in health and longevity.

In the process, we allowed the actual practice of public health to wither, and we virtually amputated the most important arm of public health—that is, the practitioners, the frontline fighters doing the difficult, controversial, underfunded, unheralded, and often tedious work of connecting the dots, and collecting irrefutable proof that ubiquitous exposures, such as to lead, can cause irreversible brain damage in children, or that pesticides sprayed on crops were killing farmworkers. I've constantly wrestled with how to bring this exquisite, beautiful science that we generated in the lab into spaces where people are suffering.

How do we do the hard work of follow-through, and turn those breakthroughs into programs and policies that make a difference to real people in real communities and are truly transformative?

More than thirty years ago, Milton Terris, an internationally known epidemiologist and a tireless advocate for the social and preventive side of medicine, warned about the harmful consequences "of the shift of epidemiological research from health departments to the schools of public health." The field began to reflect the worst tendencies of academic life, he cautioned, marked by a withdrawal from community field studies, a greater concern for collecting data and publishing papers than for preventing disease and death, and "an arrogant and elitist attitude toward the health officer. . . . We cannot remain indefinitely in our ivory towers; they may crumble around us."

We must understand the legacy of our racist medical past and our current racial and social inequities, so that we are all empowered to build a more just, and healthier, future for all. Beyond the staggering losses in quality of life and unrealized potential because of entrenched racism, doing better isn't just a moral obligation. Racism extracts an enormous financial cost that robs us all.

In May of 2020, in the midst of the pandemic lockdown, Dana Peterson was one of millions of Americans glued to their TV sets, watching in horror as George Floyd's life was snuffed out, and cities in the U.S. and around the world were convulsed by protests against racial injustice. The demonstrations resonated deeply with Peterson because they echoed her own experiences as a Black woman and economist. She was part of the diversity team at Citigroup, and her colleagues were "shell-shocked about the murder," Peterson recalled. They decided that they could contribute to these unprecedented times by using their specialized skill set to quantify the costs of racism to society and put an actual dollar figure on what we all lose when we live in an unequal society.

What they uncovered surprised even Peterson: Since 2000, in a period that included the largest economic expansion in American history, closing the racial gaps would have generated an additional $16 trillion in economic output over the past two decades. These disparities along racial fault lines in housing, education, and policing all feed into one another to restrict the access of Black Americans and other minorities to employment, higher incomes, and the ability to build wealth. There were inequities at every juncture: Segregated housing leads to unequal access to quality education because schools are funded by property taxes. It's more difficult to get loans to start a business, even Ivy League graduates are paid less, and on and on.

Their calculations revealed that equitable access to home loans could have resulted in 770,000 additional Black homeowners since 2000, which would have added $218 billion to the gross domestic product—and this didn't factor in all the items that are purchased when someone buys a home, including furniture, household items, renovations, and landscaping. And an additional 6.1 million jobs per year and $13 trillion in business revenues could have been generated over the last two decades if Black entrepreneurs had had fair and equitable access to credit.

Their analysis only covered the past twenty years and didn't include the cascade of what Peterson calls the secondary domino effects that compound over generations: If your ancestor wasn't allowed to buy a home because of predatory lending practices, the home wasn't passed on to the next generation, where the equity could have been used to buy another house, or to invest, or to send someone to college so they would have qualified for a higher-wage job. "These are historical trends, and the seeds for many of these inequities were planted hundreds of years ago, even before the United States was a country," said Peterson, who is now the chief economist at the Conference Board. "There's tons of money, trillions, that's been left on the table."

Public health must become everyone's business. We all have a role to play, whether it's demanding that our local schools fund on-site nurses, creating meal programs for kids who come to school hungry, or pushing lawmakers to enact stronger gun-safety legislation and restore women's reproductive rights in states that are abortion deserts.

Yet most Americans don't participate in civic life. Only two-thirds of those eligible to vote turn out for presidential elections, less than half cast their ballots in midterms, and the turnout in local elections is abysmal. That's a national disgrace in one of the world's oldest modern democracies, where people lost their lives fighting for the right to vote, and where elected officials hold enormous power over whether we live or die. We've paid a huge price for our complacency.

More Republicans than Democrats died in the pandemic. That's not partisanship—it's a fact. When researchers stripped away the common contributors to early death, like income, health status, and education, what stood out in stark relief was that more Republicans died because conservative lawmakers refused to enforce or outright opposed basic public health measures like lockdowns, masking, social distancing, and vaccinations.

Gun safety is another example. Two out of three Americans favor stricter gun-control laws, according to a 2023 CNN poll. Yet the gun lobby continues to have a stranglehold on conservative lawmakers, so nothing is done in the face of record numbers of people killing themselves in their lowest moments because of the easy availability of guns, and we have one mass shooting after another at concerts, synagogues, churches, and elementary schools.

The reality is that residents of blue states live *far* longer than those in red states, according to a 2023 analysis done by Colin Woodard at the Salve Regina University's Pell Center for International Relations and Public Policy in Newport, Rhode Island. And these gaps are huge. There's a difference of nearly five years of longevity between the blue states on the Pacific Coast and a swath of red states in the Deep South and what Woodard calls Greater Appalachia, which stretches from southern Pennsylvania through the Ozarks and the hill country of Texas. In southern Louisiana, the gap is nearly six years, in a lingering legacy of that region's brutal history as home to the most barbaric slaveholders in the antebellum South.

To put this into perspective, Woodard notes, "a difference of five years is like the gap separating the U.S. from decidedly unwealthy Mongolia, Belarus, or Libya, and six years gets you to impoverished El Salvador and Egypt."

What was especially striking is that the poorest, most hardscrabble counties in the predominantly blue Northeast, in places where up to 60 percent of children live in dire poverty, have higher life expectancies than the people in the richest counties in the Deep South. These enormous gaps are not the result of any of the usual suspects, like race, income, education, urbanization, or access to decent medical care, researchers found. The essential truth about life expectancy in the U.S. is that it all comes down to place. These wide disparities in longevity are the inevitable consequences of a region's history and of the harsh social policies enacted by the mostly Republican lawmakers, notes Woodard, "who have resisted investing tax dollars in public goods and health programs."

We must vote like our lives depends on it—because they do. When people vote, good things happen. Our democracy is stronger and more resilient when everyone participates and we don't leave anyone behind. The one thing all of our public health heroes had in common is that they thought about the long game. Despite the obstacles they faced and whether they were personally threatened, they were driven by science, by evidence, and by a realistic optimism that they were acting for the greater good and contributing to a better future for us all.

Every last one of them engaged in what's called "cathedral thinking." It took hundreds of years to construct those magnificent cathedrals in the Middle Ages, and most of the workers who toiled tirelessly on them over the centuries understood that they'd never see the finished product. But they laid the foundations anyway for future generations to enjoy. We need to be like those monks from the Middle Ages and prepare for the long, hard fight for ourselves, for our children, and for all the generations that will come after us.

We need to heed the words of the great John Lewis. In March of 2020, on the fifty-fifth anniversary of "Bloody Sunday" in Selma, Alabama, he stood on the Edmund Pettus Bridge, the place where he had survived a brutal beating so many decades before. "Speak up, speak out. Get in the way," he exhorted the crowd, in what would be one of the veteran Georgia congressman's final speeches before his death a few months later. "Get in good trouble. Necessary trouble, and help redeem the soul of America."

ACKNOWLEDGMENTS

IN THE SUMMER OF 2020, LIKE SO MANY AMERICANS, I FOUND MY-self sheltering in place as an invisible pathogen brought the world to a standstill. During this unprecedented crisis, I came to realize that my life's work in public health, though noble and personally gratifying, remained grossly underappreciated and misunderstood by far too many. With the encouragement of dear friends Arianna Huffington, Deborah Marcus, and Michelle Kydd Lee, I accepted the formidable challenge of writing this book. I am profoundly grateful to them and to the many individuals who made invaluable contributions to this work—a labor of respect and love for the beautiful discipline of public health.

I wish to express my deepest appreciation to Linda Marsa for her exceptional contributions to this book. Her journalistic expertise—particularly her insightful interviewing techniques—brought depth and authenticity to every narrative. Her genuine and abiding interest in public health was evident throughout each phase of our collaboration, guiding the research process and elevating the integrity of the work. I am especially grateful for her relentless curiosity and meticulous writing skills, which transformed complex ideas into accessible, compelling prose. Without her unwavering commitment and exceptional professionalism, this project would not have reached its fullest potential.

Intellectual exchanges with distinguished scholars and public health professionals significantly improved this book. I am deeply indebted to all those who generously shared their time and insights through interviews. I would like to extend special recognition to the late Caledonia (Cal) Jones, the former Manhattan borough historian, and to the Williams family—Ariel, Mareia, and Andrew Thomas Williams IV, descendants of Andrew Williams, one of the original settlers of New York City's Seneca Village. With their invaluable assistance, the story of Seneca Village comes to life, and I hope readers will appreciate how Andrew Williams managed to create a public health–forward ecosystem even under the most inhospitable circumstances. I'd also like to thank Anthony Wallace for sharing the story about his wife Dr. Chaniece Wallace's untimely death after the birth of their daughter, Charlotte.

This book would not have been possible without the contributions of numerous publishing industry professionals. I am grateful to my agents at Creative Artists Agency, Mollie Glick and David Larabell, who shepherded this project from its inception. I also appreciate the crucial role Mollie and David played in connecting me with Linda Marsa—a connection facilitated by Linda's agents, Madeleine Morel of 2M Communications and Alice Martell of the Martell Agency. Special thanks to Alice for her timely words of advice and encouragement as we navigated this book through all its developmental stages.

I am further indebted to Mollie and David for helping me transform the academic narrative of public health into a compelling and marketable proposal. Their expert guidance led to my connection with the outstanding team at Penguin Random House's One World, headed by the brilliant editor Christopher Jackson, who shaped and elevated our manuscript into the book you hold today. From the outset, Chris appreciated both the vastness of public health and the expansive human stories that bring this discipline to life. In addition to my editor, I owe a debt of gratitude to Hiab Debessai and Sun Robinson-Smith for their contributions in managing the editorial process and to Stuart Calderwood for copyediting the manuscript. I am grateful to many others at One World for stewarding the manuscript through the production processes and for their support in marketing and publicity. I wrote this book with the aspiration that I would reach as many people as possible with the stories of the radicals and renegades who fought for the health and well-being of total strangers, and how public health institutions and infrastructure helped to transform our world. To the talented teams in the publicity and marketing departments, I share my sincere thanks for helping make this dream come true.

I have benefited immeasurably from the brilliant research assistance of Jacqueline Forsyte, who tracked down journal articles, archival papers, and diary entries of figures such as W.E.B. Du Bois and Frederick Law Olmsted. I would also like to thank Howard Cohn, whose meticulous and invaluable fact-checking work strengthened this book immeasurably through careful verification of sources, dates, and details, giving the stories of public health the accuracy they deserve.

I am grateful for the scholarship and experiences of numerous intellectuals, public health warriors, and experts whose work inspired me and whom I cite throughout this book, including Jim Downs, Arne Duncan, Barbara Edelin, Margaret Humphreys, Dana Peterson, Charles Rosenberg, Kathryn Olivarius, David Satcher, Elizabeth Etheridge, Maryn McKenna, Harriet Washington, Vivian Pinn, Phillip Landrigan, Cheryl Blackmore Prince, Deborah Prothrow-Stith, David Williams, Phyllis Kanki, Mark Rosenberg, Julie Gerberding, Karen DeSalvo, Wanda Barfield, Diane Rowley, and Richard Rothstein. I am especially grateful to Alfredo Morabia for sharing his insights during our interview for this book, for his own excellent book that was an invaluable resource, and for the countless discussions we've had over the years regarding the importance of teaching the history of public health and epidemiology.

I am deeply indebted to my colleagues at Harvard University, particularly within the T.H. Chan School of Public Health. I am also deeply indebted to Annette Rossingnol for opening the door to public health for me. I am appreciative of the opportunities I've had to learn from and to study and work with dedicated scholars including Claire Mahan, Richard Monson, Earl Francis Cook, Nancy Cook, Marg Drolette, Alec Walker, Bernard Guyer, Doug Dockery, Walter Willett,

Frank Hu, Heather Baer, John Orav, Nancy Mueller, David Williams, Dimitrious Trichopoulos, Richard Monson and Noel Weiss, Pagona Lagiou, Arnold Epstein, Joseph Allen, Lee Chin, Lilian Cheung, Betty Johnson, I-Min Lee, Seth Welles, Alison Evans, Susan Hankinson, Eric Rimm, Edward Giovannucci, Cuilin Zhang, Yi Ning, Vitool Lohsoon-thorn, Shekhar Saxena, and Bizu Gelaye. I owe special thanks to Linda Brady and Marsha Lee, who created the intellectual space and time necessary for me to complete this book amid the demanding responsi-bilities of my role as Dean of the Faculty.

I would like to thank Melissa Bondy, Steve Goodman, and the many faculty members, fellows, students, and staff of Stanford Uni-versity School of Medicine's Department of Epidemiology and Popu-lation Health who welcomed me and have given me the time and space to directly re-engage in teaching, mentoring, and research after years of full-time academic administration.

Finally, I am grateful beyond words to my family for their love and unwavering support. My husband, Todd, sustained me during some of the most challenging periods of the pandemic. A brilliant engineer and natural caretaker, he provided the support I needed to tend to others' needs while managing our household as I retreated to my office during countless nights and weekends. To my son, Alex, thank you for your patience, love, and understanding. Our trav-els to Europe as the world reopened after the pandemic provided an excellent re-entry into broader life beyond these pages. To my siblings—Jacqueline, Coleen, and Noel—I thank you for your love and encouragement throughout the writing process. My sisters, both nurses, served on the front lines of the Covid pandemic, working tire-lessly to treat patients and their families with dignity and compassion. To my brother, Noel, thank you for helping spread awareness about public health at the World Economic Forum and among your col-leagues at "the bank." I am eternally grateful to my parents, Noel and Angelita Williams, for the countless sacrifices they made to ensure my place as a global citizen and scholar.

BIBLIOGRAPHY

Aggarwal, Neil Krishan. "The Legacy of James McCune Smith, MD—The First US Black Physician." *JAMA* 326, no. 22 (2021): 2245–46. https://doi.org/10.1001/jama.2021.18511.

"A Great Excitement—A Negro Major Has His Straps Cut Off." *Baltimore Clipper,* May 2, 1863. Maryland State Archives.

"Alice Hamilton Changed the World. Do You Know Her Story?" American Federation of Government Employees (AFGE), September 21, 2018. https://www.afge.org/article/alice–hamilton–changed-the-world.-do-you-know-her-story/.

"Alice Hamilton." Science History Institute. Accessed June 21, 2023. https://sciencehistory.org/education/scientific–biographies/alice–hamilton/.

American Chemical Society National Historic Chemical Landmarks. "Alice Hamilton and the Development of Occupational Medicine." American Chemical Society. Accessed June 21, 2023. https://www.acs.org/education/whatischemistry/landmarks/alicehamilton.html.

Andrews, R.J. "How Florence Nightingale Changed Data Visualization Forever." *Scientific American,* August 1, 2022. https://www.scientificamerican.com/article/how-florence-nightingale-changed-data-visualization-forever/.

Andrews, William L. "Harriet A. Jacobs (Harriet Ann), 1813–1897." Documenting the American South. Accessed July 10, 2022. https://docsouth.unc.edu/fpn/jacobs/bio.html.

Applebome, Peter. "Conversations/David Satcher; C.D.C.'s New Chief Worries as Much About Bullets as About Bacteria." *New York Times,* September 26, 1993. https://www.nytimes.com/1993/09/26/weekinreview/conversations-david-satcher-cdc-s-new-chief-worries-much-about-bullets-about.html.

Arnette, Robin. "NRDC Scientist Gives Labor Day Seminar." *Environmental Factor, National Institute of Environmental Health Sciences,* October 2008.

"Atlanta's New Professor.; W.E.B. Du Bois Appointed to the Chair of Economics and History." *New York Times,* August 17, 1897. https://www.nytimes.com/1897/08/17/archives/atlantas-new-professor-web-du-bois-appointed-to-the-chair-of.html.

Attiah, Karen. "Gun and Abortion Laws Have Made Texas a Woman's Nightmare." *Washington Post,* May 19, 2023. https://www.washingtonpost.com/opinions/2023/05/19/texas-gun-abortion-domestic-violence-gabriella-gonzalez/.

Augusta, Alexander T. "The Late Outrage upon Surgeon Augusta in Baltimore, Washington, May 15, 1863." *Christian Recorder,* May 30, 1863.

Bachmann, Gloria, and Nancy Woods. "Dr. Vivian Pinn: A Woman Pioneer & Leader." *Women's Midlife Health* 7, no. 1 (December 5, 2021): 11. https://doi.org /10.1186/s40695-021-00070-7.

Badger, Emily, Margot Sanger-Katz, Claire Cain Miller, and Eve Washington. "States with Abortion Bans Are Among Least Supportive for Mothers and Children." *New York Times,* July 28, 2022. https://www.nytimes.com/2022/07/28/upshot /abortion-bans-states-social-services.html.

Bankoff, Caroline. "What We Know About How 9/11 Has Affected New Yorkers' Health, 15 Years Later." *Intelligencer,* September 10, 2016. https://nymag.com /intelligencer/2016/09/15-years-later-how-has-9-11-affected-new-yorkers-health .html.

Barfield, Wanda. Director of the Division of Reproductive Health (DRH) within the National Center for Chronic Disease Prevention and Health Promotion. Author interview via Zoom, April 10, 2023.

Bass, Brent. Manager of Safer Homes at Forefront Suicide Prevention at the University of Washington. Author interview via Zoom, May 2, 2023.

Bassett, Mary T. "Black Americans' Poor Health Outcomes Is Proof of Wildly Overdue Unpaid Tab for Slavery." *Boston Globe,* October 4, 2022. https://www .bostonglobe.com/2022/10/04/opinion/black-americans-poor-health-outcomes -is-proof-wildly-overdue-unpaid-tab-slavery/.

Bates, Richard. "Florence Nightingale: A Pioneer of Hand Washing and Hygiene for Health." *Conversation,* March 23, 2020. http://theconversation.com/florence -nightingale-a-pioneer-of-hand-washing-and-hygiene-for-health-134270.

Beard, Rick. "City Under Siege: The New York Draft Riots." Warfare History Network, Early Spring 2016. https://warfarehistorynetwork.com/article/city -under-siege-the-new-york-draft-riots/.

"Before Central Park: The Story of Seneca Village." *Central Park Conservancy,* January 18, 2018. https://www.centralparknyc.org/articles/seneca-village.

Belluck, Pam. "Depression During and After Pregnancy Can Be Prevented, National Panel Says. Here's How." *New York Times,* February 12, 2019. https://www .nytimes.com/2019/02/12/health/perinatal-depression-maternal-counseling.html.

Bellware, Kim, and Emily Guskin. "Effects of Dobbs on Maternal Health Care Overwhelmingly Negative, Survey Shows." *Washington Post,* June 21, 2023. https://www.washingtonpost.com/politics/2023/06/21/obgyn-abortion-poll/.

Benin, Leigh, Rob Linné, Adrienne Sosin, Joel Sosinsky, Workers United (ILGWU), and HBO Documentary Films. *The New York City Triangle Factory Fire.* Charleston, South Carolina: Arcadia Publishing, 2011.

Blackmore Prince, Cheryl. Former CDC epidemiologist. Author interview via Zoom, February 24, 2023.

Boileau, John. "Alexander Thomas Augusta." *The Canadian Encyclopedia,* June 2, 2022. https://www.thecanadianencyclopedia.ca/en/article/alexander-thomas-augusta.

Bollet, Alfred J. "Politics and Pellagra: The Epidemic of Pellagra in the U.S. in the Early Twentieth Century." *Yale Journal of Biology and Medicine* 65, no. 3 (1992): 211–21.

Boots, Anna. "'The Burning Bed' Recalls the Case that Changed How Law Enforcement Treats Domestic Violence." *New Yorker,* July 9, 2020. https://www.newyorker.com/culture/video-dept/the-burning-bed-recalls-the-case-that-changed-how-law-enforcement-treats-domestic-violence.

Bor, Jacob. Epidemiologist at the Boston University School of Public Health. Author interview via Zoom, July 18, 2023.

Breiseth, Christopher N. "From the Triangle Fire to the New Deal: Frances Perkins in Action." Presented at the Commemoration of the 100th Anniversary of the Triangle Fire, New York State Museum, Albany, New York, February 25, 2011. https://web.archive.org/web/20201227215054/; https://francesperkinscenter.org/wp-content/uploads/2014/04/From-the-Triangle-Fire-to-the-New-Deal.pdf.

Brooks, David. "How the First Woman in the U.S. Cabinet Found Her Vocation." *Atlantic,* April 14, 2015. https://www.theatlantic.com/politics/archive/2015/04/frances-perkins/390003/.

———."The Terrifying Future of the American Right." *Atlantic,* November 18, 2021. https://www.theatlantic.com/ideas/archive/2021/11/scary-future-american-right-national-conservatism-conference/620746/.

Brown, DeNeen L. "'You've Got Bad Blood': The Horror of the Tuskegee Syphilis Experiment." *Washington Post,* May 16, 2017, accessed October 28, 2021. https://www.washingtonpost.com/news/retropolis/wp/2017/05/16/youve-got-bad-blood-the-horror-of-the-tuskegee-syphilis-experiment/.

Brown, DeNeen L., and Aaron Wiener. "The Racist Tuskegee Syphilis Experiment Was Exposed 50 Years Ago." *Washington Post,* July 26, 2022. https://www.washingtonpost.com/history/2022/07/26/tuskegee-syphilis-experiment-50-years/.

Brown, Stacia L. "Dispatch from Baltimore: Praying for Peace, Living Another Reality." *Nation,* April 28, 2015. https://www.thenation.com/article/archive/dispatch-baltimore-praying-peace-living-another-reality/.

Byrd, W. Michael. "An American Health Dilemma." *Journal of the National Medical Association* 78, no. 11 (1986). https://www.ncbi.nlm.nih.gov/pmc/articles/PMC2571436/pdf/jnma00290-0023.pdf.

Byrd, W. M., and L. A. Clayton. "An American Health Dilemma: A History of Blacks in the Health System." *Journal of the National Medical Association* 84, no. 2 (February 1992): 189–200.

———. "Race, Medicine, and Health Care in the United States: A Historical Survey." *Journal of the National Medical Association* 93, no. 3 Suppl (March 2001): 11S–34S.

Carstens, Andy. "Diagrammatic War, 1858." *The Scientist Digest*, no. 1 (December 2022). https://www.the-scientist.com/foundations/diagrammatic-war-1858-70702.

Changing the Face of Medicine. "Dr. Vivian W. Pinn." October 14, 2003. https://cfmedicine.nlm.nih.gov/physicians/biography_254.html.

Chotiner, Isaac. "The Interwoven Threads of Inequality and Health." *New Yorker*, April 14, 2020. https://www.newyorker.com/news/q-and-a/the-coronavirus-and-the-interwoven-threads-of-inequality-and-health.

Christiani, David. "The Triangle Factory Fire and Workplace Safety Regulations." Harvard T.H. Chan School of Public Health, March 25, 2011.

Cobb, W. Montague. "A Short History of Freedmen's Hospital." *Journal of the National Medical Association* 54, no. 3 (May 1962): 271–87.

Cohen, Elizabeth, John Bonifield, and Justin Lape. "'Something Has to Be Done': After Decades of Near-Silence from the CDC, the Agency's Director Is Speaking Up About Gun Violence." CNN, August 28, 2021. https://www.cnn.com/2021/08/27/health/cdc-gun-research-walensky/index.html.

Cohen, Jessica Kim. "Hospitals Tackling Gun Violence as a Public Health Issue." *Modern Healthcare*, July 20, 2021. https://www.modernhealthcare.com/safety-quality/hospitals-tackling-gun-violence-public-health-issue.

Cohn, Victor. "Never-Delivered U.S. Report Cites Abortion Benefits." *Washington Post*, July 11, 1981. https://www.washingtonpost.com/archive/politics/1981/07/12/never-delivered-us-report-cites-abortion-benefits/be64e6c5-840b-4aa5-82c8-01369aeaf02a/.

Collins, Dave. "Gun Violence Tests Limits of Urban Crime Prevention Groups." *San Diego Union-Tribune*, June 24, 2021. https://www.sandiegouniontribune.com/news/california/story/2021-06-24/gun-violence-tests-limits-of-urban-crime-prevention-groups.

Cooper, Kenneth J. "The Costs of Inequality: Faster Lives, Quicker Deaths." *Harvard Gazette*, March 14, 2016. https://news.harvard.edu/gazette/story/2016/03/the-costs-of-inequality-faster-lives-and-quicker-deaths/.

Coppola, Vincent. "A Plague of Politics." *Atlanta*, May 1, 1994. https://www.atlantamagazine.com/great-reads/a-plague-of-politics/.

Cox, John Woodrow, Lynh Bui, and DeNeen L. Brown. "Who Was Freddie Gray? How Did He Die? And What Led to the Mistrial in Baltimore?" *Washington Post*, December 16, 2015, accessed June 5, 2023. https://www.washingtonpost.com/local/who-was-freddie-gray-and-how-did-his-death-lead-to-a-mistrial-in-baltimore/2015/12/16/b08df7ce-a433-11e5-9c4e-be37f66848bb_story.html.

Criss, Doug, and Madeline Holcombe. "Bill Jenkins, Who Helped End the Infamous Tuskegee Syphilis Study, Has Died at Age 73." CNN, February 28, 2019. https://www.cnn.com/2019/02/27/health/bill-jenkins-obit-trnd/index.html.

Cusick, Daniel. "Past Racist Redlining Practices Increased Climate Burden on Minority Neighborhoods." *Scientific American*, January 21, 2020. https://www

.scientificamerican.com/article/past-racist-redlining-practices-increased-climate
-burden-on-minority-neighborhoods/.

D'Ambrosio, Amanda. "Black Doctor Dies After Giving Birth, Underscoring Maternal Mortality Crisis." *MedPage Today,* November 2, 2020. https://www .medpagetoday.com/obgyn/pregnancy/89462.

Dawidoff, Nicholas. "Poverty Is Violent." *Atlantic,* December 28, 2022. https:// www.theatlantic.com/ideas/archive/2022/12/new-haven-connecticut-gun-violence /672504/.

Declercq, Eugene, Emily Feinberg, and Candice Belanoff. "Racial Inequities in the Course of Treating Perinatal Mental Health Challenges: Results from Listening to Mothers in California." *Birth* 49, no. 1 (March 2022): 132–40. https://doi.org/10 .1111/birt.12584.

Delafave, Rachel. "An Empirical Assessment of Homicide and Suicide Outcomes with Red Flag Laws." *Loyola University Chicago Law Journal* 52, no. 3 (January 1, 2021): 867.

Dellinger, Matt. "Frederick Law Olmsted's War on Disease and Disunity." *New Yorker,* May 16, 2020. https://www.newyorker.com/culture/cultural-comment /frederick-law-olmsteds-war-on-disease-and-disunity.

Demsas, Jerusalem. "The Great Defenders of the Status Quo." *Atlantic,* March 16, 2023. https://www.theatlantic.com/ideas/archive/2023/03/national -environmental-policy-act-1970-nepa-regulation/673385/.

DeRienzo, Paul. "Remembering New York's Cholera Pandemic of 1832 . . . and 1849." *Village Sun,* April 22, 2020. https://thevillagesun.com/remembering-new -yorks-cholera-pandemic-of-1832and-1849.

DeSalvo, Karen, chief health officer, Google. Author interview via Zoom, March 9, 2023.

Dickey, Jay, and Mark Rosenberg. "How to Protect Gun Rights While Reducing the Toll of Gun Violence." *Washington Post,* December 25, 2015. https://www .washingtonpost.com/opinions/time-for-collaboration-on-gun-research/2015/12 /25/f989cd1a-a819-11e5-bff5-905b92f5f94b_story.html.

Dine, Sarah B. "Wartime Health Disparities and Their Aftermath." *Health Affairs* 27, no. 4 (July/August 2008): 1191–92. https://doi.org/10.1377/hlthaff.27.4 .1191.

Donnella, Leah. "How Yellow Fever Turned New Orleans into the 'City of the Dead.'" NPR, October 31, 2018. https://www.npr.org/sections/codeswitch/2018 /10/31/415535913/how-yellow-fever-turned-new-orleans-into-the-city-of-the -dead.

Donnelly, Ally. "Domestic Violence Advocates Fear 'Perfect Storm' During Coronavirus Pandemic." NBC 10 Boston, April 2, 2020. https://www.nbcboston.com /investigations/domestic-violence-advocates-fear-perfect-storm-during-pandemic /2100955/.

Downs, Jim. "Emancipation, Sickness, and Death in the American Civil War." *Lancet* 380, no. 9854 (November 10, 2012): 1640–41. https://doi.org/10.1016/S0140 -6736(12)61937-0.

———. "The Epidemics America Got Wrong." *Atlantic*, March 22, 2020. https:// www.theatlantic.com/ideas/archive/2020/03/role-apathy-epidemics/608527/.

———. "How the Origins of Epidemiology Are Linked to the Transatlantic Slave Trade." *Time*, September 2, 2021. Accessed June 20, 2023. https://time.com /6094376/transatlantic-slave-trade-disease-outbreaks-epidemiology/.

———. "Journals of Plague Years." *Lapham's Quarterly*, September 8, 2021. https://www.laphamsquarterly.org/roundtable/journals-plague-years.

———. *Maladies of Empire: How Colonialism, Slavery, and War Transformed Medicine*. Cambridge, Massachusetts: Belknap Press of Harvard University Press, 2021.

———. "Never Forget that Early Vaccines Came from Testing on Enslaved People." *STAT*, June 19, 2022. https://www.statnews.com/2022/06/19/never-forget-that -early-vaccines-came-from-testing-on-enslaved-people/.

———. *Sick from Freedom: African-American Illness and Suffering During the Civil War and Reconstruction*. New York: Oxford University Press, 2012.

———. "This Pandemic Isn't Over." *Atlantic*, June 9, 2021. https://www .theatlantic.com/ideas/archive/2021/06/pandemics-end-when-we-stop-caring -about-their-victims/619127/.

Dranginis, Anne M. "Why the Hormone Study Finally Happened." *New York Times*, July 15, 2002. https://www.nytimes.com/2002/07/15/opinion/why-the -hormone-study-finally-happened.html.

"Dr. A.T. Augusta." *Evening Star* (Washington, D.C.), October 8, 1863: 2.

Drexler, Madeline. "Racism Harms Health." Harvard T.H. Chan School of Public Health, October 24, 2013. https://www.hsph.harvard.edu/news/magazine /centennial-racism-harms-health/.

"Dr. Wilbur Michael Byrd." *Tennessean*, March 3, 2021. https://www.tennessean .com/obituaries/ten188510.

Du Bois, W. E. B. "The Freedmen's Bureau." *Atlantic Monthly*, March 1901. https://www.theatlantic.com/magazine/archive/1901/03/the-freedmens-bureau /308772.

———. "The Health and Physique of the Negro American." *American Journal of Public Health* 93, no. 2 (February 2003): 272–76. https://ajph.aphapublications .org/doi/pdfplus/10.2105/AJPH.93.2.272.

———. *The Philadelphia Negro: A Social Study*. University of Pennsylvania Press, 1899.

———. "Strivings of the Negro People." *Atlantic Monthly*, August 1897. https:// www.theatlantic.com/magazine/archive/1897/08/strivings-of-the-negro-people /305446/.

Duncan, Arne, managing director Chicago CRED. Author interview via Zoom, May 4, 2023.

———. "We Know How to Prevent Gun Violence. Now We Need to Scale It." *Stanford Social Innovation Review,* July 14, 2022. https://doi.org/10.48558 /HKA8-RF51.

Durkee, Alison. "Attacks on Abortion Providers Surged in 2021, Report Finds as Supreme Court Overturns Roe V. Wade." *Forbes,* June 24, 2022. https://www .forbes.com/sites/alisondurkee/2022/06/24/attacks-on-abortion-providers -surged-in-2021-report-finds-ahead-of-roe-v-wade-ruling/?sh=2ee895a95419.

Durkin, Erin. "September 11: Nearly 10,000 People Affected by 'Cesspool of Cancer.'" *Guardian,* September 11, 2018. https://www.theguardian.com/us-news /2018/sep/10/911-attack-ground-zero-manhattan-cancer.

Dzau, Victor J., and Mark Rosenberg. "Congress Hasn't Banned Research on Gun Violence. It Just Won't Fund It." *Washington Post,* March 21, 2018. https://www .washingtonpost.com/opinions/how-research-can-help-us-address-gun-violence /2018/03/21/ecde2128-2c4d-11e8-8ad6-fbc50284fce8_story.html.

Eddy, Matthew Daniel. "James McCune Smith: New Discovery Reveals How First African American Doctor Fought for Women's Rights in Glasgow." *Conversation,* October 8, 2021. https://theconversation.com/james-mccune-smith-new-discovery -reveals-how-first-african-american-doctor-fought-for-womens-rights-in-glasgow -166233.

Edelin, Barbara, widow of Dr. Kenneth Edelin. Author interview via Zoom, May 3, 2023.

Edelin, Kenneth C. *Broken Justice: A True Story of Race, Sex, and Revenge in a Boston Courtroom.* Pondview Press, 2008.

Ellison, Katherine, and Nina Martin. "Nearly Dying in Childbirth: Why Preventable Complications Are Growing in U.S." NPR, December 22, 2017. https://www.npr .org/2017/12/22/572298802/nearly-dying-in-childbirth-why-preventable -complications-are-growing-in-u-s.

Etheridge, Elizabeth W. *Sentinel for Health: A History of the Centers for Disease Control.* Berkeley and Los Angeles: University of California Press, 1992.

Evans, Annie, and Cameron Katz. "Redlining and Hotter Neighborhoods: How Racist Housing Policies Created Urban Heat Islands." *Teen Vogue,* April 21, 2023. https://www.teenvogue.com/story/redlining-hotter-neighborhoods.

Fairchild, Amy L., David Rosner, James Colgrove, Ronald Bayer, and Linda P. Fried. "The EXODUS of Public Health: What History Can Tell Us About the Future." *American Journal of Public Health* 100, no. 1 (January 1, 2010): 54–63. https:// doi.org/10.2105/AJPH.2009.163956.

Farmer, Paul. *Fevers, Feuds and Diamonds: Ebola and the Ravages of History.* New York: Farrar, Straus and Giroux, 2020.

Faust, Drew Gilpin. *This Republic of Suffering: Death and the American Civil War.* New York: Alfred A. Knopf, 2008.

Fee, Elizabeth, and Mary E. Garofalo. "Florence Nightingale and the Crimean War." *American Journal of Public Health* 100, no. 9 (September 2010): 1591. https://doi .org/10.2105/AJPH.2009.188607.

Fee, Elizabeth, and Theodore M. Brown. "The Unfulfilled Promise of Public Health: Déjà Vu All Over Again." *Health Affairs* 21, no. 6 (November /December 2002): 31–43. https://doi.org/10.1377/hlthaff.21.6.31.

Feiden, Karyn. "How the Legacy of Redlining Influences Climate Justice Today." *Drexel Public Health Magazine,* May 8, 2023. https://issuu.com /dornsifesphmagazine/docs/drexel-dornisfe-sph-magazine-2023/s/24226501.

Feldman, Nina, and Aneri Pattani. "Black Mothers Get Less Treatment for Their Postpartum Depression." NPR, November 29, 2019. https://www.npr.org/sections /health-shots/2019/11/29/760231688/black-mothers-get-less-treatment-for -their-postpartum-depression.

Fenton, Justin. "Criminal Indictments Filed Against Maryland Company that Targeted Baltimore Lead Paint Victims' Settlements." *Baltimore Sun,* December 22, 2021. https://www.baltimoresun.com/maryland/baltimore-city/bs-md-ci-access -funding-criminal-charges-20211222-eajvbepqofasbk5rifdztirlya-story.html.

"First Colored 'Fellow' Appointed." *New York Times,* September 30, 1896.

"First Long-Term Study of World Trade Center Rescue and Recovery Workers Shows Widespread Health Problems Ten Years After 9-11." Mount Sinai, September 6, 2011. https://www.mountsinai.org/about/newsroom/2011/first-longterm -study-of-world-trade-center-rescue-and-recovery-workers-shows-widespread-health -problems-ten-years-after-911.

Fisher, Thomas. "Frederick Law Olmsted and the Campaign for Public Health." *Places Journal,* November 15, 2010. https://doi.org/10.22269/101115.

Flanagan, Caitlin. "The Dishonesty of the Abortion Debate." *Atlantic,* December 2019. https://www.theatlantic.com/magazine/archive/2019/12/the-things -we-cant-face/600769/.

———. "The Kids Working in Factories Aren't Alright." *Atlantic,* August 2023. https://www.theatlantic.com/magazine/archive/2023/08/child-labor-us-factories /674785/.

———. "The Sanguine Sex." *Atlantic,* May 2007. https://www.theatlantic.com /magazine/archive/2007/05/the-sanguine-sex/305780/.

Fleegler, Eric W., Lois K. Lee, Michael C. Monuteaux, David Hemenway, and Rebekah Mannix. "Firearm Legislation and Firearm-Related Fatalities in the United States." *JAMA Internal Medicine* 173, no. 9 (May 13, 2013): 732–40. https://doi .org/10.1001/jamainternmed.2013.1286.

Fleming, Nic. "Asbestos Is Still Killing People." *New Republic,* March 22, 2014. https://newrepublic.com/article/117119/asbestos-still-killing-people.

"Florence Nightingale: The Pioneer Statistician." Science Museum, December 10, 2018. https://www.sciencemuseum.org.uk/objects-and-stories/florence -nightingale-pioneer-statistician.

Foege, William H. *House on Fire: The Fight to Eradicate Smallpox*. Berkeley and Los Angeles: University of California Press, 2011.

Follman, Mark. "The Uvalde Massacre Could Have Been Prevented." *Mother Jones,* May 23, 2023. https://www.motherjones.com/politics/2023/05/uvalde-robb -elementary-mass-shooting-anniversary-police-investigation-threat-assessment/.

Foner, Eric. "Abraham Lincoln: The Great Emancipator?" *British Academy* 125 (n.d.): 149–62. https://www.thebritishacademy.ac.uk/documents/2000 /pba125p149.pdf.

Fuertes, James H. *Water and Public Health: The Relative Purity of Waters from Different Sources*. New York: John Wiley, 1897. http://archive.org/details /b24764632.

Gabler, Ellen. "How 2 Industries Stymied Justice for Young Lead Paint Victims." *New York Times,* March 29, 2022. https://www.nytimes.com/2022/03/29/us /lead-poisoning-insurance-landlords.html.

General Board of Health, Medical Council. *Report of the Committee for Scientific Inquiries in Relation to the Cholera-Epidemic of 1854*. London: George E. Eyre and William Spottiswoode, 1855. https://wellcomecollection.org/works/ckquck57.

Gerberding, Julie, former CDC director. Author interview via Zoom, April 21, 2023.

Goodman, Leah McGrath. "9/11's Second Wave: Cancer and Other Diseases Linked to the 2001 Attacks Are Surging." *Newsweek,* September 7, 2016. https:// www.newsweek.com/2016/09/16/9-11-death-toll-rising-496214.html.

Goodman, Shaina. "Intimate Partner Violence Endangers Pregnant People and Their Infants." National Partnership for Women & Families, May 2021. https:// nationalpartnership.org/report/intimate-partner-violence/.

Goodwin, Michele. "Banning Abortion Doesn't Protect Women's Health." *New York Times,* July 9, 2021. https://www.nytimes.com/2021/07/09/opinion/roe -abortion-supreme-court.html.

Gore, Karenna. "The Remarkable Life of the First Woman on the Harvard Faculty." *New York Times,* August 29, 2019. https://www.nytimes.com/2019/08/29 /opinion/alice-hamilton-harvard.html.

Gould, Jeffrey, CEO of the California Maternal Quality Care Collaborative. Author interview via Zoom, April 2, 2023.

Graham, David A. "The Mysterious Death of Freddie Gray." *Atlantic,* April 22, 2015. https://www.theatlantic.com/politics/archive/2015/04/the-mysterious -death-of-freddie-gray/391119/.

Gramlich, John. "What the Data Says About Gun Deaths in the U.S." Pew Research Center, March 5, 2025. https://www.pewresearch.org/short-reads/2023/04/26 /what-the-data-says-about-gun-deaths-in-the-u-s/.

———. "What We Know About the Increase in U.S. Murders in 2020," Pew Research Center, October 27, 2021. https://www.pewresearch.org/short-reads /2021/10/27/what-we-know-about-the-increase-in-u-s-murders-in-2020/.

Greenwald, Richard, labor historian at Fairfield University. Author interview via Zoom, January 18, 2023.

Griscom, John Hoskins. *The Sanitary Condition of the Laboring Population of New York: With Suggestions for Its Improvement.* New York: Harper & Brothers, 1845. http://archive.org/details/sanitaryconditi00grisgoog.

Gross, Terry. "A 'Forgotten History' of How the U.S. Government Segregated America." NPR, May 3, 2017. https://www.npr.org/2017/05/03/526655831/a-forgotten-history-of-how-the-u-s-government-segregated-america.

Gumas, Evan D., Munira Z. Gunja, and Reginald D. Williams II. "Comparing Deaths from Gun Violence in the U.S. with Other Countries," Commonwealth Fund, October 30, 2024. https://www.commonwealthfund.org/publications/2024/oct/comparing-deaths-gun-violence-us-other-countries.

———. "The Health Costs of Gun Violence: How the U.S. Compares to Other Countries." Commonwealth Fund, April 20, 2023. https://doi.org/10.26099/a2at-gy62.

Hackett, Martine, professor of health professions at Hofstra University. Author interview via Zoom, June 22, 2023.

Haddad, Ann. "'The Destroying Angel': New York's 1832 Cholera Epidemic." Merchant's House Museum, July 20, 2016. https://merchantshouse.org/blog/cholera1832/.

Haelle, Tara. "Health Effects of 9/11 Still Plague Responders and Survivors." *Scientific American,* September 10, 2021. https://www.scientificamerican.com/article/health-effects-of-9-11-still-plague-responders-and-survivors/.

———. "'Many Tuskegees' Occur Daily in the U.S." Association of Health Care Journalists, August 8, 2022. https://healthjournalism.org/blog/2022/08/many-tuskegees-occur-daily-in-the-u-s/.

Haight, Sarah C., Nancy Byatt, Tiffany A. Moore Simas, Cheryl L. Robbins, and Jean Y. Ko. "Recorded Diagnoses of Depression During Delivery Hospitalizations in the United States, 2000–2015." *Obstetrics and Gynecology* 133, no. 6 (June 2019): 1216–23. https://doi.org/10.1097/AOG.0000000000003291.

Hamilton, Alice. *Exploring the Dangerous Trades: The Autobiography of Alice Hamilton, M.D.* Boston: Little, Brown and Company, 1943. https://archive.org/details/exploringthedang011737mbp/page/n7/mode/2up.

Harris, Paul. "How the End of Slavery Led to Starvation and Death for Millions of Black Americans." *Guardian,* June 16, 2012. https://www.theguardian.com/world/2012/jun/16/slavery-starvation-civil-war.

Hathaway, Jeanne E., Georgianna Willis, Bonnie Zimmer, and Jay G. Silverman. "Impact of Partner Abuse on Women's Reproductive Lives." *Journal of the American Medical Women's Association* (1972) 60, no. 1 (2005): 42–45.

Healy, Bernadine. "Cancer and Me." U.S. News & World Report, August 9, 2011. https://health.usnews.com/health-news/managing-your-healthcare/cancer/articles/2011/08/09/cancer-and-me.

Heller, Jean. "AP Was There: Black Men Untreated in Tuskegee Syphilis Study." Associated Press, May 10, 2017. https://apnews.com/article/business-science -health-race-and-ethnicity-syphilis-e9dd07eaa4e74052878a68132cd3803a.

Henderson, Donald Ainslie. *Smallpox—The Death of a Disease: The Inside Story of Eradicating a Worldwide Killer.* Amherst, New York: Prometheus Books, 2009.

"History of Alice Hamilton, MD." National Institute for Occupational Safety and Health. Centers for Disease Control and Prevention, June 25, 2021. https://www .cdc.gov/niosh/awards/hamilton/hamhist.html.

"History of Slavery in New York." New-York Historical Society. Accessed June 22, 2023. https://www.slaveryinnewyork.org/history.htm.

Holmes, Megan R., and June-Yung Kim. *Prenatal Exposure to Domestic Violence: Summary of Key Research Findings.* Cleveland: Case Western Reserve University, 2019. https://case.edu/socialwork/traumacenter/resources/research-briefs /prenatal-exposure-domestic-violence.

Holt, Thomas C. "W. E. B. Du Bois." Hutchins Center for African & African American Research. Accessed June 21, 2023. https://hutchinscenter.fas.harvard.edu/web -dubois.

"Home of Susan Wharton." Race and Class in Du Bois' Seventh Ward. Accessed August 7, 2022. http://www.dubois-theward.org/resources/walking-tour /locations/.

Hood, R. G. "The 'Slave Health Deficit': The Case for Reparations to Bring Health Parity to African Americans." *Journal of the National Medical Association* 93, no. 1 (January 2001): 1–5. https://pubmed.ncbi.nlm.nih.gov/12653374/.

Horn, Heather Souvaine. "A Legendary Abortion Rights Activist on What Comes After Texas." *New Republic,* September 8, 2021. https://newrepublic.com/article /163570/heather-booth-jane-collective-texas-abortion-ban.

Horton, Richard. "Offline: A Lie at the Heart of Public Health." *Lancet* 399, no. 10326 (February 19, 2022): 704. https://doi.org/10.1016/S0140 -6736(22)00312-9.

———. "Offline: The Slave Trade—Medicine's Necessary Remorse." *Lancet* 400, no. 10362 (October 29, 2022): 1499. https://doi.org/10.1016/S0140 -6736(22)02119-5.

Howard, Jeffrey T., Jessica K. Perrotte, Caleb Leong, Timothy J. Grigsby, and Krista J. Howard. "Evaluation of All-Cause and Cause-Specific Mortality by Race and Ethnicity Among Pregnant and Recently Pregnant Women in the US, 2019 to 2020." *JAMA Network Open* 6, no. 1 (January 27, 2023): e2253280. https://doi .org/10.1001/jamanetworkopen.2022.53280.

Howard, Jeffrey T., Nicole Androne, Karl C. Alcover, Alexis R. Santos-Lozada. "Trends of Heat-Related Deaths in the US, 1999–2023," *JAMA* 332, no. 14 (August 26, 2024): 1203–4. https://pmc.ncbi.nlm.nih.gov/articles /PMC11348089/.

Hoyert, Donna L. "Maternal Mortality Rates in the United States, 2020." National Center for Health Statistics, CDC, February 23, 2022. https://www.cdc.gov/nchs /data/hestat/maternal-mortality/2020/maternal-mortality-rates-2020.htm.

———. "Maternal Mortality Rates in the United States, 2021." National Center for Health Statistics, CDC, March 16, 2023. https://www.cdc.gov/nchs/data/hestat /maternal-mortality/2021/maternal-mortality-rates-2021.htm.

Humphreys, Margaret. *Marrow of Tragedy: The Health Crisis of the American Civil War.* Baltimore: Johns Hopkins University Press, 2013.

Hunter, Marcus Anthony. "Black Philly After *The Philadelphia Negro.*" *American Sociological Association* 13, no. 1 (Winter 2014): 26–31. https://journals.sagepub .com/doi/10.1177/1536504214522005.

———. "For Colored Scholars Who Consider Suicide When Our Rainbows Are Not Enuf." *Berkeley Journal of Sociology,* February 1, 2016. https://berkeleyjournal.org /2016/02/01/for-colored-scholars-who-consider-suicide-when-our-rainbows-are -not-enuf/.

Hunter, Marcus, professor of sociology and African American studies at UCLA. Author interview via Zoom, October 26, 2022.

"The Influence of the London Epidemiological Society." *Yale Journal of Biology and Medicine* 46, no. 1 (February 1973): 29–31.

Institute of Medicine Committee for the Study of the Future of Public Health. *The Future of Public Health.* Washington, D.C.: National Academies Press, 1988. https://doi.org/10.17226/1091.

Irving, Doug. "Environmental Racism: How Historic Redlining Continues to Affect Communities." *Rand Review,* June 27, 2022. https://www.rand.org/blog/rand -review/2022/06/environmental-racism-how-historic-redlining-continues.html.

Jacobs, Andrew. "Health Care Workers Still Face Daunting Shortages of Masks and Other P.P.E." *New York Times,* December 20, 2020. https://www.nytimes.com /2020/12/20/health/covid-ppe-shortages.html.

Jacobs, Harriet A. "From Savannah." *Freedmen's Record,* January 1866. https:// docsouth.unc.edu/fpn/jacobs/support2.html.

———. "Jacobs School." *Freedmen's Record,* March 1865.

———. "Life Among the Contrabands." *Liberator,* September 5, 1862. https:// docsouth.unc.edu/fpn/jacobs/support5.html.

———. "Savannah Freedmen's Orphan Asylum." *Anti-Slavery Reporter,* March 2, 1868.

Jacobs, Harriet A., and Louisa Jacobs. "Letters from Teachers of the Freedmen." *National Anti-Slavery Standard,* April 16, 1864. https://docsouth.unc.edu/fpn /jacobs/support4.html.

Jacobs, Louisa. "Louisa Jacobs." *Freedmen's Record,* March 1866.

———. "Louisa Jacobs." *Freedmen's Record,* July 1866.

Jatoi, Ismail, Hyuna Sung, and Ahmedin Jemal. "The Emergence of the Racial Disparity in U.S. Breast-Cancer Mortality." *New England Journal of Medicine* 386, no. 25 (2022): 2349–52. https://doi.org/10.1056/NEJMp2200244.

Jenkins, DeMarcus, assistant professor in the School of Social Policy and Practice at the University of Pennsylvania. Author interview via Zoom, August 29, 2023.

Johns, Jacob R. "Clinical Diphtheria: A Summary of Investigations Concerning the Diptheria-Bacillus, the Toxin and Anti-Toxin of Diphtheria, Including the Diagnosis, Prognosis, and Treatment of the Disease." *Philadelphia Monthly Medical Journal* 1 (1899): 179–212.

Johnson, Anne. "Satcher, David 1941—." Encyclopedia.com, updated June 11, 2018. https://www.encyclopedia.com/people/history/us-history-biographies /david-satcher.

Johnson, Greg. "The Times and Life of W. E. B. Du Bois at Penn." *Penn Today,* February 22, 2019. https://penntoday.upenn.edu/news/times-and-life-web-du -bois-penn.

Johnson, Steven. *Extra Life: A Short History of Living Longer.* New York: Riverhead Books, 2021.

Jones, Cal, Borough of Manhattan historian emeritus. Author interview via Zoom, June 23, 2022.

Jones, Jonathan S., Civil War historian, James Madison University. Author interview via Zoom, June 24, 2022.

Jones, Jonathan S. "Lessons Learned—and Forgotten—from the Horrific Epidemics of the U.S. Civil War." *STAT,* April 18, 2021. https://www.statnews.com/2021/04 /18/lessons-learned-forgotten-horrific-epidemics-us-civil-war/.

Jones, Tom. "Confederates' Lost Cause Still Cripples the South's Economy." MLK50: Justice Through Journalism, July 27, 2017. http://mlk50.com/2017/07 /27/confederates-lost-cause-still-cripples-the-souths-economy/.

"Joseph Goldberger & the War on Pellagra." Office of NIH History & Stetten Museum. National Institutes of Health. Accessed June 20, 2023. https://history .nih.gov/pages/viewpage.action?pageId=8883184.

Kanki, Phyllis, professor of Health Sciences, Harvard T.H. Chan School of Public Health, Department of Immunology and Infectious Diseases. Author interview via Zoom, July 29, 2021.

Kaufman, Alexander C. "UN Says Environmental Racism in Louisiana's Cancer Alley Must End." *Grist,* March 5, 2021. https://grist.org/justice/united-nations -environmental-racism-cancer-alley-louisiana/.

Kellermann, A. L., F. P. Rivara, N. B. Rushforth, J. G. Banton, D. T. Reay, J. T. Francisco, A. B. Locci, J. Prodzinski, B. B. Hackman, and G. Somes. "Gun Owner-ship as a Risk Factor for Homicide in the Home." *New England Journal of Medicine* 329, no. 15 (October 7, 1993): 1084–91. https://doi.org/10.1056 /NEJM199310073291506.

Kennedy-Moulton, Kate, Sarah Miller, Petra Persson, Maya Rossin-Slater, Laura Wherry, and Gloria Aldana. "Maternal and Infant Health Inequality: New Evidence from Linked Administrative Data." Working Paper Series. National Bureau of Economic Research, November 2022. https://doi.org/10.3386/w30693.

Kennedy, Robert C. "Dr. Elizabeth Blackwell." Hobart and William Smith Colleges. https://www.hws.edu/about/history/elizabeth-blackwell/nyt-harpers.aspx.

Kilgoe, Ashley. "Addressing the Increased Risk of Postpartum Depression for Black Women." National Alliance on Mental Illness, July 26, 2021. https://www.nami.org /Blogs/NAMI-Blog/July-2021/Addressing-the-Increased-Risk-of-Postpartum -Depression-for-Black-Women.

Kisner, Jordan. "The Lockdown Showed How the Economy Exploits Women. She Already Knew." *New York Times Magazine,* February 17, 2021. https://www .nytimes.com/2021/02/17/magazine/waged-housework.html.

Kivisto, Aaron J., and Peter Lee Phalen. "Effects of Risk-Based Firearm Seizure Laws in Connecticut and Indiana on Suicide Rates, 1981–2015." *Psychiatric Services* 69, no. 8 (June 2018): 855–62. https://doi.org/10.1176/appi.ps.201700250.

Klass, Perri. "How Science Conquered Diphtheria, the Plague Among Children." *Smithsonian Magazine,* October 2021. https://www.smithsonianmag.com/science -nature/science-diphtheria-plague-among-children-180978572/.

Klein, Christopher. "How Pandemics Spurred Cities to Make More Green Space for People." History.com, April 27, 2020. https://www.history.com/news/cholera -pandemic-new-york-city-london-paris-green-space.

Kliff, Sarah, Claire Cain Miller, and Larry Buchanan. "Childbirth Is Deadlier for Black Families Even When They're Rich, Expansive Study Finds." *New York Times,* February 12, 2023. https://www.nytimes.com/interactive/2023/02/12/upshot /child-maternal-mortality-rich-poor.html.

Kliff, Sarah, and Margot Sanger-Katz. "Bottleneck for U.S. Coronavirus Response: The Fax Machine." *New York Times,* July 13, 2020. https://www.nytimes.com /2020/07/13/upshot/coronavirus-response-fax-machines.html.

Ko, Lisa. "Unwanted Sterilization and Eugenics Programs in the United States." PBS, January 29, 2016. https://www.pbs.org/independentlens/blog/unwanted -sterilization-and-eugenics-programs-in-the-united-states/.

Kostyal, K.M. "Behind the Lines: Olmsted at War." HistoryNet, April 28, 2015. https://www.historynet.com/behind-the-lines-olmsted-at-war/.

Krieger, Nancy. *Epidemiology and the People's Health: Theory and Context.* New York: Oxford University Press, 2011.

———. "Shades of Difference: Theoretical Underpinnings of the Medical Controversy on Black/White Differences in the United States, 1830–1870." *International Journal of Health Services* 17, no. 2 (April 1987): 259–78. https://journals.sagepub .com/doi/10.2190/DBY6-VDQ8-HME8-ME3R.

Landrigan, Philip, director of the Program for Global Public Health and the Common Good at Boston College. Author interview via Zoom, February 16, 2023.

Landrigan, Philip. "Nine Years Later: Health Effects in World Trade Center Responders, with Philip Landrigan." *Podcasts: The Researcher's Perspective* 2010, no. 1 (January 2010): ehp.trp090110. https://doi.org/10.1289/ehp.trp090110.

Langer, Emily. "Kenneth C. Edelin, Physician in Noted Abortion Case, Dies at 74." *Washington Post,* January 1, 2014. https://www.washingtonpost.com/national /kenneth-c-edelin-physician-in-noted-abortion-case-dies-at-74/2014/01/01 /45adf9d6-723a-11e3-8b3f-b1666705ca3b_story.html.

Lankford, Adam, Krista G. Adkins, and Eric Madfis. "Are the Deadliest Mass Shootings Preventable? An Assessment of Leakage, Information Reported to Law Enforcement, and Firearms Acquisition Prior to Attacks in the United States," 2019. https://ir.ua.edu/handle/123456789/8642.

Le Strat, Yann, Caroline Dubertret, and Bernard Le Foll. "Prevalence and Correlates of Major Depressive Episode in Pregnant and Postpartum Women in the United States." *Journal of Affective Disorders* 135, no. 1–3 (December 2011): 128–38. https://doi.org/10.1016/j.jad.2011.07.004.

Leavitt, Noah. "Uncommon Ground: Harvard Chan Researchers and Utah Gun-Rights Advocates Are Forging a Rare Partnership in the Quest to Prevent Firearm Suicides." Harvard Public Health. Harvard T.H. Chan School of Public Health, September 13, 2018. https://www.hsph.harvard.edu/magazine/magazine_article /uncommon-ground/.

Leemis, R.W., N. Friar, S. Khatiwada, M.S. Chen, M. Kresnow, S.G. Smith, S. Caslin, and K.C. Basile. "The National Intimate Partner and Sexual Violence Survey: 2016/2017 Report on Intimate Partner Violence." Atlanta: National Center for Injury Prevention and Control, Centers for Disease Control and Prevention, 2022.

"Letter from University of Pennsylvania to W. E. B. Du Bois, August 15, 1896." Robert S. Cox Special Collections and University Archives Research Center, University of Massachusetts Amherst. Accessed June 21, 2023. https://credo.library .umass.edu/view/full/mums312-b004-i335.

Levine, Lucie. " 'The Lungs of the City': Frederick Law Olmsted, Public Health, and the Creation of Central Park." The Gotham Center for New York City History, July 30, 2020. https://www.gothamcenter.org/blog/the-lungs-of-the-city-frederick -law-olmsted-public-health-and-the-creation-of-central-park.

Lewis, David Levering. *W. E. B. Du Bois: A Biography 1868–1963.* New York: Henry Holt and Company, 2009.

"Life Story: Elizabeth Blackwell (1821–1910)." Women & the American Story. https://wams.nyhistory.org/a-nation-divided/civil-war/elizabeth-blackwell/.

Lindsey, Bryan, senior director at the National Foundation for the CDC. Author interview via Zoom, February 28, 2023.

Linker, Beth. "On the Borderland of Medical and Disability History: A Survey of the Fields." *Bulletin of the History of Medicine* 87, no. 4 (2013): 499–535.

Liptak, Adam, J. David Goodman, and Sabrina Tavernise. "Supreme Court, Breaking Silence, Won't Block Texas Abortion Law." *New York Times,* September 1,

2021. https://www.nytimes.com/2021/09/01/us/supreme-court-texas-abortion
.html.

Liu, Korbin, Marilyn Moon, Margaret Sulvetta, and Juhi Chawla. "International
Infant Mortality Rankings: A Look Behind the Numbers." *Health Care Financing
Review* 13, no. 4 (Summer 1992): 105–18. https://pmc.ncbi.nlm.nih.gov/articles
/PMC4193257.

Lopez, German. "How to Dramatically Reduce Gun Violence in American Cities."
Vox, July 12, 2019. https://www.vox.com/policy-and-politics/2019/7/12
/20679091/thomas-abt-bleeding-out-urban-gun-violence-book-review.

Lord, Alexandra M. "As AIDS Epidemic Raged, a Rogue Reagan Official Taught
America the Truth." *Washington Post,* June 8, 2023. https://www.washingtonpost
.com/history/2023/06/04/aids-epidemic-reagan-everett-koop/.

MacGillis, Alec. "When Law Enforcement Alone Can't Stop the Violence." *New
Yorker,* January 30, 2023. https://www.newyorker.com/magazine/2023/02/06
/when-law-enforcement-alone-cant-stop-the-violence.

Marcus, Adam. "William Carter Jenkins." *Lancet* 393, no. 10180 (April 13, 2019):
1498. https://doi.org/10.1016/S0140-6736(19)30804-9.

Markel, Howard. "Celebrating the Life of Alice Hamilton, Founding Mother of
Occupational Medicine." PBS News, September 22, 2015. https://www.pbs.org
/newshour/health/celebrating-life-alice-hamilton-founding-mother-occupational
-medicine.

———. "How the Triangle Shirtwaist Factory Fire Transformed Labor Laws and
Protected Workers' Health." PBS News, March 31, 2021. https://www.pbs.org
/newshour/nation/how-the-triangle-shirtwaist-factory-fire-transformed-labor-laws
-and-protected-workers-health.

———. "In 1850, Ignaz Semmelweis Saved Lives with Three Words: Wash Your
Hands." PBS News, May 15, 2015. https://www.pbs.org/newshour/health/ignaz
-semmelweis-doctor-prescribed-hand-washing.

Markowitz, Gerald, and David Rosner. " 'Cater to the Children': The Role of the
Lead Industry in a Public Health Tragedy, 1900–1955." *American Journal of Public
Health* 90, no. 1 (January 2000): 36–46.

———. *Deceit and Denial: The Deadly Politics of Industrial Pollution.* Berkeley and
Los Angeles: University of California Press, 2002.

———. *Lead Wars: The Politics of Science and the Fate of America's Children.*
Berkeley and Los Angeles: University of California Press, 2013.

———. "Standing Up to the Lead Industry: An Interview with Herbert Needleman." *Public Health Reports* 120, no. 3 (May–June 2005). https://pmc.ncbi.nlm
.nih.gov/articles/instance/1497712/pdf/16134577.pdf.

Martin, Douglas. "A Village Dies, A Park Is Born." *New York Times,* January 31,
1997. https://www.nytimes.com/1997/01/31/arts/a-village-dies-a-park-is-born
.html.

Martin, Michel. "Racism Is Literally Bad for Your Health." NPR, October 28, 2017. https://www.npr.org/2017/10/28/560444290/racism-is-literally-bad-for-your-health.

Martin, Nina, and Renee Montagne. "Black Mothers Keep Dying After Giving Birth. Shalon Irving's Story Explains Why." NPR, December 7, 2017. https://www.npr.org/2017/12/07/568948782/black-mothers-keep-dying-after-giving-birth-shalon-irvings-story-explains-why.

———. "The Last Person You'd Expect to Die in Childbirth." NPR, May 12, 2017. https://www.npr.org/2017/05/12/527806002/focus-on-infants-during-childbirth-leaves-u-s-moms-in-danger.

———. "U.S. Has the Worst Rate of Maternal Deaths in the Developed World." NPR, May 12, 2017. https://www.npr.org/2017/05/12/528098789/u-s-has-the-worst-rate-of-maternal-deaths-in-the-developed-world.

"Maryland: Integration of Intimate Partner Violence Screening into Women's Health Services." Centers for Disease Control and Prevention, April 22, 2022. https://www.cdc.gov/prams/state-success-stories/Maryland.html.

Masur, Louis P. "Olmsted's Southern Landscapes." *New York Times,* July 9, 2011. https://archive.nytimes.com/opinionator.blogs.nytimes.com/2011/07/09/olmsteds-southern-landscapes/.

Maturen, Stephen, and Riley D. Champine. "Racist Housing Policies Have Created Some Oppressively Hot Neighborhoods." *National Geographic,* September 2, 2020. https://www.nationalgeographic.com/science/article/racist-housing-policies-created-some-oppressively-hot-neighborhoods.

Maxmen, Amy. "Inequality's Deadly Toll." *Nature,* April 28, 2021. https://www.nature.com/immersive/d41586-021-00943-x/index.html.

———. "The Radical Plan for Vaccine Equity," *Nature,* July 13, 2022. https://www.nature.com/immersive/d41586-022-01898-3/index.html.

———. "These 7 Radical Changes Would Fortify the U.S. Against the Next Pandemic," *Washington Post,* May 11, 2023. https://www.washingtonpost.com/opinions/2023/05/10/prevent-next-pandemic-steps/.

McCoy, Terrence. "Freddie Gray's Life a Study on the Effects of Lead Paint on Poor Blacks." *Washington Post,* April 29, 2015. https://www.washingtonpost.com/local/freddie-grays-life-a-study-in-the-sad-effects-of-lead-paint-on-poor-blacks/2015/04/29/0be898e6-eea8-11e4-8abc-d6aa3bad79dd_story.html.

McDonell-Parry, Amelia, and Justine Barron. "Death of Freddie Gray: 5 Things You Didn't Know." *Rolling Stone,* April 12, 2017. https://www.rollingstone.com/culture/culture-features/death-of-freddie-gray-5-things-you-didnt-know-129327/.

McDougle, Leon, professor of family medicine at The Ohio State University. Author interview via Zoom, November 2, 2022.

McFadden, Robert D. "Bernadine P. Healy, a Pioneer at National Institutes of Health, Dies at 67." *New York Times,* August 8, 2011. https://www.nytimes.com/2011/08/09/us/09healy.html.

McFarlane, Judith, Ann Malecha, Kathy Watson, Julia Gist, Elizabeth Batten, Iva Hall, and Sheila Smith. "Intimate Partner Sexual Assault Against Women: Frequency, Health Consequences, and Treatment Outcomes." *Obstetrics and Gynecology* 105, no. 1 (January 2005): 99–108. https://doi.org/10.1097/01.AOG.0000146641 .98665.b6.

McFarling, Usha Lee. "In Counties with More Black Doctors, Black People Live Longer, 'Astonishing' Study Finds." *STAT,* April 14, 2023. https://www.statnews .com/2023/04/14/black-doctors-primary-care-life-expectancy-mortality/.

McGhee, Heather. *The Sum of Us: What Racism Costs Everyone and How We Can Prosper Together.* New York: One World, 2021.

McGill, Ralph. "W. E. B. Du Bois." *Atlantic,* November 1965.

McGreevy, Nora. "How Redlining Made City Neighborhoods Hotter." *Smithsonian Magazine,* September 9, 2020. https://www.smithsonianmag.com/smart-news /how-redlining-made-city-neighborhoods-hotter-180975754/.

McKenna, Maryn. *Beating Back the Devil: On the Front Lines with the Disease Detectives of the Epidemic Intelligence Service.* New York: Free Press, 2004.

McLeod, Kari S. "Our Sense of Snow: The Myth of John Snow in Medical Geography." *Social Science and Medicine* 50 (2000): 923–35.

McNamara, Robert. "The Cholera Epidemic of 1832: As Immigrants Were Blamed, Half of New York City Fled in Panic." *ThoughtCo,* updated May 1, 2025. https:// www.thoughtco.com/the-cholera-epidemic-1773767.

Michaels, David, and Robert Bullard. "Environmental Justice Is Essential in the Workplace and at Home." *Nation,* October 22, 2021. https://www.thenation.com /article/economy/workplace-environmental-justice/.

Montagne, Renee. "To Keep Women from Dying in Childbirth, Look to California." NPR, July 29, 2018. https://www.npr.org/2018/07/29/632702896/to -keep-women-from-dying-in-childbirth-look-to-california.

Moore, Wes, and Erica L. Green. *Five Days: The Fiery Reckoning of an American City.* New York: One World, 2020.

Morabia, Alfredo, epidemiologist at the Mailman School of Public Health, Columbia University. Author interview via Zoom, November 14, 2022.

————. *Enigmas of Health and Disease: How Epidemiology Helps Unravel Scientific Mysteries.* New York: Columbia University Press, 2014.

Morgan, Thomas M. "The Education and Medical Practice of Dr. James McCune Smith (1813–1865), First Black American to Hold a Medical Degree." *Journal of the National Medical Association* 95, no. 7 (July 2003): 603–14. https://pubmed.ncbi .nlm.nih.gov/12911258.

Morrall, Andrew. "The Science of Gun Policy: A Critical Synthesis of Research Evidence on the Effects of Gun Policies in the United States." *Rand Health Quarterly* 8, no. 1 (2018): 5.

Morton, Carol Cruzan. "Gun Advocates Take the Lead in Embracing Suicide Prevention Message." *Oregonian,* November 28, 2020. https://www.oregonlive.com/pacific-northwest-news/2020/11/gun-advocates-take-the-lead-in-embracing-suicide-prevention-message.html.

Muncy, Robyn, labor historian at the University of Maryland. Author interview via Zoom, January 25, 2023.

Muncy, Robyn. "First Measured Century: Robyn Muncy Interview." PBS. Accessed June 20, 2023. https://www.pbs.org/fmc/interviews/muncy.htm.

Mydans, Seth. "When Is an Abortion Not an Abortion?" *Atlantic,* May 1975. https://www.theatlantic.com/past/docs/issues/95sep/abortion/myda.htm.

Nakayama, Don K. "Contraband Hospital, Freedmen's Hospital, and Alexander Augusta." *American Surgeon* 88, no. 6 (June 2022): 1046–50. https://doi.org/10.1177/00031348211067992.

National Institutes of Health. "Dr. Alexander T. Augusta: Patriot, Officer, Doctor." Binding Wounds, Pushing Boundaries: African Americans in Civil War Medicine. https://www.nlm.nih.gov/exhibition/bindingwounds/pdfs/BioAugustaOB571.pdf.

National Park Service. "Olmsted and the United States Sanitary Commission," February 3, 2022. https://www.nps.gov/articles/000/olmsted-and-the-united-states-sanitary-commission.htm.

Newkirk II, Vann R. "Fighting Environmental Racism in North Carolina." *New Yorker,* January 16, 2016. https://www.newyorker.com/news/news-desk/fighting-environmental-racism-in-north-carolina.

Newmark, Jill. "Contraband Hospital, 1862–1863: Health Care for the First Freedpeople." Black Past, March 28, 2012. https://www.blackpast.org/african-american-history/contraband-hospital-1862-1863-heath-care-first-freedpeople/.

Newsome, Melba. "We Learned the Wrong Lessons from the Tuskegee 'Experiment.'" *Scientific American,* March 31, 2021. https://www.scientificamerican.com/article/we-learned-the-wrong-lessons-from-the-tuskegee-experiment/.

Nielsen, David. "Disarming Dangerous Persons: How Connecticut's Red Flag Law Saves Lives without Jeopardizing Constitutional Protections." *Quinnipiac Health Law Journal* 23 (2020): 253.

Norsigian, Judy. "Our Bodies Ourselves and the Women's Health Movement in the United States: Some Reflections." *American Journal of Public Health* 109, no. 6 (June 2019): 844–46. https://doi.org/10.2105/AJPH.2019.305059.

Northwestern Neighborhood & Network Initiative. "Reaching and Connecting: Preliminary Results from Chicago CRED's Impact on Gun Violence Involvement." Institute for Policy Research, Northwestern University, August 25, 2021. https://www.ipr.northwestern.edu/documents/reports/ipr-n3-rapid-research-reports-cred-impact-aug-25-2021.pdf.

Norton, Ruth Ann, president and CEO of the Green & Healthy Homes Initiative. Author interview via Zoom, June 23, 2023.

Nowell, Cecilia. "Homicide Is a Leading Cause of Death in Pregnant People, a New Study Finds. Black Women Are at Greatest Risk." *Washington Post,* December 6, 2021. https://www.washingtonpost.com/gender-identity/homicide-is-a-leading -cause-of-death-in-pregnant-people-a-new-study-finds-black-women-are-at-greatest -risk/.

Nuriddin, Ayah. "The Black Politics of Eugenics." Nursing Clio, June 1, 2017. https://nursingclio.org/2017/06/01/the-black-politics-of-eugenics/.

Oeur, Freeden Blume. "Fever Dreams: W. E. B. Du Bois and the Racial Trauma of COVID-19 and Lynching." *Ethnic and Racial Studies* 44, no. 5 (2021): 735–45.

Olivarius, Kathryn, historian at Stanford University. Author interview via Zoom, June 16, 2022.

Orleck, Annelise. "And the Virus Rages On: 'Contingent' and 'Essential' Workers in the Time of COVID-19." *International Labor and Working-Class History* 99 (April 2021): 1–14. https://doi.org/10.1017/S0147547920000174.

———. "Clara Lemlich Shavelson." Jewish Women's Archive, December 31, 1999. https://jwa.org/encyclopedia/article/shavelson-clara-lemlich.

Orleck, Annelise, labor historian at Dartmouth College. Author interview via Zoom, January 19, 2023.

———. "Rose Schneiderman." Jewish Women's Archive, December 31, 1999. https://jwa.org/encyclopedia/article/schneiderman-rose.

Ostfeld, Jackie. "The Outdoors Are Great, But Not for All." *The Hill,* March 26, 2021. https://thehill.com/opinion/energy-environment/545067-the-outdoors-are -great-but-not-for-all/.

Parker, George F. "Circumstances and Outcomes of a Firearm Seizure Law: Marion County, Indiana, 2006–2013." *Behavioral Sciences & the Law* 33, no. 2–3 (June 2015): 308–22. https://doi.org/10.1002/bsl.2175.

Persaud, Nav, Alanna McKnight, and Heather Butts. "Dr Alexander Augusta Sought Medical Education in Canada But Became a Medical Educator in America after the Civil War." *Canadian Medical Education Journal* 12, no. 6 (December 2021): 100–102. https://doi.org/10.36834/cmej.72666.

Peterson, Dana, chief economist at The Conference Board. Author interview via Zoom, June 21, 2021.

Pinn, Vivian, former director of the Office of Research on Women's Health at the NIH. Author interview via Zoom, April 7, 2023.

———. "Perspectives from a Pathologist: My Journey on the Path to Women's Health Research, Sex and Gender Policy, and Practice Implications." *Annual Review of Pathology: Mechanisms of Disease* 13 (January 2018): 1–25. https://www .annualreviews.org/content/journals/10.1146/annurev-pathol-020117-044020.

"Pioneering Research of First Published African American Doctor Revealed." *EurekAlert!,* October 12, 2021. https://www.eurekalert.org/news-releases /931259.

Piper, Kelsey. "Smallpox Used to Kill Millions of People Every Year. Here's How Humans Beat It." *Vox,* May 8, 2022. https://www.vox.com/future-perfect /21493812/smallpox-eradication-vaccines-infectious-disease-covid-19.

Prothrow-Stith, Deborah, dean for the College of Medicine at Charles R. Drew University of Medicine and Science. Author interview via Zoom, August 30, 2023.

———. "Deaths Among Pregnant Women and New Mothers Rose Sharply During Pandemic." *New York Times,* January 27, 2023. https://www.nytimes.com/2023 /01/27/health/pregnancy-maternity-women-deaths.html.

Rabin, Roni Caryn. " 'How Did We Not Know?' Gun Owners Confront a Suicide Epidemic." *New York Times,* November 17, 2020. https://www.nytimes.com/2020 /11/17/health/suicide-guns-prevention.html.

Reid, Richard M. "Black Doctors: Challenging the Barriers." In *African Canadians in Union Blue: Enlisting for the Cause in the Civil War.* Vancouver: UBC Press, 2014, 146–76.

Reilly, Robert F. "Medical and Surgical Care During the American Civil War, 1861–1865." *Baylor University Medical Center Proceedings* 29, no. 2 (April 2016): 138–42. https://www.tandfonline.com/doi/abs/10.1080/08998280.2016 .11929390.

Reimer, Terry. "Smallpox and Vaccination in the Civil War." National Museum of Civil War Medicine, November 9, 2004. https://www.civilwarmed.org/surgeons -call/small_pox/.

Renkl, Margaret. "The South's Republicans Talk About Freedom While People Die." *New York Times,* September 6, 2021. https://www.nytimes.com/2021/09/06 /opinion/south-republicans-vaccines-climate-change.html.

Rentz, Catherine. "Freddie Gray Remembered as Jokester Who Struggled to Leave Drug Trade." *Baltimore Sun,* updated July 1, 2019. https://www.baltimoresun.com /2015/11/22/freddie-gray-remembered-as-jokester-who-struggled-to-leave-drug -trade/.

Researching Black History at the National Archives: The Dr. Alexander T. Augusta Workshop. Washington, D.C.: National Archives Tour Office, Office of the Public Programs, 1994.

Reynolds, P. Preston. "UVA and the History of Race: Eugenics, the Racial Integrity Act, Health Disparities." *UVA Today,* January 9, 2020. https://news.virginia.edu /content/uva-and-history-race-eugenics-racial-integrity-act-health-disparities.

Ringenberg, Matthew C., William C. Ringenberg, and Joseph D. Brain. *The Education of Alice Hamilton: From Fort Wayne to Harvard.* Bloomington: Indiana University Press, 2019.

Robeznieks, Andis. "Why eGFR-Reporting Change Helps Tackle Kidney Disease Inequities." American Medical Association, May 19, 2021. https://www.ama-assn .org/delivering-care/population-care/why-egfr-reporting-change-helps-tackle -kidney-disease-inequities.

Robinson, Henry S. "Anderson Ruffin Abbott, MD, 1837–1913." *Journal of the National Medical Association* 72, no. 7 (July 1980): 713.

Rochman, Susan, and Lauren Davitt. "Colon Cancer Screening Can Erase Disparities in Outcomes." Kaiser Permanente, February 24, 2022. https://about .kaiserpermanente.org/content/internet/kp/kpcomms/en/news/colon-cancer -screening-can-erase-disparities-in-outcomes.html.

Roeder, Amy. "The Education of Occupational Health Pioneer Alice Hamilton." Harvard T.H. Chan School of Public Health, February 11, 2020. https://www .hsph.harvard.edu/news/features/education-of-alice-hamilton/.

Rogers, Lindsay Smith. "The Racial Inequities of Kidney Disease." Johns Hopkins Bloomberg School of Public Health, September 3, 2020. https://publichealth.jhu .edu/2020/the-racial-inequities-of-kidney-disease.

Rogers, Simon. "Florence Nightingale, Datajournalist: Information Has Always Been Beautiful." *Guardian,* August 13, 2010. https://www.theguardian.com/news /datablog/2010/aug/13/florence-nightingale-graphics.

Rosenberg, Alyssa. "How Many Dead Moms Will It Take to Stop America's Maternal Mortality Epidemic?" *Washington Post,* June 20, 2023. https://www.washingtonpost .com/opinions/2023/06/20/tori-bowie-maternal-mortality-fixes/.

Rosenberg, Charles E. *The Cholera Years: The United States in 1832, 1849, and 1866.* Chicago and London: University of Chicago Press, 1962.

Rosenberg, Mark L., former CDC epidemiologist. Author interview via Zoom, May 2, 2023.

———. "This Myth About Guns Is Killing Us." *Knowable Magazine,* June 20, 2022. https://knowablemagazine.org/article/health-disease/2022/this-myth -about-guns-killing-us.

———. "What's Missing from the Gun Debate." POLITICO, February 18, 2018. https://www.politico.com/magazine/story/2018/02/18/whats-missing-from-the -gun-debate-217022/.

Rosenberg, Mark L., and Mary Ann Fenley, eds. *Violence in America: A Public Health Approach.* New York: Oxford University Press, 1991.

Rosner, David, professor of history at the Mailman School of Public Health, Columbia University. Author interview via Zoom, November 18, 2022.

Rosner, David. "'Spanish Flu, or Whatever It Is. . . .': The Paradox of Public Health in a Time of Crisis." *Public Health Reports* 124, supplement 3 (April 2010): 38–47. https://pmc.ncbi.nlm.nih.gov/articles/PMC2862333/.

Rosner, David, and Gerald Markowitz. "A 'Gift of God'?: The Public Health Controversy over Leaded Gasoline During the 1920s." *American Journal of Public Health* 75, no. 4 (April 1985): 344–52.

———. "A Short History of Occupational Safety and Health in the United States." *American Journal of Public Health* 110, no. 5 (May 2020): 622–28. https://doi .org/10.2105/AJPH.2020.305581.

Roth, Alisa. "An Epidemic of Violence We Never Discuss." *New York Times,* June 7, 2019. https://www.nytimes.com/2019/06/07/books/review/rachel-louise -snyder-no-visible-bruises.html.

Rothstein, Richard. *The Color of Law: A Forgotten History of How Our Government Segregated America.* New York: Liveright, 2017.

Roubein, Rachel. "What Does a 19th-Century Federal Law Have to Do with Abortion?" *Washington Post,* March 21, 2023. https://www.washingtonpost.com /politics/2023/03/21/what-does-19th-century-federal-law-have-do-with -abortion/.

Rowley, Diane, former CDC epidemiologist. Author interview via Zoom, February 16, 2023.

Ruane, Michael E. "A Brief History of the Enduring Phony Science that Perpetuates White Supremacy." *Washington Post,* April 30, 2019. https://www.washingtonpost .com/local/a-brief-history-of-the-enduring-phony-science-that-perpetuates-white -supremacy/2019/04/29/20e6aef0-5aeb-11e9-a00e-050dc7b82693_story.html.

Rudúlph, Heather Wood. "Why We Need 'Our Bodies Ourselves' Now More than Ever." *Dame Magazine,* April 13, 2018. https://www.damemagazine.com/2018 /04/13/why-we-need-our-bodies-ourselves-now-more-than-ever/.

Ruths, Mitali Banerjee. "The History of Medicine: The Lesson of John Snow and the Broad Street Pump." *American Medical Association Journal of Ethics* 11, no. 6 (June 2009): 470–72.

Sacks, Jeffrey J., James A. Mercy, George W. Ryan, and R. Gibson Parrish. "Guns in the Home, Homicide, and Suicide." *JAMA* 272, no. 11 (September 21, 1994): 847–48. https://doi.org/10.1001/jama.1994.03520110025011.

Safi, Michael, and Dominic Rushe. "Rana Plaza, Five Years On: Safety of Workers Hangs in Balance in Bangladesh." *Guardian,* April 24, 2018. https://www .theguardian.com/global-development/2018/apr/24/bangladeshi-police-target -garment-workers-union-rana-plaza-five-years-on.

Santora, Tyler. "Whiter Neighborhoods Get More Park Space, a New Report Shows." *Audubon,* May 27, 2021. https://www.audubon.org/news/whiter -neighborhoods-get-more-park-space-new-report-shows.

Sarkar, N. N. "The Impact of Intimate Partner Violence on Women's Reproductive Health and Pregnancy Outcome." *Journal of Obstetrics and Gynaecology* 28, no. 3 (2008): 266–71. https://doi.org/10.1080/01443610802042415.

Satcher, David. *My Quest for Health Equity: Notes on Learning While Leading.* Baltimore: Johns Hopkins University Press, 2020.

Schell, Terry L., Matthew Cefalu, Beth Ann Griffin, Rosanna Smart, and Andrew R. Morral. "Changes in Firearm Mortality Following the Implementation of State Laws Regulating Firearm Access and Use." *Proceedings of the National Academy of Sciences* 117, no. 26 (June 15, 2020): 14906–10. https://doi.org/10.1073/pnas .1921965117.

Schell, Terry L., Samuel Peterson, Brian G. Vegetabile, Adam Scherling, Rosanna Smart, and Andrew R. Morral. "State-Level Estimates of Household Firearm Ownership." RAND, April 22, 2020. https://www.rand.org/pubs/tools/TL354.html.

Schifman, Jonathan. "How New York City Found Clean Water." *Smithsonian,* November 25, 2019. https://www.smithsonianmag.com/history/how-new-york -city-found-clean-water-180973571/.

Schoendorf, Kenneth C., Carol J. R. Hogue, Joel C. Kleinman, and Diana Rowley. "Mortality Among Infants of Black as Compared with White College-Educated Parents." *New England Journal of Medicine* 326, no. 23 (June 4, 1992): 1522–26. https://doi.org/10.1056/NEJM199206043262303.

Schultz, Myron. "Rudolf Virchow." *Emerging Infectious Diseases* 14, no. 9 (September 2008): 1480–81. https://doi.org/10.3201/eid1409.086672.

Seelye, Katharine Q. "Bill Jenkins, Who Tried to Halt Tuskegee Syphilis Study, Dies at 73." *New York Times,* February 25, 2019. https://www.nytimes.com/2019/02 /25/obituaries/bill-jenkins-dead.html.

Seligson, Susan. "Governor, Colleagues Pay Tribute to Kenneth Edelin." *Bostonia,* January 28, 2014. https://www.bu.edu/bostonia/2014/governor-colleagues-pay -tribute-to-kenneth-edelin/.

Seneca Village Project. "History of the Community." Accessed June 21, 2023. https://projects.mcah.columbia.edu/seneca_village/htm/history.htm.

"Severe Maternal Morbidity after Delivery Discharge among U.S. Women, 2010–2014 | CDC." Centers for Disease Control and Prevention, December 16, 2021. https://www.cdc.gov/reproductivehealth/maternalinfanthealth/smm/smm-after -delivery-discharge-among-us-women/index.htm.

"Severe Maternal Morbidity in the United States." Centers for Disease Control and Prevention, February 2, 2021. https://www.cdc.gov/reproductivehealth /maternalinfanthealth/severematernalmorbidity.html.

Shaban, Hamza. "How Racism Creeps Into Medicine." *Atlantic,* August 29, 2014. https://www.theatlantic.com/health/archive/2014/08/how-racism-creeps-into -medicine/378618/.

Shane, Scott, Nikita Stewart, and Ron Nixon. "Hard But Hopeful Home to 'Lot of Freddies.'" *New York Times,* May 3, 2015. https://www.nytimes.com/2015/05 /03/us/sandtown-winchester-baltimore-home-to-a-lot-of-freddie-grays.html.

Shao, Elena. "Cleaner Air Helps Everyone. It Helps Black Communities a Lot." *New York Times,* March 24, 2023. https://www.nytimes.com/2023/03/24 /climate/air-pollution-pm25-health-effects.html.

Shattuck, Lemuel. *Report of the Sanitary Commission of Massachusetts, 1850.* Cambridge, Massachusetts: Harvard University Press, 1948. http://archive.org /details/reportofsanitary00shat.

Shryock, Richard H. "The Early American Public Health Movement." *American Journal of Public Health and the Nation's Health* 27, no. 10 (October 1937): 965–71. https://ajph.aphapublications.org/doi/abs/10.2105/AJPH.27.10.965.

Sigmund, Pete. "NYC's Central Park: An American Masterpiece." Construction Equipment Guide, July 27, 2006. https://www.constructionequipmentguide.com /nycs-central-park-an-american-masterpiece/7148.

Smart, Rosanna, Terry L. Schell, Matthew Cefalu, and Andrew R. Morral. "Impact on Nonfirearm Deaths of Firearm Laws Affecting Firearm Deaths: A Systematic Review and Meta-Analysis." *American Journal of Public Health* 110, no. 10 (October 2020): e1–9. https://doi.org/10.2105/AJPH.2020.305808.

Smith, Harrison. "Bill Jenkins, Epidemiologist Who Tried to End Tuskegee Syphilis Study, Dies at 73." *Washington Post,* February 27, 2019. https://www .washingtonpost.com/local/obituaries/bill-jenkins-epidemiologist-who-tried-to-end -tuskegee-syphilis-study-dies-at-73/2019/02/27/2319e142-3aa2-11e9-a06c -3ec8ed509d15_story.html.

Snow, John. *Cholera and the Water Supply in the South Districts of London in 1854.* London: T. Richards, 1856. http://archive.org/details/b22299257.

———. *On the Mode of Communication of Cholera.* London: John Churchill, 1849. http://archive.org/details/b30383158.

———. *On the Mode of Communication of Cholera.* London: John Churchill, 1855. http://archive.org/details/b28985266.

Solis, Hilda L. "What the Triangle Shirtwaist Fire Means for Workers Now." *Washington Post,* March 18, 2011. https://www.washingtonpost.com/opinions /what-the-triangle-shirtwaist-fire-means-for-workers-now/2011/03/15/ABVAFIs_ story.html.

Spencer, Jane, and Christina Jewett. "12 Months of Trauma: More than 3,600 US Health Workers Died in Covid's First Year." KFF Health News, April 8, 2021. https://kffhealthnews.org/news/article/us-health-workers-deaths-covid-lost-on-the -frontline/.

Stafford, Ned. "Kenneth C Edelin." *British Medical Journal* 348 (February 17, 2014): g411. https://doi.org/10.1136/bmj.g411.

Standback, Jevon, life coach Chicago CRED. Author interview via Zoom, May 4, 2023.

Staples, Brent. "The Death of the Black Utopia." *New York Times,* November 28, 2019. https://www.nytimes.com/2019/11/28/opinion/seneca-central-park-nyc .html.

St. Fleur, Nicholas, Abena Asare, Hannah Thomas, Monique Fitzgerald, Robert Bullard, and Dennis Nix. "'A Textbook Case of Environmental Racism': The Battle Over the Brookhaven Landfill." *Color Code,* May 22, 2023. Accessed June 22, 2023. https://www.statnews.com/2023/05/22/north-bellport-new-york-brookhaven -landfill-environmental-racism/.

St. Fleur, Nicholas, and Martine Hackett. "Welcome to Long Island." *Color Code,* May 8, 2023. Accessed June 22, 2023. https://www.statnews.com/2023/05/08 /long-island-segregation-suburban-health/.

Stolberg, Sheryl Gay. "A Nation Challenged: The Disease; Anthrax Threats Points to Limits in Health Systems." *New York Times,* October 14, 2001. https://www .nytimes.com/2001/10/14/us/nation-challenged-disease-anthrax-threats-points -limits-health-systems.html.

Sullivan, Patricia. "Bernadine Healy, NIH and Red Cross Leader, Dies at 67." *Washington Post,* August 8, 2011. https://www.washingtonpost.com/local /obituaries/bernadine-healy-nih-and-red-cross-leader-dies-at-67/2011/08/08 /gIQAywhA3I_story.html.

Swanson, Jeffrey, Michael Norko, Hsiu-Ju Lin, Kelly Alanis-Hirsch, Linda Frisman, Madelon Baranoski, Michele Easter, Allison Robertson, Marvin Swartz, and Richard Bonnie. "Implementation and Effectiveness of Connecticut's Risk-Based Gun Removal Law: Does It Prevent Suicides?" *Law and Contemporary Problems* 80, no. 2 (May 12, 2017): 179–208.

Swanson, Jeffrey W., Michele M. Easter, Kelly Alanis-Hirsch, Charles M. Belden, Michael A. Norko, Allison G. Robertson, Linda K. Frisman, Hsiu-Ju Lin, Marvin S. Swartz, and George F. Parker. "Criminal Justice and Suicide Outcomes with Indiana's Risk-Based Gun Seizure Law." *Journal of the American Academy of Psychiatry and the Law* 47, no. 2 (June 2019): 18–97. https://doi.org/10.29158 /JAAPL.003835-19.

Tabuchi, Hiroko, and Nadja Popovich. "People of Color Breathe More Hazardous Air. The Sources Are Everywhere." *New York Times,* April 28, 2021. https://www .nytimes.com/2021/04/28/climate/air-pollution-minorities.html.

Taddonio, Patrice. "Depleted National Stockpile Contributed to COVID PPE Shortage." *Frontline,* October 6, 2020. https://www.pbs.org/wgbh/frontline /article/depleted-national-stockpile-contributed-to-covid-ppe-shortage/.

Talbot, Margaret. "Matters of Privacy." *New Yorker,* September 29, 2014. https:// www.newyorker.com/podcast/comment/matters-of-privacy.

———. "The Radical Women Who Paved the Way for Free Speech and Free Love." *New Yorker,* July 19, 2021. https://www.newyorker.com/magazine/2021/07/26 /the-radical-women-who-paved-the-way-for-free-speech-and-free-love.

Taylor, Keeanga-Yamahtta. "The Black Plague." *New Yorker,* April 16, 2020. https://www.newyorker.com/news/our-columnists/the-black-plague.

Terris, Milton. "The Changing Relationships of Epidemiology and Society: The Robert Cruikshank Lecture." *Journal of Public Health Policy* 6, no. 1 (March 1985): 15–36. https://doi.org/10.2307/3342015.

———. "The Society for Epidemiologic Research (SER) and the Future of Epidemi- ology." *American Journal of Epidemiology* 136, no. 8 (October 15, 1992): 909–15. https://doi.org/10.1093/oxfordjournals.aje.a116563.

Theerman, Paul. "From Central Park to the Front Lines: Frederick Law Olmsted and the Sanitary Commission." Center for the History of Medicine and Public Health, The New York Academy of Medicine Library Blog, April 26, 2016. https:// nyamcenterforhistory.org/2016/04/26/from-central-park-to-the-front-lines -frederick-law-olmsted-and-the-sanitary-commission/.

Thomas, Dana. "Why Won't We Learn from the Survivors of the Rana Plaza Disaster?" *New York Times,* April 24, 2018. https://www.nytimes.com/2018/04/24/style/survivors-of-rana-plaza-disaster.html.

Titford, Michael. "Rudolf Virchow: Cellular Pathologist." *Laboratory Medicine* 41, no. 5 (May 2010): 311–12. https://doi.org/10.1309/LM3GYQTY79CPYLBI.

Tolentino, Jia. "Is Abortion Sacred?" *New Yorker,* July 16, 2022. https://www.newyorker.com/culture/essay/is-abortion-sacred.

Traub, Alex. "Dr. LeRoy Carhart, Fierce Defender of Abortion Rights, Dies at 81." *New York Times,* April 30, 2023. https://www.nytimes.com/2023/04/30/obituaries/dr-leroy-carhart-fierce-defender-of-abortion-rights-dies-at-81.html.

Treisman, Rachel. "One Way to Prevent Gun Violence? Treat It as a Public Health Issue." NPR, May 12, 2023. https://www.npr.org/2023/05/12/1173141518/gun-violence-prevention-public-health.

"The Triangle Shirtwaist Factory Fire." Occupational Safety and Health Administration, United States Department of Labor. https://www.osha.gov/aboutosha/40-years/trianglefactoryfire.

Truman, Harry S. "Special Message to the Congress Recommending a Comprehensive Health Program." Harry S. Truman Library and Museum, November 19, 1945. https://www.trumanlibrary.gov/library/public-papers/192/special-message-congress-recommending-comprehensive-health-program.

Tulchinsky, Theodore H. "Chapter 5—John Snow, Cholera, the Broad Street Pump; Waterborne Diseases Then and Now." In *Case Studies in Public Health,* 77–99. Academic Press, 2018. https://doi.org/10.1016/B978-0-12-804571-8.00017-2.

Tuthill, Kathleen. "John Snow and the Broad Street Pump: On the Trail of an Epidemic." UCLA Department of Epidemiology Fielding School of Public Health. Accessed June 20, 2023. https://www.ph.ucla.edu/epi/snow/snowcricketarticle.html.

"University of Pennsylvania Condition of the Negroes of Philadelphia, Ward Seven, ca. 1896." W. E. B. Du Bois Papers, Robert S. Cox Special Collections and University Archives Research Center, University of Massachusetts Amherst. Accessed June 21, 2023. http://credo.library.umass.edu/view/full/mums312-b004-i337.

Van Brocklin, Elizabeth. "What Gun Violence Prevention Looks Like When It Focuses on the Communities Hurt the Most." *The Trace,* July 10, 2019. https://www.thetrace.org/2019/07/gun-violence-prevention-communities-of-color-funding/.

Varela, Natalia Vega, Nancy L. Cohen, Neisha Opper, Myriam Shiran, and Clare Weber. "The State of Reproductive Health in the United States: The End of Roe and the Perilous Road Ahead for Women in the Dobbs Era." Gender Equity Policy Institute, January 19, 2023. https://thegepi.org/state-of-reproductive-health-united-states/.

Vermeer, Danielle. "Redlining and Environmental Racism." University of Michigan School for Environment and Sustainability, August 16, 2021. https://seas.umich.edu/news/redlining-and-environmental-racism.

Villarosa, Linda. "Myths About Physical Racial Differences Were Used to Justify Slavery—and Are Still Believed by Doctors Today." *New York Times Magazine,* August 14, 2019. https://www.nytimes.com/interactive/2019/08/14/magazine /racial-differences-doctors.html.

———. *Under the Skin: The Hidden Toll of Racism on American Lives and on the Health of Our Nation.* New York: Doubleday, 2022.

Vinten-Johansen, Peter, Howard Brody, Nigel Paneth, Stephen Rachman, and Michael Rip. *Cholera, Chloroform, and the Science of Medicine: A Life of John Snow.* New York: Oxford University Press, 2003. http://archive.org/details /cholerachlorofor00pete.

Virchow, Rudolf Carl. "Report on the Typhus Epidemic in Upper Silesia. 1848." *American Journal of Public Health* 96, no. 12 (December 2006): 2102–5. https:// pubmed.ncbi.nlm.nih.gov/17123938/.

Von Drehle, David. *Triangle: The Fire that Changed America.* New York: Grove Press, 2003.

Wald, Chelsea. "Waste Not: A Brief History of the Urban Sewer System." Lit Hub, April 15, 2021. https://lithub.com/waste-not-a-brief-history-of-the-urban-sewer -system/.

Wallace, Anthony, husband of the late Dr. Chaniece Wallace. Author interview via Zoom, April 11, 2023.

Warsh, Marie, historian, Central Park Conservancy. Author interview via Zoom, July 7, 2022.

———. "How the Landscape of Seneca Village Can Reveal Its History." *Central Park Conservancy,* February 1, 2021. https://www.centralparknyc.org/articles/how -the-landscape-of-seneca-village-can-reveal-its-history.

———. "How Public Health Influenced the Creation, Purpose, and Design of Central Park," *Central Park Conservancy,* June 26, 2020. https://www .centralparknyc.org/articles/how-public-health-influenced-the-creation-purpose-and -design-of-central-park.

Washington, Harriet A. *Medical Apartheid: The Dark History of Medical Experimentation on Black Americans from Colonial Times to the Present.* New York: Anchor Books, 2006.

Weil, D. S., and D. Hemenway. "Loaded Guns in the Home. Analysis of a National Random Survey of Gun Owners." *JAMA* 267, no. 22 (June 10, 1992): 3033–37.

"When Men Murder Women: An Analysis of 2020 Homicide Data." Violence Policy Center, October 2020. https://vpc.org/when-men-murder-women/.

Wilford, John Noble. "How Epidemics Helped Shape the Modern Metropolis." *New York Times,* April 15, 2008. https://www.nytimes.com/2008/04/15/health /15iht-15chol.11988148.html.

Wilkerson, Isabel. "From Jan. 6 to Tyre Nichols, American Life Is Still Defined by Caste." *Time,* February 2, 2023. https://time.com/6252144/american-life-caste -isabel-wilkerson/.

Williams, Ariel, great granddaughter of Andrew Williams. Author interview via Zoom, June 24, 2022.

Williams, David R., professor of Public Health and Professor of African and African American Studies at Harvard University. Author interview via Zoom, July 21, 2021.

———. "Stress Was Already Killing Black Americans. Covid-19 Is Making It Worse." *Washington Post*, May 13, 2020. https://www.washingtonpost.com /opinions/2020/05/13/stress-was-already-killing-black-americans-covid-19-is -making-it-worse/.

Williams, David R., and Michelle Sternthal. "Understanding Racial-Ethnic Dispari- ties in Health: Sociological Contributions." *Journal of Health and Social Behavior* 51, no. 1 supplement (2010): S15–27. https://doi.org/10.1177 /0022146510383838.

Williams, Mareia, descendant of Andrew Williams. Author interview via Zoom, June 24, 2022.

Williams, Michelle A. "2021 Climate Disasters Foreshadow Future Challenges for Public Health." *The Hill*, September 5, 2021. https://thehill.com/opinion /healthcare/570890-2021-climate-disasters-foreshadow-future-challenges-for-public -health/.

Williams, Nikesha Elise. "This Father Had to Turn His Pain into Purpose After Losing His Wife in Childbirth." SheKnows, February 16, 2023. https://www .sheknows.com/health-and-wellness/articles/2553864/father-black-maternal -mortality-advocate/.

Williams, Thomas Elias, descendant of Andrew Williams. Author interview via Zoom, June 23, 2022.

Willsher, Kim. "Story of Cities #12: Haussmann Rips Up Paris—and Divides France to This Day." *Guardian*, March 31, 2016. https://www.theguardian.com/cities /2016/mar/31/story-cities-12-paris-baron-haussmann-france-urban-planner -napoleon.

Wilusz, Luke. "Man Charged with Hitting CPD Officer with Car While Fleeing Fernwood Traffic Stop." *Chicago Sun-Times*, October 27, 2019. https://chicago .suntimes.com/crime/2019/10/27/20934436/jevon-standbak-charged-hitting -cpd-officer-car-fernwood-traffic-stop-103rd.

Witte, Griff. "He Had Changed His Life. He Died Trying to Change Others." *Washington Post*, August 2, 2022. https://www.proquest.com/docview /2697205257/citation/E58BB65ACBDC436BPQ/1.

"Women of the U.S. Sanitary Commission." History of American Women. Accessed June 20, 2023. https://www.womenhistoryblog.com/2015/02/women-of-the-u-s -sanitary-commission.html.

Woodard, Colin. "The Surprising Geography of Gun Violence." POLITICO, April 23, 2023. https://www.politico.com/news/magazine/2023/04/23 /surprising-geography-of-gun-violence-00092413.

Woodruff, Judy. "Why Are Black Mothers and Infants Far More Likely to Die in U.S. from Pregnancy-Related Causes?" *PBS NewsHour,* April 18, 2018. https://www.pbs.org/newshour/show/why-are-black-mothers-and-infants-far-more-likely-to-die-in-u-s-from-pregnancy-related-causes.

Woods, Baynard. "Korryn Gaines: Police Killing Highlights Baltimore's Lead Poisoning Crisis." *Guardian,* August 5, 2016. https://www.theguardian.com/us-news/2016/aug/05/korryn-gaines-baltimore-lead-poisoning-crisis.

Wright, Matthew. "How America's 'First Black Middle Class Village' Was Destroyed to Make Way for Central Park." *New York Daily Mail,* March 9, 2017. http://www.dailymail.co.uk/~/article-4293744/index.html.

Yadlapalli, Aswini, and Shams Rahman. "Years After the Rana Plaza Tragedy, Bangladesh's Garment Workers Are Still Bottom of the Pile." *Conversation,* April 22, 2021. http://theconversation.com/years-after-the-rana-plaza-tragedy-bangladeshs-garment-workers-are-still-bottom-of-the-pile-159224.

Yong, Ed. "How Public Health Took Part in Its Own Downfall." *Atlantic,* October 23, 2021. https://www.scribd.com/article/535011089/How-Public-Health-Took-Part-In-Its-Own-Downfall.

Yost, Paula. "Agent Orange Study Called Botched or Rigged." *Washington Post,* July 11, 1989. https://www.washingtonpost.com/archive/politics/1989/07/12/agent-orange-study-called-botched-or-rigged/6e34800b-0901-4b70-ad89-5468df4332af/.

Zhang, Sarah. "The Plan to Stop Every Respiratory Virus at Once." *Atlantic,* September 7, 2021. https://www.theatlantic.com/health/archive/2021/09/coronavirus-pandemic-ventilation-rethinking-air/620000/.

Zhong, Raymond, and Nadja Popovich. "How Air Pollution Across America Reflects Racist Policy from the 1930s." *New York Times,* March 9, 2022. https://www.nytimes.com/2022/03/09/climate/redlining-racism-air-pollution.html.

NOTES

INTRODUCTION

ix   **"Of all the forms of inequality, injustice in health is the most shock-ing"** See Martin Luther King Jr., speech to the Medical Committee for Human Rights, Chicago, March 25, 1966. Available at: https://pnhp.org/news/dr-martin-luther-king-on-health-care-injustice/.

x   **how disruptive Nestlé's formula marketing campaigns** See Stephen Solomon, "The Controversy Over Infant Formula," *New York Times Magazine,* December 6, 1981. Available at: https://www.nytimes.com/1981/12/06/magazine/the-controversy-over-infant-formula.html.

xi   **more than 122 years to pay** See Catherine Porter et al., "The Ransom: How a French Bank Captured Haiti," *New York Times,* May 20, 2022. Available at: https://www.nytimes.com/2022/05/20/world/french-banks-haiti-cic.html.

xi   **cost Haiti as much as $115 billion** See Matt Apuzzo et al., "The Ransom: The Root of Haiti's Misery: Reparations to Enslavers," *New York Times,* May 20, 2022. Available at: https://www.nytimes.com/2022/05/20/world/americas/haiti-history-colonized-france.html.

xii   **eradicated tetanus in regions of Haiti** See W.L. Berggren, "Administration and Evaluation of Rural Health Services. I. A Tetanus Control Program in Haiti," *American Journal of Tropical Medicine and Hygiene* 23, no. 5 (September 1974): 936–49. Available at: https://pubmed.ncbi.nlm.nih.gov/4217569/.

xii   **we couldn't honestly encourage them to breastfeed** See Alison Mildon et al., "Protecting Both Infant and Mother: Perceptions of Infant Feeding Practices in Rural Haiti," *Journal of Global Health Reports* 6 (October 22, 2022). Available at: https://www.joghr.org/article/38736-protecting-both-infant-and-mother-perceptions-of-infant-feeding-practices-in-rural-haiti.

xiv   **W.C. Fields, and Groucho Marx** See Bayside Historical Society/John Golden Estate. Available at: https://www.baysidehistorical.org/vintage-postcards/john-golden-estate.

xiv   **dozens of Nobel laureates** See "List of Nobel laureates affiliated with Princeton University as alumni or faculty." Wikipedia. Available at: https://en.wikipedia.org/wiki/List_of_Nobel_laureates_affiliated_with_Princeton_University_as_alumni_or_faculty.

xv   **Eric Wieschaus . . . Nobel Prize** See NobelPrize.org, "The Nobel Prize in
        Physiology or Medicine 1995." Available at: https://www.nobelprize.org
        /prizes/medicine/1995/wieschaus/biographical/.

xv   **Annette Rossignol** See Annette Rossignol, *Principles and Practice of
        Epidemiology: An Engaged Approach,* McGraw Hill, 2007).

xv   **Clare Mahan** See https://prabook.com/web/clare_maureen.mahan
        /3458387.

xvi   **Life expectancy has nearly doubled** See Saloni Dattanim et al., "Life
        Expectancy," Our World in Data, 2023. Available at: https://ourworld
        indata.org/life-expectancy.

xvi   **child deaths have dropped by half** See UNICEF, "Under-Five Mortal-
        ity," UNICEF Data, updated March 2025. Available at: https://data
        .unicef.org/topic/child-survival/under-five-mortality/.

xvi   **toilet . . . has been credited with saving a billion lives** See "How the
        Toilet Changed History," *Be Smart,* PBS, February 14, 2017. Available at:
        https://www.pbs.org/video/how-the-toilet-changed-history-brjgoe/.

xvi   **adding nearly two decades to life expectancy** See Caroline Kantis,
        "Around the World in Twenty-Five Toilets," *Think Global Health,* Novem-
        ber 12, 2021. Available at: https://www.thinkglobalhealth.org/article
        /around-world-twenty-five-toilets.

xvi   **are largely responsible for the modern, technologically advanced
        world** See Jeff Desjardines, "These Discoveries Saved Billions of Lives,"
        World Economic Forum, March 28, 2018. Available at: https://www
        .weforum.org/stories/2018/03/the-50-most-important-life-saving
        -breakthroughs-in-history/.

xvi   **densely populated urban metropolises** See Craig Spencer, "How to Lose
        a Century of Progress," *Atlantic,* June 30, 2023. Available at: https://
        www.theatlantic.com/ideas/archive/2023/06/covid-public-health
        -successes/674568/.

xvii   **pandemic . . . failure of public health** See Steffie Woolhandler et al.,
        "Public Policy and Health in the Trump Era," *Lancet* 397, no. 10275
        (February 10, 2021): 705–53. Available at: https://www.thelancet.com
        /journals/lancet/article/PIIS0140-6736(20)32545-9/fulltext.

xvii   **more than a million American lives** See Sachin Silva et al., "Assessing the
        Impact of One Million COVID-19 Deaths in America: Economic and Life
        Expectancy Losses," *Scientific Reports* 13, no. 3065 (February 22, 2023).
        Available at: https://doi.org/10.1038/s41598-023-30077-1.

xvii   **more than 120,000 medical professionals** See "Health and Care Worker
        Deaths During Covid-19," World Health Organization, October 20, 2021.
        Available at: https://www.who.int/news/item/20-10-2021-health-and
        -care-worker-deaths-during-covid-19.

xvii   **drastic shortages of protective gear** Ibid.

xvii   **will grow up in families torn by grief** See Dan Keating and Akilah
        Johnson, "The Pandemic Marks Another Grim Milestone: 1 in 500
        Americans Have Died of Covid-19," *Washington Post,* September 15,
        2021. Available at: https://www.washingtonpost.com/health/interactive
        /2021/1-in-500-covid-deaths/.

xviii   **dominated political debate for a century** See Amy L. Fairchild et al.,
        "The EXODUS of Public Health: What History Can Tell Us About the

Future," *American Journal of Public Health* 100, no. 1 (January 1, 2010): 54–63. Available at: https://doi.org/10.2105/AJPH.2009.163956.

xviii **far more on health care than any other nation** See Emma Wager, Shameek Rakshit, and Cynthia Cox, "What Drives Health Spending in the U.S. Compared to Other Countries?" Peterson-KFF Health System Tracker, August 2, 2024. Available at: https://www.healthsystemtracker .org/brief/what-drives-health-spending-in-the-u-s-compared-to-other -countries/.

xviii **much lower than those of other industrialized nations** See Shameek Rakshit and Matthew McGough, "How Does U.S. Life Expectancy Compare to Other Countries?" Peterson-KFF Health System Tracker, January 31, 2025. Available at: https://www.healthsystemtracker.org /chart-collection/u-s-life-expectancy-compare-countries/.

xix **on a once-unimaginable scale** See Spencer, "How to Lose a Century of Progress."

xx **in the public health infrastructure and its workforce** See Y Natalia Alfonso et al., "US Public Health Neglected: Flat or Declining Spending Left States Ill Equipped to Respond to COVID-19," *Health Affairs* 40, no. 4 (April 2021): 664–71. Available at: https://www.pmc.ncbi.nlm.nih .gov/articles/PMC9890672/.

xxi **because there was no room in the morgues** See Woolhandler, "Public Policy and Health in the Trump Era." See also Richard Pérez-Peña and Donald G. McNeil Jr., "W.H.O. Warned Trump About Coronavirus Early and Often," *New York Times,* April 16, 2020. Available at: https://www .nytimes.com/2020/04/16/health/WHO-Trump-coronavirus.html.

xxi **administration actively discouraged masking** See Ed Yong, "How the Pandemic Defeated America," *Atlantic,* September 2020. Available at: https://www.theatlantic.com/magazine/archive/2020/09/coronavirus -american-failure/614191/.

xxi **health that persists to this day** See Jacob Bor, David U. Himmelstein, and Steffie Woolhandler, "Trump's Policy Failures Have Exacted a Heavy Toll on Public Health," *Scientific American,* March 5, 2021. Available at: https://www.scientificamerican.com/article/trumps-policy-failures-have -exacted-a-heavy-toll-on-public-health1/.

xxi **championing this ill-advised policy** See Melody Schreiber, "Trump Pick for US Health Agency Proposed 'Herd Immunity' During Covid," *Guardian,* November 26, 2024. Available at: https://www.theguardian .com/us-news/2024/nov/26/nih-trump-bhattacharya-covid.

xxi **Public health has become a "tool for authoritarian power"** See "Lockdowns, Mandates and the Future of Public Health," Brownstone Institute Inaugural Conference, NTD Newsroom, November 13, 2021. Available at: https://www.ntd.com/lockdowns-mandates-and-the-future -of-public-health-brownstone-institute-inaugural-conference_700976.html.

xxii **grim distinction of leading the world in Covid deaths** See Woolhandler, "Public Policy and Health in the Trump Era."

xxii **suppressing data on the purported origins of the epidemic** See Benjamin Mazer, "Revenge of the COVID Contrarians," *Atlantic,* November 25, 2024. Available at: https://www.theatlantic.com/health /archive/2024/11/covid-revenge-administration/680790/.

xxii   **"public health, or on-the-ground common-sense experience"** See
          Kenichi Serino, "Emails Detail Trump Administration's Fight with Own
          Medical Experts over COVID Advice," PBS News, December 23, 2021.
          Available at: https://www.pbs.org/newshour/health/emails-detail-trump
          -administrations-fight-with-own-medical-experts-over-covid-advice.

xxiii   **Fluoride vastly improves dental health** See "Fluoride & Dental Health,"
          National Institute of Dental and Craniofacial Research. Available at:
          https://www.nidcr.nih.gov/health-info/fluoride.

xxiii   **in the case of the yellow fever vaccine** See CDC, "Yellow Fever Vaccine:
          What You Need to Know," April 1, 2020. Available at: https://www.cdc
          .gov/vaccines/hcp/current-vis/yellow-fever.html.

xxiii   **Guillain-Barré syndrome** See eds. Kathleen Stratton et al., *Adverse Effects
          of Vaccines: Evidence and Causality* (Washington, D.C.: National Academies
          Press, 2011). Available at: https://www.ncbi.nlm.nih.gov/books
          /NBK190024/.

xxiii   **which translates to about six lives a minute** See Andrew J. Shattock et
          al., "Contribution of Vaccination to Improved Survival and Health: Model-
          ling 50 Years of the Expanded Programme on Immunization," *Lancet* 403,
          no. 10441 (2024): 2307–16. Available at: https://www.pubmed.ncbi.nlm
          .nih.gov/38705159/.

xxiii   **"If you are unsure"** See Michael Okuda on X: "Go to a cemetery. Notice
          all the graves of dead babies from before the 1960s, from before people
          started vaccinating their kids? Notice how few infant deaths since then?
          That's because vaccinations work." https://t.co/VyzR1xk2pu.

xxiii   **fueled mistrust in our institutions** See Mazer, "Revenge of the COVID
          Contrarians."

xxiv   **number-one killer in this country** See "Firearm Mortality: Death Data
          Maps," CDC, National Center for Health Statistics: Stats of the States,
          updated August 20, 2025. Available at: https://www.cdc.gov/nchs/state
          -stats/deaths/firearms.html.

xxiv   **gross overspending on acute-care hospitalizations** See Jon Niccum,
          "Economist Pinpoints When Hospitalizations Increase Health Care Costs
          But Don't Prevent Death," KU News, February 4, 2020. Available at:
          https://www.news.ku.edu/news/article/2020/02/03/economist
          -pinpoints-when-diagnosis-doesnt-justify-increased-health-care-costs-or.

xxiv   **equitable health care for everyone** See Donald M. Berwick, "*Salve
          Lucrum*: The Existential Threat of Greed in US Health Care," *JAMA* 329,
          no. 8 (January 30, 2023). Available at: https://www.jamanetwork.com
          /journals/jama/fullarticle/2801097.

xxiv   **billionaire oligarchs are in charge of key federal agencies** See Laura
          Mannweiler, "All the President's Billionaires: The Extraordinary Wealth in
          Trump's Administration," U.S. News & World Report, June 4, 2025.
          Available at: https://www.usnews.com/news/national-news/articles/how
          -many-billionaires-are-in-trumps-administration-and-what-is-their-worth.

xxv   **which are predominantly Black and poor** See Tristan Baurick, Lylla
          Younes, and Joan Meiners, "Welcome to 'Cancer Alley,' Where Toxic Air Is
          About to Get Worse," ProPublica, October 30, 2019. Available at:
          https://www.propublica.org/article/welcome-to-cancer-alley-where-toxic
          -air-is-about-to-get-worse.

xxv   **seventy-two countries . . . have universal health insurance** See OECD, "Indicator Overview: Country Dashboards and Major Trends," *Health at a Glance 2023*. Available at: https://www.oecd.org/en/publications/health -at-a-glance-2023_7a7afb35-en/full-report/indicator-overview-country -dashboards-and-major-trends_d4962905.html#chapter-d1e843 -3c7a7758e7.

CHAPTER ONE: EVERY LIFE MATTERS

3   **more than one out of every ten babies** See *Population Index* 4, no. 3 (July 1938): 192–204. Table 4. Available at: https://www.jstor.org/stable /i353869.

4   **plagued by severe economic hardship** See Martin Thomas, "The Political Economy of Colonial Violence in Interwar Jamaica," paper for Terror and the Making of Modern Europe Conference, Stanford University, April 2008. Available at: https://web.stanford.edu/dept/france-stanford /Conferences/Terror/Thomas.pdf.

4   **so deficient in calories and vital nutrients** See "IV. The Crown Colony Period," *Food and Nutrition Bulletin* 2, no. 2 (1980). Available at: https://journals.sagepub.com/doi/abs/10.1177/156482658000 200204.

4   **in 1934, infant mortality rates in the U.S.** See Robert M. Woodbury, "Infant Mortality in the United States," *Annals of the American Academy of Political and Social Science* 188, no. 1 (November 1936): 94–106. Available at: https://www.jstor.org/stable/1020363.

4   **most rapid health improvement in our nation's history** See David Cutler and Grant Miller, "The Role of Public Health Improvements in Health Advances: The Twentieth-Century United States," *Demography* 42, no. 1 (February 2005): 1–22. Available at: https://pubmed.ncbi.nlm.nih .gov/15782893/.

5   **taken another seven decades to reduce infant mortality** See "Infant Mortality Rate for Jamaica," World Bank via Federal Reserve Bank of St. Louis, updated April 16, 2025. Available at: https://fred.stlouisfed.org /series/SPDYNIMRTINJAM.

5   **near-miraculous doubling of life expectancy** See Aaron O'Neill, "Annual Life Expectancy at Birth in the United States, from 1850 to 2023, with Projections Until 2100," Statista, July 31, 2025. Available at: https:// www.statista.com/statistics/1040079/life-expectancy-united-states-all -time/.

6   **Wisconsin miners, and Black field hands** See Charles E. Rosenberg, *The Cholera Years: The United States in 1832, 1849, and 1866* (Chicago and London: University of Chicago Press, 1962), 1.

7   **an enduring social commitment to collective health** Ibid., 2.

7   **contributed to the collapse of the Roman Empire** See Edward Watts, "What Rome Learned from the Deadly Antonine Plague of 165 A.D.," *Smithsonian*, April 28, 2020. Available at: https://www.smithsonianmag .com/history/what-rome-learned-deadly-antonine-plague-165-d -180974758/.

7   **Plague of Justinian . . . claimed the lives of nearly 10 percent** See Elizabeth Kolbert, "Pandemics and the Shape of Human History," *New*

Yorker, March 30, 2020. Available at: https://www.newyorker.com
/magazine/2020/04/06/pandemics-and-the-shape-of-human-history.
See also "Pandemics that Changed History," History.com, February 27,
2019, updated July 2, 2025. Available at: https://www.history.com
/articles/pandemics-timeline.

7   **Black Death . . . led to the end of feudalism** See "Pandemics that
Changed History." See also Kolbert, "Pandemics and the Shape of Human
History." See also Pat Lee Shipman, "The Bright Side of the Black Death,"
American Scientist 102, no. 6 (November–December 2014): 410.
Available at: https://www.americanscientist.org/article/the-bright-side-of
-the-black-death.

7   **1518, the first smallpox outbreak** See Kolbert, "Pandemics and the
Shape of Human History."

7   **isolation of the sick and quarantining the exposed** See Institute of
Medicine Committee for the Study of the Future of Public Health, *The
Future of Public Health* (Washington, D.C.: The National Academies Press,
1988), 57–58. Available at: https://doi.org/10.17226/1091.

8   **yellow fever epidemic swept through the city** See Sarah Pruitt, "When
the Yellow Fever Outbreak of 1793 Sent the Wealthy Fleeing Philadelphia,"
History.com, June 11, 2020. Available at: https://www.history.com
/articles/yellow-fever-outbreak-philadelphia.

8   **like smallpox, typhus, measles, and scarlet fever** See David Rosner,
" 'Spanish Flu, or Whatever It Is. . . .': The Paradox of Public Health in a
Time of Crisis," *Public Health Reports* 124, supplement 3 (April 2010): 40.
Available at: https://pmc.ncbi.nlm.nih.gov/articles/PMC2862333/.

8   **rancid water that spread the contagions** See "Plagues & Epidemics,"
Plumbing & Mechanical Magazine, July 1, 1988. Available at: https://
theplumber.com/plagues-epidemics/.

8   **squalid living conditions** See Richard H. Shryock, "The Early American
Public Health Movement," *American Journal of Public Health and the
Nation's Health* 27, no. 10 (October 1937): 965–71. Available at: https://
ajph.aphapublications.org/doi/abs/10.2105/AJPH.27.10.965.

8   **more than half of all working-class children** See Institute of Medicine,
The Future of Public Health, 59.

8   **waves of diphtheria, scarlet fever, influenza, and measles** See Rosner,
" 'Spanish Flu, or Whatever It Is. . . ,' " 40.

8   **even the poorest rural regions** See Shryock, "The Early American Public
Health Movement," 966.

9   **their bodies racked by excruciatingly painful spasms** See Rosenberg,
The Cholera Years, 1–3.

9   **at least 10,000 imperial troops** See "Plagues & Epidemics," which traces
how cholera spread from the Ganges to Europe.

9   **Cholera ultimately claimed more than 31,000 lives** See "Cholera in
Sunderland," UK Parliament. Available at: Cholera in Sunderland—UK
Parliament.

10   **responsible for enforcing sanitary regulations** See Rosenberg, *The
Cholera Years,* 17–20, which describes New York's unsanitary conditions.

10   **had been breached** Ibid., 21.

10   **banned all ships from docking in the New York harbor** Ibid., 22.

11   **even in the face of armed militias** Ibid., 24.

11   **before boarding ferries to New York** See Ann Haddad, "'The Destroy-ing Angel': New York's 1832 Cholera Epidemic," Merchant's House Museum, July 20, 2016. Available at: https://merchantshouse.org/blog /cholera1832/.

11   **These physicians all came to the same conclusion** See Rosenberg, *The Cholera Years,* 25–26.

11   **more than 100,000 residents fled** Ibid., 27–28.

12   **even the most basic sanitary practices or cleanliness** Ibid., 33–34. See also John Noble Wilford, "How Epidemics Helped Shape the Modern Metropolis," *New York Times,* April 15, 2008. Available at: https://www .nytimes.com/2008/04/15/health/15iht-15chol.11988148.html.

12   **If they became ill, it was their own fault** See Rosenberg, *The Cholera Years,* 29.

12   **one historian observed, the attitude was: "Who cares?"** See Shryock, "The Early American Public Health Movement," 966.

12   **five emergency hospitals in schools** See Ann Haddad, "'The Destroying Angel.'"

12   **more than one hundred new cases** See Rosenberg, *The Cholera Years,* 32.

12   **ended in September** Ibid., 35.

12   **Most of the victims were poor immigrants** See Wilford, "How Epidem-ics Helped Shape the Modern Metropolis."

13   **New York would simply dry up** See Jonathan Schifman, "How New York City Found Clean Water," *Smithsonian,* November 25, 2019. Available at: https://www.smithsonianmag.com/history/how-new-york-city-found -clean-water-180973571/.

13   **in a result that would forever change the city** Ibid.

13   **an enormous infrastructure investment** See Leslie Nemo, "Aqueduct Met New York City's Need for Clean Water in 1842," *Civil Engineering,* March 1, 2023, for a detailed description of the logistics entailed in building the aqueduct. Available at: https://www.asce.org/publications -and-news/civil-engineering-source/civil-engineering-magazine/issues /magazine-issue/article/2023/03/aqueduct-met-new-york-citys-need-for -clean-water-in-1842.

13   **made the jump to Manhattan in May of 1849** See Rosenberg, *The Cholera Years,* 101–6.

14   **the poor, living in dire circumstances, were the most vulnerable** See Institute of Medicine, *The Future of Public Health,* 58–59.

14   **appointing district medical officers** See ibid., 59–60 for a full description of Chadwick's work.

15   **The Great Stink** See Christopher Klein, "How Pandemics Spurred Cities to Make More Green Space for People," History.com, April 27, 2020. Available at: https://www.history.com/articles/cholera-pandemic-new -york-city-london-paris-green-space.

15   **cobbled streets, which were soon filled with café terraces** See Kim Willsher, "Story of Cities #12: Haussmann Rips Up Paris—and Divides France to this Day," *Guardian,* March 31, 2016. Willsher provides a detailed description of Bonaparte's transformation of Paris. Available at: https://www.theguardian.com/cities/2016/mar/31/story-cities-12-paris

-baron-haussmann-france-urban-planner-napoleon. See also Klein, "How Pandemics Spurred Cities."

16   **led several states to establish sanitary commissions** See Institute of Medicine, *The Future of Public Health*, 61.

16   **The Sanitary Movement led to wide-ranging urban reforms** Ibid., 60–62.

16   **Even the pigs were relieved of their duties** See Gwynn Guilford, "The Hogs that Created America's First Urban Working Class," *Quartz*, updated July 20, 2022. Available at: https://qz.com/1025640/hogs.

16   **the rapidly industrializing and expanding metropolis** See Pete Sigmund, "NYC's Central Park: An American Masterpiece," Construction Equipment Guide, June 27, 2006. Available at: https://www .constructionequipmentguide.com/NYCs-Central-Park-An-American -Masterpiece/7148/. See also Seneca Village Project, "History of the Community." Available at: https://projects.mcah.columbia.edu/seneca _village/htm/history.htm.

17   **where the rich and poor met on common ground** See Sigmund, "NYC's Central Park."

18   **informed his visions for a majestic urban oasis** See Charles E. Beveridge, "Frederick Law Olmsted Sr.," June 22, 2023. Available at: https:// olmsted.org/frederick-law-olmsted-sr/.

18   **the park was finally completed in 1876** See Sigmund, "NYC's Central Park." See also Lucie Levine, "'The Lungs of the City': Frederick Law Olmsted, Public Health, and the Creation of Central Park," The Gotham Center for New York City History, July 30, 2020. Available at: https:// www.gothamcenter.org/blog/the-lungs-of-the-city-frederick-law-olmsted -public-health-and-the-creation-of-central-park.

18   **So much for "uplifting" the poor** Ibid.

19   **salutary urban oasis that Olmsted envisioned** Ibid.

19   **generated by the Sanitary Movement** See Brent Staples, "The Death of the Black Utopia," *New York Times*, November 28, 2019. Available at: https://www.nytimes.com/2019/11/28/opinion/seneca-central-park -nyc.html.

20   **healthier than crowded downtown** Ibid. See also "Before Central Park: The Story of Seneca Village," *Central Park Conservancy*, January 18, 2018. See also author interview with Marie Warsh, historian, Central Park Conservancy, July 7, 2022.

20   **a "shantytown" and a "n****r village"** See Staples, "The Death of the Black Utopia."

20   **equivalent to about $3,600 today** See Matthew Wright, "How America's 'First Black Middle Class Village' Was Destroyed to Make Way for Central Park," *New York Daily Mail*, March 9, 2017. Available at: https://www .dailymail.co.uk/news/article-4293744/Seneca-Village-destroyed-make -way-Central-Park.html. See also Staples, "The Death of the Black Utopia." See also "Before Central Park." See also author interviews with Cal Jones, Manhattan historian emeritus, June 23, 2022; Ariel Williams, June 24, 2022, and Mareia Williams, June 24, 2022, descendants of Andrew Williams.

20   **Seneca Village may have even been a railroad stop** See Marie Warsh interview.

21   **rustic middle-class hamlet of mostly free Blacks** See "Before Central Park."

21   **they even built the wall on Wall Street** See "History of Slavery in New York," New-York Historical Society. Available at: https://www .slaveryinnewyork.org/history.htm.

21   **abducting both free Black people and fugitive slaves** See Jonathan Daniel Wells, "The So-Called 'Kidnapping Club' Featured Cops Selling Free Black New Yorkers into Slavery," *Smithsonian*, October 14, 2020. Available at: https://www.smithsonianmag.com/history/so-called -kidnapping-club-featured-new-york-cops-selling-free-blacks-slavery -180976055/. See also Staples, "The Death of the Black Utopia."

22   **most whites refused to work next to them** See Staples, "The Death of the Black Utopia."

22   **rebellion was finally quelled by the local militia** See James Sullivan, "The Anti-Abolition Riots (1834)," BlackPast, February 7, 2020. Available at: https://blackpast.org/african-american-history/the-anti-abolition-riots -1834/.

22   **they thought would be a home for their family** See author interviews with Cal Jones, Ariel Williams, and Mareia Williams.

22   **a major crosstown thoroughfare** See Marie Warsh, "How the Landscape of Seneca Village Can Reveal Its History," Central Park Conservancy, February 1, 2021. Available at: https://www.centralparknyc.org/articles /how-the-landscape-of-seneca-village-can-reveal-its-history. See also "History of the Community."

23   **half of them owned their own homes** See "Before Central Park."

23   **wasn't satisfied with the paltry $2,335** See Wright, "How America's 'First Black Middle Class Village' Was Destroyed."

23   **he began to rebuild** See author interview with Cal Jones.

23   **up to 60 percent of our health is determined** See Emily Orminski, "Your Zip Code Is More Important than Your Genetic Code," National Community Reinvestment Coalition, June 30, 2021. Available at: https:// ncrc.org/your-zip-code-is-more-important-than-your-genetic-code/.

24   **stress, and even mortality** See Kirsten Weir, "Nurtured by Nature," APA *Monitor on Psychology* 51, no. 3 (April/May 2020): 50. Available at: https://www.apa.org/monitor/2020/04/nurtured-nature.

24   **according to a 2021 report by the Trust for Public Land** See Ronda Chapman et al., "Parks and an Equitable Recovery," Trust for Public Land, May 27, 2021. Available at: https://www.tpl.org/parks-and-an-equitable -recovery-parkscore-report.

24   **the least vegetation** See Jackie Ostfeld, "The Outdoors Are Great, But Not for All," *The Hill*, March 26, 2021. Available at: https://thehill.com /opinion/energy-environment/545067-the-outdoors-are-great-but-not -for-all/.

CHAPTER TWO: WAR CHANGES EVERYTHING

28   **filthy, and overcrowded streets, a breeding ground for infectious diseases** See Jim Downs, *Sick from Freedom: African-American Illness and Suffering During the Civil War and Reconstruction* (Oxford University Press, 2012), 30–31.

28   **amputated limbs of wounded soldiers** See "Medical Care, Battle
Wounds, and Disease," *The Civil War Society's Encyclopedia of the Civil War*
(Wing Books, 1997). Available at: https://acwscots.co.uk/Shotguns
/civilwarmedicine.htm.

28   **claimed hundreds of thousands of lives** See Jonathan S. Jones, "Lessons
Learned—and Forgotten—from the Horrific Epidemics of the U.S. Civil
War," *STAT*, April 18, 2021. Available at: https://www.statnews.com
/2021/04/18/lessons-learned-forgotten-horrific-epidemics-us-civil-war.
See also author interview with Jonathan S. Jones via Zoom, June 24, 2022.

28   **outbreaks of dysentery, typhoid fever** See Jones, "Lessons Learned." See
also author interview with Jonathan S. Jones.

29   **the Union's medical corps had only eighty-seven men** See "Caring for
the Men: The History of Civil War Medicine," Shotgun's Home of the
American Civil War. Available at: https://acwscots.co.uk/Shotguns
/medicinehistory.htm.

29   **a handful of useful medications in their kit** See Margaret Humphreys,
Marrow of Tragedy: The Health Crisis of the American Civil War (Baltimore: Johns Hopkins University Press, 2013), 8–9.

29   **a rapid centralization of the state through the army** Ibid., 9–13. See
also author interview with Jonathan S. Jones.

29   **even individual reformers had been unable to do** See author interview
with Stanford University historian Kathryn Olivarius on June 17, 2022. Dr.
Olivarius is also author of *Necropolis: Disease, Power, and Capitalism in the
Cotton Kingdom* (Harvard University Press, 2022).

29   **relegated to inferior care, if they received care at all** See author
interview with Jonathan S. Jones.

29   **distributing lifesaving supplies . . . to soldiers** See "Women of the U.S.
Sanitary Commission," History of American Women, February 2015.
Available at: https://www.womenhistoryblog.com/2015/02/women-of
-the-u-s-sanitary-commission.html. See also "Life Story: Elizabeth Blackwell (1821–1910)," Women & the American Story. Available at: https://
wams.nyhistory.org/a-nation-divided/civil-war/elizabeth-blackwell/.

30   **a hospital she founded . . . in 1857** See "Women of the U.S. Sanitary
Commission."

30   **four thousand women . . . to form the Women's Central Association**
See Robert C. Kennedy, "Dr. Elizabeth Blackwell," Hobart and William
Smith Colleges. Available at: https://www.hws.edu/about/history
/elizabeth-blackwell/nyt-harpers.aspx.

30   **WCAR played an instrumental role in relief efforts** See "Women of the
U.S. Sanitary Commission." See also Pamela D. Toler, "How the United
States Sanitary Commission Elbowed Women to One Side in the American
Civil War," History in the Margins, April 25, 2020. Available at: https://
www.historyinthemargins.com/2020/04/25/how-the-united-states
-sanitary-commission-elbowed-women-to-one-side-in-the-american-civil
-war/.

30   **women served as paid nurses** See Humphreys, *Marrow of Tragedy*, 10.

30   **money to provide financial support** See "Women of the U.S. Sanitary
Commission."

30   **a national sanitary commission** Ibid.

31   **they enlisted male colleagues to argue their case** Ibid. See also Toler, "How the United States Sanitary Commission Elbowed Women."

31   **like a "fifth wheel to the coach"** See K.M. Kostyal, "Behind the Lines: Olmsted at War." HistoryNet, April 28, 2015. Available at: https://www .historynet.com/behind-the-lines-olmsted-at-war/.

31   **became secretary general of the commission** See Paul Theerman, "From Central Park to the Front Lines: Frederick Law Olmsted and the Sanitary Commission," Center for the History of Medicine and Public Health, The New York Academy of Medicine Library Blog, April 26, 2016. Available at https://nyamcenterforhistory.org/2016/04/26/from-central-park-to-the -front-lines-frederick-law-olmsted-and-the-sanitary-commission/. See also Matt Dellinger, "Frederick Law Olmsted's War on Disease and Disunity," *New Yorker,* May 16, 2020. Available at: https://www.newyorker.com /culture/cultural-comment/frederick-law-olmsteds-war-on-disease-and -disunity.

31   **dismayed by the chaos, "inefficiency and misery"** See Kostyal, "Behind the Lines."

31   **the necessity of sanitary measures** Ibid. See also Theerman, "From Central Park to the Front Lines."

32   **the Southern rebellion would be put down quickly** See Theerman, "From Central Park to the Front Lines."

32   **the "lethargic, paralytic, ossified" Medical Bureau** See Kostyal, "Behind the Lines."

32   **set the stage for his tireless work** Ibid. See also Dellinger, "Frederick Law Olmsted's War."

33   **the Peninsula Campaign, turned into a war of attrition** See Kostyal, "Behind the Lines."

33   **the war had created "a veritable republic of suffering"** Ibid.

33   **Congress appointed a new surgeon general** See "Dr. William Hammond, Surgeon General," National Museum of Civil War Medicine, July 18, 2022. Available at: https://www.civilwarmed.org/dr-william-hammond -surgeon-general.

34   **"And they started to bring in new younger doctors"** See author interview with Jonathan S. Jones.

34   **Modernized medical care led to a dramatic decrease** See Pat Leonard, "William Hammond and the End of the Medical Middle Ages," *New York Times,* April 27, 2012. Available at: https://archive.nytimes.com /opinionator.blogs.nytimes.com/2012/04/27/william-hammond-and -the-end-of-the-medical-middle-ages/.

34   **It took attending to other social determinants** See "Dr. William Hammond, Surgeon General."

34   **Supply lines became more efficient** See Leonard, "William Hammond and the End of the Medical Middle Ages."

34   **later worked on other Arctic expeditions** See "Dr. Isaac Israel Hayes," American Battlefield Trust. Available at: https://www.battlefields.org /learn/biographies/dr-isaac-israel-hayes. See also Humphreys, *Marrow of Tragedy,* 156–59.

34   **the buildings were constructed within forty days** See "Daughters of Charity Nursed Civil War Soldiers at West Philadelphia Hospital," Catholic

Historical Research Center of the Archdiocese of Philadelphia, March 24, 2011. Available at: https://chrc-phila.org/sisters-of-charity-nursed-wounded-civil-war-soldiers-at-west-philadelphia-hospital/. See also Humphreys, *Marrow of Tragedy*, 157.

35   **contained a total of 4,500 beds in canvas tents** Ibid., 155.

35   **cost more than $200,000** Ibid., 157.

35   **emptied waste directly into a sewer** Ibid.

35   **more than a dozen pharmacists who devised systems** See Humphreys, *Marrow of Tragedy*, 157–58, for a complete description of Satterlee Hospital.

35   **nearly a hundred Roman Catholic nuns** Ibid., 159.

35   **only 1,100 of them died, an extraordinary achievement** See "Satterlee General Hospital," American Battlefield Trust, August 18, 2021, updated May 2, 2024. Available at: https://www.battlefields.org/learn/articles/satterlee-general-hospital.

35   **sharply restricting the number of amputations** See "Dr. Isaac Israel Hayes."

35   **catastrophic public health crisis** See Humphreys, *Marrow of Tragedy*, 153–68.

35   **400 Union Army hospitals . . . 400,000 beds** See Robert F. Reilly, "Medical and Surgical Care During the American Civil War, 1861–1865," *Baylor University Medical Center Proceedings* 29, no. 2 (April 2016): 138–42. Available at: https://www.tandfonline.com/doi/abs/10.1080/08998280.2016.11929390.

36   **"hours before they received supplies from other quarters"** See Kostyal, "Behind the Lines."

36   **Battle of Antietam** See Dellinger, "Frederick Law Olmsted's War."

36   **"and other nice articles of nutriment"** Ibid.

36   **"I would rather have Mr. Olmsted's fame"** See Kostyal, "Behind the Lines."

36   **The Union Army benefited** See Humphreys, *Marrow of Tragedy*, 8.

36   **sanitary principles championed by Florence Nightingale** Ibid., 69.

37   **the South prided itself on being a mostly rural land** Ibid., 185.

37   **raise the standards of medical care** Ibid., 184–85.

37   **Confederates lacked the infrastructure** Ibid., 208–9.

37   **Sanitary Commission pushed hard for needed changes** Ibid., 9.

37   **they were better built to withstand the onslaught** See Kathryn Olivarius, "The Dangerous History of Immunoprivilege," *New York Times*, April 12, 2020. Available at: https://www.nytimes.com/2020/04/12/opinion/coronavirus-immunity-passports.html. See also author interview with Kathryn Olivarius.

37   **Frederick Law Olmsted witnessed this firsthand** See Louis P. Masur, "Olmsted's Southern Landscapes," *New York Times*, July 9, 2011. Available at: https://archive.nytimes.com/opinionator.blogs.nytimes.com/2011/07/09/olmsteds-southern-landscapes/.

38   **"self-perpetuating mechanism of dehumanization"** Ibid.

38   **"of the common comforts and consolations of civilized life"** Ibid.

39   **quarantined themselves far from the malaria-riddled wetlands** See Frederick Law Olmsted, *A Journey in the Seaboard Slave States: With*

Remarks on Their Economy (New York: Dix & Edwards, 1856), 418–19. Available at: https://archive.org/details/journeyinseaboarolms.

39   **to fend for themselves in the swamps and rice fields** See Special Correspondence of the N.Y. Daily Times, "The South Letters on the Productions, Industry and Resources of the Southern States," *New-York Daily Times,* August 9, 1853, 2.

39   **before lapsing into a coma** See Leah Donnella, "How Yellow Fever Turned New Orleans into the 'City of the Dead.'" NPR, October 31, 2018. Available at: https://www.npr.org/sections/codeswitch/2018/10/31/415535913/how-yellow-fever-turned-new-orleans-into-the-city-of-the-dead.

39   **killing about half of those who became infected** See Olivarius, "The Dangerous History of Immunoprivilege."

39   **the number-one destination for Europeans** See Kathryn Olivarius, *Necropolis: Disease, Power, and Capitalism in the Cotton Kingdom* (Harvard University Press, 2022), 6–11.

39   **enslaved Black people . . . fared the worst** Ibid., 194–202.

40   **"he survived yellow fever and very nearly died"** See author interview with Kathryn Olivarius.

40   **because people feared they would die** See Olivarius, "The Dangerous History of Immunoprivilege."

40   **"yourself and your position in society"** See author interview with Kathryn Olivarius. See also Olivarius, *Necropolis,* 121–29.

40   **let the workers become sickened and acclimated** See author interview with Kathryn Olivarius. See also Olivarius, *Necropolis,* 122–35; and Olivarius, "The Dangerous History of Immunoprivilege."

41   **"because they believed that nothing could stop yellow fever"** See author interview with Kathryn Olivarius.

41   **to protect the health of their valuable property** See Donnella, "How Yellow Fever Turned New Orleans."

42   **"an engine of wealth creation for every medical professional"** See Olivarius, *Necropolis,* 122–27.

42   **instituted a rigid program of garbage disposal** Ibid., 231–34.

42   **"the Union army cleaned up the city"** See author interview with Kathryn Olivarius.

43   **rank near the bottom or dead last** See Tom Jones, "Confederates' Lost Cause Still Cripples the South's Economy," MLK50: Justice Through Journalism, July 27, 2017. Available at: https://mlk50.com/2017/07/27/confederates-lost-cause-still-cripples-the-souths-economy/.

43   **largely immigrant workforce toiling in slaughterhouses** Ibid.

43   **the refusal of red states . . . to take the Medicaid expansion** See "Status of State Medicaid Expansion Decisions," Kaiser Family Foundation, August 26, 2025. Available at: https://www.kff.org/medicaid/status-of-state-medicaid-expansion-decisions/.

44   **coverage mandates that had protected the poor** See Noah Weiland, "Hundreds of Thousands Have Lost Medicaid Coverage Since Pandemic Protections Expired," *New York Times,* May 26, 2023. Available at: https://www.nytimes.com/2023/05/26/us/politics/medicaid-coverage-pandemic-loss.html.

44   **11,000 newborns lost health insurance** See Mary Hennigan, "1 in 5
         Arkansas Children Lost Medicaid During 'Unwinding' Process, Report
         Finds," *Arkansas Advocate,* May 2, 2024. Available at: https://arkansas
         advocate.com/2024/05/02/arkansas-quick-medicaid-unwinding-left-1-in
         -5-children-uninsured-report-finds/.

45   **the workforce that their labor-intensive economy relied upon** See Eric
         Foner, "Abraham Lincoln: The Great Emancipator?" *The British Academy*
         125 (n.d.): 149–62. Available at: https://www.thebritishacademy.ac.uk
         /documents/2000/pba125p149.pdf.

45   **no provisions were made to supply them** See Paul Harris, "How the
         End of Slavery Led to Starvation and Death for Millions of Black Ameri-
         cans," *Guardian,* June 16, 2012. Available at: https://www.theguardian
         .com/world/2012/jun/16/slavery-starvation-civil-war.

45   **"caused inordinate suffering"** See "An Interview with Professor Jim
         Downs," Oxford African American Studies Center, January 2013. Available
         at: https://oxfordaasc.com/page/2861.

46   **they were met, at best, with apathy and negligence** See Harris, "How
         the End of Slavery Led to Starvation." See also Humphreys, *Marrow of
         Tragedy,* 73–74.

46   **"become dependent on federal aid and assistance"** See Downs, *Sick
         from Freedom,* 56.

48   **Downs speculated, "he died from a broken heart"** Ibid. The story of
         the Miller family is recounted on pages 18–21.

48   **typified the suffering of the roughly 500,000 freed slaves** See Eric
         Willis, "The Forgotten: The Contraband of America and the Road to
         Freedom," National Trust for Historic Preservation, June 19, 2017.
         Available at: https://savingplaces.org/stories/the-forgotten-the
         -contraband-of-america-and-the-road-to-freedom.

48   **ignored it because it was largely seen as a "Black epidemic"** See Jim
         Downs, "The Epidemics America Got Wrong," *Atlantic,* March 22, 2020.
         Available at: https://www.theatlantic.com/ideas/archive/2020/03/role
         -apathy-epidemics/608527/. See also Jim Downs, "This Pandemic Isn't
         Over," *Atlantic,* June 9, 2021. Available at: https://www.theatlantic.com
         /ideas/archive/2021/06/pandemics-end-when-we-stop-caring-about
         -their-victims/619127/.

48   **"authorities will but take the proper steps to check it"** See Downs,
         "This Pandemic Isn't Over."

49   **The disease claimed at least 60,000 lives** Ibid.

49   **to provide resources for newly freed people** See Downs, *Sick from
         Freedom,* 52.

49   **like William Lloyd Garrison, the famed abolitionist** See Harriet A.
         Jacobs, "Life Among the Contrabands," *Liberator,* September 5, 1862, 3;
         posted on *Encyclopedia Virginia.* Available at: https://encyclopediavirginia
         .org/primary-documents/life-among-the-contrabands-harriet-a-jacobs
         -september-5-1862/.

49   **people were suffering grievously** Ibid.

50   **" 'Is this freedom?' "** Ibid.

50   **contraband camps throughout the occupied South** See Willis, "The
         Forgotten."

50   **homed about 40,000 people** See Don K. Nakayama, "Contraband
          Hospital, Freedmen's Hospital, and Alexander Augusta," *American Surgeon*
          88, no. 6 (June 2022): 1046. Available at: https://doi.org/10.1177
          /00031348211067992.

50   **fresh water, and a waste-disposal system** See Jill Newmark, "Contraband
          Hospital, 1862–1863: Healthcare for the First Freedpeople," Black Past,
          March 28, 2012. Available at: https://www.blackpast.org/african
          -american-history/contraband-hospital-1862-1863-heath-care-first
          -freedpeople/.

51   **until the Civil War broke out in 1861** See John Boileau, "Alexander
          Thomas Augusta," *The Canadian Encyclopedia*, June 2, 2022. Available at:
          https://www.thecanadianencyclopedia.ca/en/article/alexander-thomas
          -augusta.

51   **but was turned away once more** Ibid.

51   **competence from his colleagues in Toronto** See "Dr. Alexander Au-
          gusta," Ford's Theatre, National Historic Site District of Columbia,
          National Park Service. Available at: https://www.nps.gov/foth/learn
          /historyculture/alexander-augusta.htm. See also Boileau, "Alexander
          Thomas Augusta."

52   **the medical board president was enraged** See Richard M. Reid, *African
          Canadians in Union Blue: Enlisting for the Cause in the Civil War* (Van-
          couver: UBC Press, 2014), 160.

52   **first Black executive officer in charge** See Boileau, "Alexander Thomas
          Augusta." See also Cate Lineberry, "Breaking Medicine's Color Barrier,"
          New York Times, June 21, 2013. Available at: https://archive.nytimes.com
          /opinionator.blogs.nytimes.com/2013/06/21/breaking-medicines-color
          -barrier/. See also Michael Williams, "Meet the U.S. Army's First Black
          Surgeon: Alexander Augusta," HistoryNet, January 12, 2022. Available at:
          https://www.historynet.com/meet-the-u-s-armys-first-black-surgeon
          -alexander-augusta/.

52   **later convicted of assault** See Lineberry, "Breaking Medicine's Color
          Barrier." See also Williams, "Meet the U.S. Army's First Black Surgeon."

52   **several plainclothes police officers** See Reid, *African Canadians in Union
          Blue,* 160–61. See also Nakayama, "Contraband Hospital," 1048.

52   **"where it is considered a virtue to mob colored people"** See Alexander
          Augusta, Letter to editor, *National Republican,* May 15, 1863, in *The Black
          Abolitionist Papers,* vol. V (University of North Carolina Press, 1985).

52   **The army stopped commissioning Black physicians** See Reid, *African
          Canadians in Union Blue,* 162–63.

52   **he recruited several of his colleagues** See Nakayama, "Contraband
          Hospital," 1048.

52   **This cadre of surgeons formed the nucleus** See Newmark, "Contraband
          Hospital, 1862–1863."

53   **he worked at Lincoln Hospital in Savannah** See Reid, *African Canadi-
          ans in Union Blue,* 171. See also Boileau, "Alexander Thomas Augusta."

53   **"The hospital was the city poor-house"** Harriet A. Jacobs, "From
          Savannah," *Freedman's Record,* January 1866, 3–4; posted by Document-
          ing the American South. Available at: https://docsouth.unc.edu/fpn
          /jacobs/support2.html.

53   **promoted to the rank of lieutenant colonel** See Williams, "Meet the U.S. Army's First Black Surgeon."

53   **the first Black to be on the faculty of a medical school** See "Dr. Alexander Augusta."

53   **In a photo taken in 1869 of the inaugural medical faculty** Ibid.

53   **Augusta was buried with full military honors** See Reid, *African Canadians in Union Blue,* 172. See also Boileau, "Alexander Thomas Augusta."

53   **Roughly two-thirds of them died from diseases** See Humphreys, *Marrow of Tragedy,* 24.

53   **eight out of ten men there died from disease** Ibid.

53   **one in four Confederate soldiers died or were incapacitated** Ibid., 8.

54   **spared thousands of soldiers** Ibid., 9–10.

54   **long before the discovery of germs** Ibid., 271–89.

54   **became standard practice** Ibid., 272.

54   **according to Charles Rosenberg** See Rosenberg, *The Cholera Years,* 193.

54   **about 40,000 of them perished** See Sarah B. Dine, "Wartime Health Disparities and Their Aftermath," *Health Affairs* 27, no. 4 (July /August 2008): 1192. Available at: https://www.healthaffairs.org/doi /10.1377/hlthaff.27.4.1191.

54   **It wasn't until the Korean War** Ibid., 1192.

55   **a quarter of the approximately four million freed slaves** See Harris, "How the End of Slavery Led to Starvation."

55   **"dying by the scores"** See Willis, "The Forgotten."

55   **and offering them legal assistance** See W. E. B. Du Bois, "The Freed-men's Bureau," *Atlantic Monthly,* March 1901, 357. Available at: https:// www.theatlantic.com/magazine/archive/1901/03/the-freedmens-bureau /308772/.

55   **sixty hospitals and asylums were in operation** Ibid., 360.

55   **embittered former plantation owners** Ibid., 364.

56   **"vast problems of race and social condition"** Ibid., 354.

56   **"in large part foredoomed to failure"** Ibid., 359–60.

CHAPTER THREE: PUBLIC HEALTH'S MOST CELEBRATED ACT OF CIVIL DISOBEDIENCE

59   **namely that microscopic agents were responsible** See Alfredo Morabia, *Enigmas of Health and Disease: How Epidemiology Helps Unravel Scientific Mysteries* (New York: Columbia University Press, 2014), 50–53.

59   **by drinking or eating foods prepared with tainted water** Ibid., 50.

59   **During an earlier cholera outbreak, in 1848** See Theodore H. Tulchin-sky, "John Snow, Cholera, the Broad Street Pump; Waterborne Diseases Then and Now," *Case Studies in Public Health* (2018): 80. Available at: https://pmc.ncbi.nlm.nih.gov/articles/PMC7150208/.

60   **"all the surrounding houses were quite free from it"** See John Snow, *On the Mode of Communication of Cholera* (London: John Churchill, 1849), 6, 12–13, 21–23. Available at: http://archive.org/details /b30383158.

60   **could be stopped by simple sanitary measures** Ibid., 26.

60   **where sewage was dumped** See Tulchinsky, "John Snow," 82.

61   **realized immediately that this was a natural experiment** See Morabia,
        Enigmas of Health and Disease, 52.

61   **"the disease was between thirteen and fourteen times as fatal"** See
        John Snow, *Cholera and the Water Supply in the South Districts of London in
        1854* (London: T. Richards, 1856), 5–7. Available at: https://www
        .gutenberg.org/cache/epub/66507/pg66507-images.html.

61   **most of them clustered around a water-well pump** See Tulchinsky,
        "John Snow," 80–81. See also Morabia, *Enigmas of Health and Disease,* 52.

61   **Snow removed the handle himself** See Tulchinsky, "John Snow," 82.

62   **Snow compared two distinct but evenly matched groups** See Morabia,
        Enigmas of Health and Disease, 52. See also author interview with Alfredo
        Morabia, November 14, 2022.

62   **So, in one act, the scientific and methodological bases** See Tulchinsky,
        "John Snow," 83. See also author interview with Alfredo Morabia.

64   **it was probably not spread by fetid gases in the air** See Morabia,
        Enigmas of Health and Disease, 32–36.

64   **the first woman elected to the Royal Statistical Society** See R.J.
        Andrews, "How Florence Nightingale Changed Data Visualization
        Forever," *Scientific American,* August 1, 2022. Available at: https://www
        .scientificamerican.com/article/how-florence-nightingale-changed-data
        -visualization-forever/. See also Richard Bates, "Florence Nightingale: A
        Pioneer of Hand Washing and Hygiene for Health," *Conversation,*
        March 23, 2020. Available at: https://theconversation.com/florence
        -nightingale-a-pioneer-of-hand-washing-and-hygiene-for-health-134270.

64   **her father hired a mathematics tutor** See Iris Veysey, "A Statistical
        Campaign: Florence Nightingale and Harriet Martineau's *England and
        Her Soldiers,*" *Science Museum Group Journal* (Spring 2016). Available at:
        https://journal.sciencemuseum.ac.uk/article/nightingale-and-martineau/.

64   **She exhibited her exceptional talents early** See Kerri Lee Alexander,
        "Florence Nightingale," National Women's History Museum, 2019.
        Available at: https://www.womenshistory.org/education-resources
        /biographies/florence-nightingale.

64   **her efforts to improve sanitary conditions** See Alexander, "Florence
        Nightingale."

65   **they were horrified by what they saw** See "Florence Nightingale: The
        Pioneer Statistician," Science Museum, December 10, 2018. Available at:
        https://www.sciencemuseum.org.uk/objects-and-stories/florence
        -nightingale-pioneer-statistician.

65   **There were six dead dogs under one window** See Jim Downs, *Maladies
        of Empire: How Colonialism, Slavery, and War Transformed Medicine*
        (Belknap Press of Harvard University Press, 2021), 97.

65   **Worse yet, medical records were woefully inadequate** See Veysey, "A
        Statistical Campaign."

65   **Careful documentation with statistics** See Downs, *Maladies of Empire,* 96.

66   **checking on patients by lamplight** Ibid., 91–93.

66   **while they languished in squalid camps** Ibid., 95.

66   **where they would work best at keeping cholera in check** See Institute
        of Medicine, *The Future of Public Health,* 61–62.

67   **when deliveries were performed by doctors** See Dr. Howard Markel, "In

1850, Ignaz Semmelweis Saved Lives with Three Words: Wash Your Hands," PBS News, May 15, 2015. Available at: https://www.pbs.org /newshour/health/ignaz-semmelweis-doctor-prescribed-hand-washing.

67   **invisible particles that the doctors carried from the autopsy suite** Ibid.

67   **Another twenty years would pass** See Nicholas Kadar et al., "Ignaz Semmelweis: The 'Savior of Mothers': On the 200th Anniversary of His Birth," *American Journal of Obstetrics and Gynecology* 219, no. 6 (December 2018): 519–22. Available at: https://doi.org/10.1016/j.ajog.2018 .10.036.

67   **remains an important pillar of public health** See Markel, "In 1850, Ignaz Semmelweis Saved Lives."

68   **New methods of controlling or even preventing the spread** See Ritu Lakhtakia, "The Legacy of Robert Koch: Surmise, Search, Substantiate," *Sultan Qaboos University Medical Journal* 14, no. 1 (February 2014): e37–41. Available at: https://pubmed.ncbi.nlm.nih.gov/24516751/.

68   **Almost overnight, life expectancy increased** See O'Neill, "Annual Life Expectancy at Birth in the United States."

68   **Now doctors just had to find the infectious pathogen** See Milton Terris, "The Changing Relationships of Epidemiology and Society: The Robert Cruikshank Lecture," *Journal of Public Health Policy* 6, no. 1 (March 1985): 15–36. Available at: https://doi.org/10.2307/3342015.

69   **yellow fever had been vanquished** See Patrick Feng, "Major Walter Reed and the Eradication of Yellow Fever," Army Historical Foundation. Available at https://armyhistory.org/major-walter-reed-and-the -eradication-of-yellow-fever/.

69   **their offspring would survive into adulthood** Ibid., 63–66.

69   **"it was a glorious ten years"** See Institute of Medicine, *The Future of Public Health,* 64.

69   **the city invested in water sanitation** Ibid., 65–66.

70   **more than 500 tuberculosis clinics** Ibid., 66.

70   **interventions shifted from being community-based** Ibid., 64–66. See also Fairchild, "The EXODUS of Public Health."

70   **Chapin believed that public health should focus** See Institute of Medicine, *The Future of Public Health,* 64–65. See also Fairchild, "The EXODUS of Public Health."

71   **diverse scientific disciplines that come together** See Fairchild, "The EXODUS of Public Health."

71   **American Public Health Association** Elizabeth Fee and Theodore Brown, "The Unfulfilled Promise of Public Health: Déjà Vu All Over Again," *Health Affairs* 21, no. 6 (November/December 2002): 31–43. Available at: https://doi.org/10.1377/hlthaff.21.6.31.

71   **became the province of experts** See Institute of Medicine, *The Future of Public Health,* 59–65.

71   **resulted in major victories in the conquest of diseases** See Fairchild, "The EXODUS of Public Health."

72   **rather than on the big-picture** Ibid.

72   **neglecting to investigate other factors** See Terris, "The Changing Relationships of Epidemiology and Society." See also Ed Yong, "How Public Health Took Part in Its Own Downfall," *Atlantic,* October 23,

2021. Available at: https://www.theatlantic.com/health/archive/2021/10/how-public-health-took-part-its-own-downfall/620457/.

73 **Left untreated, pellagra can affect the nervous system** See Alfred Jay Bollet, "Politics and Pellagra: The Epidemic of Pellagra in the U.S. in the Early Twentieth Century," *The Yale Journal of Biology and Medicine* 65, no. 3 (1992): 211–21. Available at: https://pmc.ncbi.nlm.nih.gov/articles/PMC2589605/.

73 **Pellagra was rare in the United States** Ibid.

73 **the incidence began to skyrocket in the U.S.** Ibid., 211.

73 **and 40 percent of them had died of the disease** See Alfredo Morabia, "Joseph Goldberger's Research on the Prevention of Pellagra," *Journal of the Royal Society of Medicine* 101, no. 11 (November 2008): 566–68. Available at: https://pubmed.ncbi.nlm.nih.gov/19029358/.

73 **it is estimated that the epidemic of pellagra** See Bollet, "Politics and Pellagra," 214.

73 **pellagra could become a "national calamity"** Ibid.

73 **a hospital in Atlanta dedicated to the care** Ibid.

73 **The fact that the disease was strongly linked with poverty** Ibid.

74 **He was fighting a diphtheria outbreak in Detroit** Ibid., 216.

74 **he had never seen an infectious disease** Ibid.

74 **was convinced the disease could be eradicated** Ibid., 216–17.

75 **one inmate complained. Others asked to be shot** See "Joseph Goldberger & the War on Pellagra," *Office of NIH History and Stetten Museum*. See also Bollet, 217.

75 **disease could be prevented by a more nutritional diet** See Bollet, 217.

76 **"improving the diet of impoverished citizens"** Ibid., 215.

76 **He died in 1929 before the key element was identified** Ibid., 217.

76 **Degermination came into routine use in 1901** Ibid., 219.

77 **ensure that foods weren't adulterated** See Fee and Brown, "The Unfulfilled Promise of Public Health," 35.

77 **Because of Baker's unstinting efforts** See "Dr. Sara Josephine Baker: A Lasting Legacy in Public Health," Women in Medicine Legacy Foundation, June 20, 2024. Available at: https://www.wimlf.org/blog/dr-sara-josephine-baker-a-lasting-legacy-in-public-health.

77 **"public need over private greed"** See Fee and Brown, "The Unfulfilled Promise of Public Health," 36.

77 **condemned as "socialized medicine"** Ibid., 37.

77 **A swelling backlash against the reforms** Ibid., 35–37.

77 **the Sheppard–Towner Act** See Institute of Medicine, *The Future of Public Health*, 67.

78 **were all stripped of funding** See Fee and Brown, "The Unfulfilled Promise of Public Health," 37.

78 **the same horrific living conditions** Ibid., 35.

78 **Conservative politicians fanned the flames** Ibid.

78 **"otherize" foreigners by painting them as insidious carriers** Ibid.

78 **most of whom were deported** Ibid., 36–37.

79 **This is a stark illustration** See Jacob Wallace et al., "Excess Death Rates for Republican and Democratic Registered Voters in Florida and Ohio During the COVID-19 Pandemic," *JAMA Internal Medicine* 183, no. 9

(September 1, 2023): 916–23. Available at: https://pubmed.ncbi.nlm.nih
.gov/37486680/.

79   **only 3.3 cents of the medical dollar** See Fee and Brown, "The Unfulfilled Promise of Public Health," 38.

79   **"the great public health surge"** Ibid., 37.

CHAPTER FOUR: W.E.B. DU BOIS, THE MYTH OF RACIAL INFERIORITY, AND THE SLAVE HEALTH DEFICIT

80   **"The slave health deficit has never been made up"** See W. Michael Byrd
and Linda A. Clayton, *An American Health Dilemma: A Medical History of
African Americans and the Problem of Race: Beginnings to 1900* (New York:
Routledge, 2000), 9.

80   **what could be done to improve their situation** See Greg Johnson, "The
Times and Life of W. E. B. Du Bois at Penn," *Penn Today,* February 22,
2019. Available at: https://penntoday.upenn.edu/news/times-and-life
-web-du-bois-penn. See also "Letter from University of Pennsylvania to
W. E. B. Du Bois, August 15, 1896," Robert S. Cox Special Collections
and University Archives Research Center, University of Massachusetts
Amherst. Available at: https://credo.library.umass.edu/view/full
/mums312-b004-i335.

80   **thwarted the city's Black residents** See Johnson, "The Times and Life of
W. E. B. Du Bois at Penn."

81   **a representative from the University of Pennsylvania** Ibid.

81   **what was causing all the troubles** Ibid.

81   **"a virus to be quarantined"** See David Levering Lewis, *W. E. B. Du Bois:
A Biography 1868–1963* (New York: Henry Holt and Company, 2009),
134–35.

81   **Du Bois set out to prove them wrong** See W. E. B. Du Bois, *The
Philadelphia Negro* (University of Pennsylvania Press, 1899), 3–8.

82   **often largely responsible for communities** See Johnson, "The Times and
Life of W. E. B. Du Bois at Penn."

82   **provided a three-dimensional glimpse** See Du Bois, *The Philadelphia
Negro,* 56–60.

83   **"choice . . . is the antidote for exploitation"** See Matthew Desmond,
Poverty, by America (New York: Crown Publishing, 2023), 146.

83   **with an appreciation of the social determinants of health** See Nancy
Krieger, *Epidemiology and the People's Health: Theory and Context* (New
York: Oxford University Press, 2011), 105–9.

83   **in the College Settlement House** See Johnson, "The Times and Life of
W. E. B. Du Bois at Penn."

83   **surrounded by "an atmosphere of dirt, drunkenness"** See Marcus
Anthony Hunter, "Black Philly After *The Philadelphia Negro*," *American
Sociological Association* 13, no. 1 (Winter 2014): 26–31. Available at:
https://journals.sagepub.com/doi/10.1177/1536504214522005.

83   **numbered 43,000 in a city of more than one million** See Johnson,
"The Times and Life of W. E. B. Du Bois at Penn."

83   **forced to live in unsafe and unsanitary homes** See Du Bois, *The
Philadelphia Negro,* 90–92.

84   **which probably enabled him to gain his freedom** See Johnson, "The
          Times and Life of W. E. B. Du Bois at Penn." See also Thomas C. Holt,
          "W. E. B. Du Bois," Hutchins Center for African & African American
          Research, Harvard University. Available at: https://hutchinscenter.fas
          .harvard.edu/web-dubois.

84   **became the class valedictorian** See Johnson, "The Times and Life of
          W. E. B. Du Bois at Penn."

84   **"and all its dazzling opportunities were theirs"** See W. E. B. Du Bois,
          "Strivings of the Negro People," *Atlantic Monthly,* August 1897, 194.
          Available at: https://www.theatlantic.com/magazine/archive/1897/08
          /strivings-of-the-negro-people/305446/.

85   **the United States and the African slave trade** See Holt, "W. E. B. Du
          Bois."

85   **"authority capable of offsetting the abolitionists'"** See Nancy Krieger,
          "Shades of Difference: Theoretical Underpinnings of the Medical Contro-
          versy on Black/White Differences in the United States, 1830–1870," *Inter-
          national Journal of Social Determinants of Health and Health Services* 17,
          no. 2 (April 1987): 259–78. Available at: https://journals.sagepub.com
          /doi/10.2190/DBY6-VDQ8-HME8-ME3R.

85   **challenging the so-called scientific basis of slavery** Ibid.

86   **Cartwright was considered a legitimate scientist** See Bill Bynum,
          "Discarded Diagnoses," *Lancet* 356, no. 9241 (November 4, 2000): 1615.
          Available at: https://www.sciencedirect.com/science/article/pii
          /S0140673605744688?via%3Dihub. See also Michael Coard, "Drapeto-
          mania: Compliant Blacks Sane, Resisting Blacks Insane," *Philadelphia
          Tribune,* March 15, 2019. Available at: https://www.phillytrib.com
          /commentary/drapetomania-compliant-blacks-sane-resisting-blacks-insane
          /article_0087a2d0-1acb-5364-870c-1205212e0a13.html.

86   **"the African is incapable of self-care"** See Peter Whoriskey, "The Bogus
          U.S. Census Numbers Showing Slavery's 'Wonderful Influence' on the
          Enslaved," *Washington Post,* October 17, 2020. Available at: https://www
          .washingtonpost.com/history/2020/10/17/1840-census-slavery
          -insanity/.

86   **Dr. Samuel Forry . . . demonstrated** See Krieger, "Shades of Difference."
          See also James W. Trent Jr., *Inventing the Feeble Mind: A History of
          Intellectual Disability in the United States* (New York: Oxford University
          Press, 1995), 56–58. See also Michael E. Ruane, "A Brief History of the
          Enduring Phony Science that Perpetuates White Supremacy," *Washington
          Post,* April 30, 2019. Available at: https://www.washingtonpost.com/local
          /a-brief-history-of-the-enduring-phony-science-that-perpetuates-white
          -supremacy/2019/04/29/20e6aef0-5aeb-11e9-a00e-050dc7b82693
          _story.html. See also Linda Villarosa, "Myths About Physical Racial
          Differences Were Used to Justify Slavery—and Are Still Believed by
          Doctors Today," *New York Times Magazine,* August 14, 2019. Available at:
          https://www.nytimes.com/interactive/2019/08/14/magazine/racial
          -differences-doctors.html.

86   **treat insubordination as proof** See Krieger, "Shades of Difference," 266.

86   **the pro-slavery argument seemed to win the day** Ibid.

87   **was James McCune Smith** See Kelly Harris, "Foreshadowing Du Bois: James McCune Smith and the Shaping of Nineteenth Century Black Social Scientists," *Du Bois Review: Social Science Research on Race* 22, no. 1 (May 13, 2024): 154–70. Available at: https://www.cambridge.org/core /journals/du-bois-review-social-science-research-on-race/article /foreshadowing-du-bois/AC5646EF7C60E05E69D60CA418939222.

87   **"that attained by the Europe-American population"** See Thomas M. Morgan, "The Education and Medical Practice of Dr. James McCune Smith (1813–1865), First Black American to Hold a Medical Degree," *Journal of the National Medical Association* 95, no. 7 (July 2003): 603–14. Available at: https://pubmed.ncbi.nlm.nih.gov/12911258/. See also Neil Krishan Aggarwal, "The Legacy of James McCune Smith, MD—The First Black US Physician," *JAMA* 326, no. 22 (2021): 2245–46. Available at: https://jamanetwork.com/journals/jama/fullarticle/2786889.

87   **his intellectual gifts were obvious** See Aggarwal, "The Legacy of James McCune Smith."

88   **a medical degree the following year** Ibid.

88   **took steps toward justice at great personal cost** See Matthew Daniel Eddy, "James McCune Smith: New Discovery Reveals How First African American Doctor Fought for Women's Rights in Glasgow," *Conversation,* October 8, 2021. Available at: https://theconversation.com/james -mccune-smith-new-discovery-reveals-how-first-african-american-doctor -fought-for-womens-rights-in-glasgow-166233. See also "Pioneering Research of First Published African American Doctor Revealed," *EurekAlert!,* October 12, 2021. Available at: https://www.eurekalert.org /news-releases/931259.

88   *Notes on the State of Virginia,* **in which he questioned** See Thomas Jefferson, "Query XIV," *Notes on the State of Virginia,* 1787. Available at: https://avalon.law.yale.edu/18th_century/jeffvir.asp.

88   **the most damaging and enduring instance** See Ibram X. Kendi, *Stamped from the Beginning: The Definitive History of Racist Ideas in America* (New York: Nation Books, 2016), 94–96.

89   **and not because of some innate weakness** See Morgan, "The Education and Medical Practice of Dr. James McCune Smith," 604.

89   **Rudolf Virchow . . . spearheaded** See Myron Schultz, "Rudolf Virchow," *Emerging Infectious Diseases* 14, no. 9 (September 2008): 1480–81. Available at: https://doi.org/10.3201/eid1409.086672. See also George Rosen, *A History of Public Health* (Baltimore: Johns Hopkins University Press, 1993), 152–54.

89   **poor diets . . . had made the people more vulnerable to illness** See Rudolf Virchow, "Report on the Typhus Epidemic in Upper Silesia. 1848," *American Journal of Public Health* 96, no. 12 (December 2006): 2102–5. Available at: https://pubmed.ncbi.nlm.nih.gov/17123938/.

89   **build the scaffolding of his nation's modern public health system** See Schultz, "Rudolf Virchow." See also Rosen, *A History of Public Health.* See also Morabia, *Enigmas of Health and Disease,* 61–64.

90   **the man who would become his intellectual heir** See Aggarwal, "The Legacy of James McCune Smith."

90   **was later championed by Adolf Hitler** See Lisa Ko, "Unwanted Steriliza-

tion and Eugenics Programs in the United States," PBS, January 29, 2016. Available at: https://www.pbs.org/independentlens/blog/unwanted -sterilization-and-eugenics-programs-in-the-united-states/.

90   **other "undesirables" in the 1940s** See P. Preston Reynolds, "UVA and the History of Race: Eugenics, the Racial Integrity Act, Health Dispari- ties," *UVA Today,* January 9, 2020. Available at: https://news.virginia.edu /content/uva-and-history-race-eugenics-racial-integrity-act-health -disparities.

91   **"knowledge based on scientific investigation"** See Johnson, "The Times and Life of W. E. B. Du Bois at Penn."

91   **about 86 percent of school-age children attended** Ibid.

91   **with approximately 2,500 households in his investigation** See Lewis, *W. E. B. Du Bois,* 135–36.

91   **and other publications to corroborate his work** See Johnson, "The Times and Life of W. E. B. Du Bois at Penn."

91   **at a rate two times higher than their white neighbors** See Du Bois, *The Philadelphia Negro,* 144–47.

91   **before the age of fifteen as their white counterparts** Ibid., 147.

91   **primarily due to social, not biological factors** Ibid., 139.

92   **in an older part of the city that lacked indoor plumbing** Ibid., 150.

92   **makeshift latrines in hallways** See Johnson, "The Times and Life of W. E. B. Du Bois at Penn."

92   **against the dampness and cold** See Du Bois, *The Philadelphia Negro,* 140. See also W. E. B. Du Bois, "The Health and Physique of the Negro American," *American Journal of Public Health* 93, no. 2 (February 2003): 274–75. Available at: https://ajph.aphapublications.org/doi/pdfplus/10 .2105/AJPH.93.2.272.

92   **skin color was not the cause of their poor health** See Du Bois, *The Philadelphia Negro,* 139.

92   **compared to 49.6 years for whites** See W.M. Byrd and L.A. Clayton, "An American Health Dilemma: A History of Blacks in the Health System," *Journal of the National Medical Association* 84, no. 2 (February 1992), 195. Available at: https://pubmed.ncbi.nlm.nih.gov/1602519/.

92   **"human suffering has been viewed"** See Du Bois, *The Philadelphia Negro,* 151.

93   **in all its beauty, culture, possibilities, and messy splendor** See Johnson, "The Times and Life of W. E. B. Du Bois at Penn."

93   **"Imagine if you actually fulfilled your duty"** See author interview via Zoom with Marcus Anthony Hunter, a professor of sociology and African American studies at UCLA, October 26, 2022.

93   **"the road to success is to have a white face?"** See Lewis, *W. E. B. Du Bois,* 149.

94   **collapsed right before Christmas** See Hunter, "Black Philly After *The Philadelphia Negro.*"

94   **in a cruel twist of fate** Lewis, *W. E. B. Du Bois,* 267–70.

95   **"into bitter loathing" . . . she never truly forgave him** Ibid., 153–54, 164.

95   **was the decades-long culmination of the movement** See Holt, "W. E. B. Du Bois."

95   **since arriving in the United States from Africa** See Byrd and Clayton, "An American Health Dilemma," 189–200.

96   **"sometimes cruel health system"** See W. Michael Byrd, "An American Health Dilemma," *Journal of the National Medical Association* 78, no. 11 (November 1986): 1025–26.

96   **awarded the Bronze Star** See "Dr. Wilbur Michael Byrd," *Tennessean,* March 3, 2021. Available at: https://www.tennessean.com/obituaries /ten188510.

96   **might have been controlled if caught earlier** See Anna Flagg, "The Black Mortality Gap, and a Document Written in 1910," *New York Times,* August 30, 2021. Available at: https://www.nytimes.com/2021/08/30 /upshot/black-health-mortality-gap.html.

96   **inspired changes in governmental policies** Ibid.

97   **followed by a "breaking-in period"** See R.G. Hood, "The 'Slave Health Deficit': The Case for Reparations to Bring Health Parity to African Americans," *Journal of the National Medical Association* 93, no. 1 (January 2001): 2–3. Available at: https://pubmed.ncbi.nlm.nih.gov /12653374/.

97   **and created a segregated health system** See Krieger, "Shades of Difference."

97   **William Welch and . . . William Osler** See Kenneth M. Ludmerer, *Learning to Heal: The Development of American Medical Education* (New York: Basic Books, 1985), 65–68.

98   **But their seemingly noble efforts** See Angus Rae, "Osler Vindicated: the ghost of Flexner laid to rest," *Canadian Medical Association Journal* 164, no. 13 (June 26, 2001): 1860–61. Available at: https://pmc.ncbi.nlm.nih .gov/articles/PMC81198/.

98   **Flexner was an unlikely choice** See Thomas P. Duffy, "The Flexner Report—100 Years Later," *Yale Journal of Biology and Medicine* 84, no. 3 (September 2011): 269–76. Available at: https://pmc.ncbi.nlm.nih.gov /articles/PMC3178858/.

98   **he had no medical background** See Ibid., 271.

98   **He was also a virulent and unapologetic racist** See Abraham Flexner, *Medical Education in the United States and Canada: A Report to the Carnegie Foundation for the Advancement of Teaching* (Boston: Merrymount Press, 1910), Introduction and Chapter XI. Available at: https:// archive.org/details/medicaleducation00flexiala/mode/2up.

98   **His research reflected his prejudices** See Flagg, "The Black Mortality Gap."

98   **paving the way for medicine to be firmly based on science** See Flexner, *Medical Education in the United States and Canada,* 15–22. See also Flagg, "The Black Mortality Gap."

98   **remedies that often did more harm than good** See Duffy, "The Flexner Report," 269–76.

99   **drastically reduced the number of Black doctors** See Hood, "The 'Slave Health Deficit,'" 3.

100   **"It started us down a road that is hard to undo"** See Elizabeth Hlavinka, "Racial Bias in Flexner Report Permeates Medical Education

Today," *MedPage Today,* June 18, 2020. Available at: https://www
.medpagetoday.com/publichealthpolicy/medicaleducation/87171.

100   **more willing to follow doctors' orders** See John E. Snyder et al., "Black
        Representation in the Primary Care Physician Workforce and Its Associa-
        tion with Population Life Expectancy and Mortality Rates in the US,"
        JAMA Network Open 6, no. 4 (April 14, 2023), 1–14. Available at:
        https://pubmed.ncbi.nlm.nih.gov/37058307/. See also Usha Lee McFar-
        ling, "In Counties with More Black Doctors, Black People Live Longer,
        'Astonishing' Study Finds," *STAT,* April 14, 2023. Available at: https://
        www.statnews.com/2023/04/14/black-doctors-primary-care-life
        -expectancy-mortality/.

100   **they listen more closely and sympathetically** See McFarling, "In
        Counties with More Black Doctors."

101   **Michael Bloomberg, who donated $600 million** See Anemona Harto-
        collis and Alan Blinder, "Historically Black Medical Schools Land a $600
        Million Donation," *New York Times,* August 6, 2024. Available at:
        https://www.nytimes.com/2024/08/06/us/donation-historically-black
        -medical-schools-bloomberg.html.

102   **"It was just this amazing feel-good celebration"** See author interview
        via Zoom with Dr. Deborah Prothrow-Stith, dean and professor of
        medicine for the Charles R. Drew University College of Medicine,
        September 6, 2023.

102   **and suffer from more than 59,000 excess deaths** See Byrd and Clayton,
        "An American Health Dilemma," 190–91.

102   **that doesn't fully account for the disparities** See Lindsay Smith Rogers,
        "The Racial Inequities of Kidney Disease," Johns Hopkins Bloomberg
        School of Public Health, September 3, 2020. Available at: https://
        publichealth.jhu.edu/2020/the-racial-inequities-of-kidney-disease.

102   **kidneys seemed healthier than they really were** See Andis Robeznieks,
        "Why eGFR-Reporting Change Helps Tackle Kidney Disease Inequities,"
        American Medical Association, May 19, 2021. Available at: https://www
        .ama-assn.org/public-health/population-health/why-egfr-reporting
        -change-helps-tackle-kidney-disease-inequities.

103   **Black Americans were misdiagnosed** See author interview via Zoom with
        Dr. Leon McDougle on November 2, 2022. Dr. McDougle is a professor
        of family and community medicine at The Ohio State University College of
        Medicine and former president of the National Medical Association.

103   **deaths of Black women . . . rose for decades** See Neal A. Chatterjee,
        Yulei He, and Nancy L. Keating, "Racial Differences in Breast Cancer Stage
        at Diagnosis in the Mammography Era," *American Journal of Public
        Health* 103, no. 1 (January 2013): 170–76. Available at: https://pmc.ncbi
        .nlm.nih.gov/articles/PMC3518347/.

103   **mortality rates of Black women** See Sandy McDowell, "Breast Cancer
        Incidence Still Rises and Death Rate Still Declines," American Cancer
        Society, October 2, 2024. Available at: https://www.cancer.org/research
        /acs-research-news/breast-cancer-incidence-still-rises-and-death-rate-still
        -declines.html.

104   **The study, which was published in 2022** See Chyke A. Doubeni et al.,

"Association Between Improved Colorectal Screening and Racial Dispari-ties," *New England Journal of Medicine* 386, no. 8 (February 23, 2022): 796–98. Available at: https://www.nejm.org/doi/full/10.1056/NEJMc2112409.

104   **"can eliminate health disparities"** See "Colon Cancer Screening Can Erase Disparities in Outcomes," Kaiser Permanente, February 24, 2022. Available at: https://www.prnewswire.com/news-releases/colon-cancer-screening-can-erase-disparities-in-outcomes-301485664.html.

104   **"how that shapes our opportunities to be healthy"** Author interview with Dr. David Williams via Zoom, July 21, 2021.

105   **neglected or inadequately treated** See Michel Martin, "Racism Is Literally Bad for Your Health," NPR, October 28, 2017. Available at: https://www.npr.org/2017/10/28/560444290/racism-is-literally-bad-for-your-health.

105   **where sixty—or even eighty—is genuinely the new forty** See Dan Buettner and Sam Skemp, "Blue Zones: Lessons from the World's Longest Lived," *American Journal of Lifestyle Medicine* 10, no. 5 (July 7, 2016): 318–21. Available at: https://pubmed.ncbi.nlm.nih.gov/30202288/.

106   **cultivating a culture of healthy living** See Ansel Oliver, "Loma Linda's Longevity Legacy," Loma Linda University Health, April 5, 2018. Available at: https://news.llu.edu/health-wellness/loma-linda-s-longevity-legacy.

106   **than poor white women who are high school dropouts** See Samuel H. Fishman et al., "Race/Ethnicity, Maternal Educational Attainment, and Infant Mortality in the United States," *Biodemography Social Biology* 66, no. 1 (January–March 2020): 1–26. Available at: https://pubmed.ncbi.nlm.nih.gov/33682572/.

107   **constant hypervigilance to guard against perceived threats** See David R. Williams, "Stress Was Already Killing Black Americans. Covid-19 Is Making It Worse," *Washington Post*, May 13, 2020. Available at: https://www.washingtonpost.com/opinions/2020/05/13/stress-was-already-killing-black-americans-covid-19-is-making-it-worse/.

107   **problems in relationships** Ibid.

107   **for a year. Year in and year out** See author interview with David R. Williams.

CHAPTER FIVE: DANGEROUS TRADES : FROM THE TRIANGLE SHIRTWAIST FACTORY FIRE TO THE WORLD TRADE CENTER COLLAPSE

109   **The blaze spread so fast that 146 workers** See David Von Drehle, *Triangle: The Fire that Changed America* (New York: Grove Press, 2003), 3–5. See also History.com editors, "Triangle Shirtwaist Factory Fire," History.com, December 2, 2009. Available at: https://www.history.com/topics/early-20th-century-us/triangle-shirtwaist-fire. See also Dr. Howard Markel, "How the Triangle Shirtwaist Factory Fire Transformed Labor Laws and Protected Workers' Health," PBS News, March 31, 2021. Available at: https://www.pbs.org/newshour/health/how-the-triangle-shirtwaist-factory-fire-transformed-labor-laws-and-protected-workers-health.

110   **lined the streets as the funeral procession** See "Paying Tribute to Triangle Fire Victims," *American Experience*, PBS. Available at: https://

www.pbs.org/wgbh/americanexperience/features/triangle-fire-paying
-tribute-triangle-fire-victims/.

110   **The Triangle Commission . . . found horrific conditions** See "Remembering the 1911 Triangle Factory Fire," Cornell University ILR School
Kheel Center. Available at: https://trianglefire.ilr.cornell.edu/.

110   **reforms became the template** Ibid. See also Markel, "How the Triangle
Shirtwaist Factory Fire Transformed Labor Laws."

111   **"Women had to burn to death for this to happen"** See author interview with labor historian Dr. Richard Greenwald via Zoom, January 19,
2023.

111   **18,000 to 21,000 workers died** See Norman Root and Deborah
Sebastian, "BLS Develops Measure of Job Risk by Occupation," *Monthly
Labor Review,* October 1981. Available at: https://www.bls.gov/opub
/mlr/1981/10/art4full.pdf.

111   **were tied to outbreaks in meatpacking plants** See Charles A. Taylor et
al., "Livestock Plants and COVID-19 Transmission," *PNAS* 117, no. 50
(November 19, 2020): 31706–15. Available at: https://www.pnas.org
/doi/10.1073/pnas.2010115117.

112   **"as class conflict and horrendous poverty"** See David Brooks, "The
Terrifying Future of the American Right," *Atlantic,* November 18, 2021.
Available at: https://www.theatlantic.com/ideas/archive/2021/11/scary
-future-american-right-national-conservatism-conference/620746/.

113   **not worth the cost of protection** See Matthew C. Ringenberg et al., *The
Education of Alice Hamilton: From Fort Wayne to Harvard* (Bloomington:
Indiana University Press, 2019), 53–54.

113   **called it an age of "triumphant ruthlessness"** See Alice Hamilton,
Exploring the Dangerous Trades (Boston: Little, Brown and Company,
1943), 1–3. Available at: https://archive.org/details/exploringthedang
011737mbp/page/n7/mode/2up. See also Karenna Gore, "The Remarkable Life of the First Woman on the Harvard Faculty," *New York Times,*
August 29, 2019. Available at: https://www.nytimes.com/2019/08/29
/opinion/alice-hamilton-harvard.html.

113   **Her struggles echo the battles faced** See Susan Ware, *Beyond Suffrage:
Women in the New Deal* (Harvard University Press, 1981), 84–87.

113   **she accepted a job teaching pathology** See Judah Ginsberg, "Alice
Hamilton and the Development of Occupational Medicine," American
Chemical Society, September 21, 2002. Available at: https://www.acs.org
/content/dam/acsorg/education/whatischemistry/landmarks
/alicehamilton/alice-hamilton-and-the-development-of-occupational
-medicine-commemorative-booklet.pdf.

114   **the two women became lifelong friends** Ibid. See also Ringenberg, *The
Education of Alice Hamilton,* 65.

114   **Hamilton opened a well-baby clinic** See Ginsberg, "Alice Hamilton and
the Development of Occupational Medicine."

114   **clear connection between working conditions** See Ringenberg, *The
Education of Alice Hamilton,* 51.

114   **regulations had already been in place** Ibid., 51, 60.

114   **The use of white phosphorus . . . caused "phossy jaw"** See U.S.
Department of Labor, "Industrial Poisons Used in the Manufacture of

Matches," *Bulletin of the United States Bureau of Labor Statistics,* no. 120, 1913. Available at: https://fraser.stlouisfed.org/title/bulletins-us-bureau-labor-statistics-62/industrial-poisons-used-manufacture-matches-3880.

115   **If the infection spread** See Alice Hamilton, "The Poisonous Occupations in Illinois." Excerpted from *Exploring the Dangerous Trades,* History Matters. Available at: https://historymatters.gmu.edu/d/105/.

115   **forced to live on a liquid diet** See Ringenberg, *The Education of Alice Hamilton,* 52–53.

115   **uncovered more than 150 cases of phossy jaw** Ibid., 55.

115   **Lead exposures were the culprit** See Gerald Markowitz and David Rosner, *Deceit and Denial: The Deadly Politics of Industrial Pollution* (Berkeley and Los Angeles: University of California Press, 2002), 96–102.

115   **of grisly deaths in mines or factories** See Ringenberg, *The Education of Alice Hamilton,* 51.

116   **thirty-five employees had been stricken with lead poisoning** See Hamilton, "The Poisonous Occupations in Illinois."

116   **if workers thought their jobs were too hazardous** See Ringenberg, *The Education of Alice Hamilton,* 52–53.

116   **accounted for their higher susceptibility** Ibid., 44–45.

116   **Hamilton took it upon herself** See Hamilton, *Exploring the Dangerous Trades,* 115–21.

116   **In 1910, she was appointed** See Ringenberg, *The Education of Alice Hamilton,* 54, 60.

116   **Her research into pollutants in Chicago's factories** See Barbara Sicherman, *Alice Hamilton: A Life in Letters* (Chicago: University of Illinois Press, 1984), 144–47.

117   **the basic techniques of public health** See Mark Aldrich, "History of Workplace Safety in the United States, 1880–1970," Economic History Association. Available at: https://eh.net/encyclopedia/history-of-workplace-safety-in-the-united-states-1880-1970/.

117   **in working-class neighborhoods** See Hamilton, *Exploring the Dangerous Trades,* 129. See also Ringenberg, *The Education of Alice Hamilton,* 67.

117   **how the severe injuries workers sustained** See Hamilton, *Exploring the Dangerous Trades,* 168–72.

117   **toxic metals that cause permanent disability** Ibid., 120.

117   **'Well, I suppose that is about the size of it'** Ibid.

118   **"was rife among the immigrants"** See Markowitz and Rosner, *Deceit and Denial,* 103–8.

118   **"to make sure of getting the healthiest men"** See Hamilton, *Exploring the Dangerous Trades,* 152.

118   **"a little thing like lead colic attracts no attention"** Ibid., 151, 152.

118   **"contribute all the money that their surgical and medical care costs"** Ibid., 152.

118   **plants produced shells and mines** See Elizabeth D. Schafer, *Exploding Danger: Women and Factory Work in World War I, Journal of American History,* vol. 77, no. 1 (June 1990): 125–46. Available at: https://doi.org/10.2307/2078649.

119   **which became poisonous death traps** See Hamilton, *Exploring the Dangerous Trades,* 184–85.

119   **"visit the plants I knew and pick up gossip"** Ibid., 184.

119   **locals called them "canaries"** See Debbie Nathan, "Working on the Bomb," *The Texas Observer,* July 27, 2007. Available at: https://www .texasobserver.org/working-on-the-bomb/.

119   **During a visit to the plant** See Hamilton, *Exploring the Dangerous Trades,* 184.

119   **Because a plant owner's mind is "fixed only on profits"** Ibid., 188–89.

119   **"such deaths as due to 'natural causes'"** Ibid., 189.

120   **making explosives that the factory's smokestacks pumped** Ibid., 188.

120   **she was able to identify the perpetrator** See Hamilton, *Exploring the Dangerous Trades,* 188.

120   **poisoning mainly occurs from contact** See R.A. Kehoe, "Occupational Poisoning in the Manufacture of TNT," *Public Health Reports,* vol. 34, no. 48 (November 29, 1919), 2701–6. Available at: https://www.ncbi .nlm.nih.gov/pmc/articles/PMC1995361/.

121   **bathe to wash off any TNT residue** Ibid., 195–96.

121   **"in this dark picture of a return to barbarism"** Ibid., 199.

121   **the best candidate, by far, was a woman** See "Alice Hamilton Becomes First Woman on Harvard Faculty," *Harvard Gazette,* September 6, 2021. Available at: https://news.harvard.edu/gazette/story/2021/09/alice -hamilton-broke-barriers-at-harvard/.

121   **she worked closely with FDR's labor secretary** See Kirstin Downey, *The Woman Behind the New Deal: The Life and Legacy of Frances Perkins* (New York: Anchor Books, 2009), 117–20.

121   **A kindred spirit, Perkins had been part** See William T. Moye, "BLS and Alice Hamilton: Pioneers in Industrial Health," *Monthly Labor Review,* June 1986, 27. Available at: https://www.bls.gov/opub/mlr/1986/06 /art4full.pdf.

122   **"knowing there was no help"** See David Brooks, "How the First Woman in the U.S. Cabinet Found Her Vocation," *Atlantic,* April 14, 2015. Available at: https://www.theatlantic.com/politics/archive/2015/04 /frances-perkins/390003/. See also Hilda L. Solis, "What the Triangle Shirtwaist Fire Means for Workers Now," *Washington Post,* March 18, 2011. Available at: https://www.washingtonpost.com/opinions/what-the-triangle -shirtwaist-fire-means-for-workers-now/2011/03/15/ABVAFIs_story.html.

122   **March 25, 1911, said Perkins** See Jane LaTour, *Sisters in the Brother- hoods: Working Women Organizing for Equality in New York City* (New York: Palgrace Macmillan, 2008), 25–28. See also Brooks, "How the First Woman in the U.S. Cabinet Found Her Vocation."

122   **the "Uprising of 20,000"** See Annelise Orleck, *Common Sense and a Little Fire: Women and Working-Class Politics in the United States, 1900– 1965* (University of North Carolina Press, 1995), 28–31. See also "Tri- angle Shirtwaist Fire," AFL-CIO. Available at: https://aflcio.org/about /history/labor-history-events/triangle-shirtwaist-fire.

123   **"Women often had their fingers punctured"** Author interview via Zoom with Robyn Muncy on January 26, 2023. See also Robyn Muncy, quoted in "The Triangle Fire: A Turning Point in Labor History," *NPR Weekend Edition,* March 23, 2011. Available at: https://www.npr.org/2011/03 /23/134755262/the-triangle-fire-a-turning-point-in-labor-history.

123 **joined the picket lines and recruited her socialite friends** See Daniel E. Bender, *Sweated Work, Weak Bodies: Anti-Sweatshop Campaigns and Languages of Labor* (New Brunswick, New Jersey: Rutgers University Press, 2004), 89–91.

123 **"Mink Brigades," a reference to the costly coats** See Ella Wagner, "Mink Brigade," National Park Service. Available at: https://www.nps.gov /people/mink-brigade.htm.

123 **"visible to the middle class"** See author interview with Richard Greenwald via Zoom, January 18, 2023. See also Richard Greenwald, quoted in "Triangle Fire," *American Experience*, PBS, aired January 30, 2018. Available at: https://www.pbs.org/wgbh/americanexperience/films /triangle/.

124 **the Wagner Act, which established** See "National Labor Relations Act (1935)," National Archives. Available at: https://www.archives.gov /milestone-documents/national-labor-relations-act.

124 **Schneiderman later served in Roosevelt's brain trust** See Rose Schneiderman, *All for One* (New York: Paul S. Eriksson, 1967). Available at: https://archive.org/details/allforone00schn.

125 **Perkins threw herself into the job** See Brooks, "How the First Woman in the U.S. Cabinet Found Her Vocation." See also Downey, *The Woman Behind the New Deal*, 168–72.

125 **But all that changed after he contracted polio** See Brooks, "How the First Woman in the U.S. Cabinet Found Her Vocation."

125 **one of the most consequential job interviews** Ibid. See Downey, *The Woman Behind the New Deal*, 197–99.

126 **sweatshops never really went away** See author interview with Richard Greenwald.

127 **Labor officials estimate that more than half** See Alexia Fernández Campbell, "Sweatshops in the US? 'Made in America' Label Doesn't Mean Much," *Atlantic*, May 22, 2017. Available at: https://www.theatlantic .com/business/archive/2017/05/sweatshops-in-the-us/527781/.

127 **violate health and safety regulations** See "The Garment Sector in the United States," Verité, October 2015. Available at: https://verite.org/wp -content/uploads/2023/10/GarmentSectorUS-WhitePaper-102215-Final .pdf.

128 **More than 1,100 people perished** See Sarah Labowitz and Dorothée Baumann-Pauly, "Beyond the Tip of the Iceberg," NYU Stern Center for Business and Human Rights, April 2015. Available at: https://bhr.stern .nyu.edu/wp-content/uploads/2024/02/beyond_the_tip_of_the_iceberg _report-1.pdf.

128 **no compensation for their life-altering injuries** See Dana Thomas, "Why Won't We Learn from the Survivors of the Rana Plaza Disaster?" *New York Times*, April 24, 2018. Available at: https://www.nytimes.com /2018/04/24/style/survivors-of-rana-plaza-disaster.html.

128 **"mass industrial homicide"** See Michael Safi and Dominic Rushe, "Rana Plaza, Five Years On: Safety of Workers Hangs in Balance in Bangladesh," *Guardian*, April 24, 2018. Available at: https://www.theguardian.com /global-development/2018/apr/24/bangladeshi-police-target-garment -workers-union-rana-plaza-five-years-on.

128   **"after a month of highly embarrassing media coverage"** See Thomas, "Why Won't We Learn?"

128   **more than 97,000 workplace hazards** Ibid.

128   **2018 study by the Center for Global Workers' Rights** Ibid.

128   **"Like the Triangle fire, Rana Plaza was a turning point"** See author interview with Annelise Orleck, January 19, 2023.

128   **operate under the regulatory radar in Bangladesh** See Thomas, "Why Won't We Learn?"

129   **unionization rates plummeted** See "Union Members Summary," U.S. Bureau of Labor Statistics, January 28, 2025. Available at: https://www .bls.gov/news.release/union2.nr0.htm.

129   **"Right to work" laws . . . were passed** See Jake Rosenfeld, *What Unions No Longer Do* (Harvard University Press, 2014), 101–5.

129   **was stocked with industry appointees** See Ian Kullgren, "Trump's NLRB Appointees Deliver for Business," POLITICO, January 11, 2019. Available at: https://www.politico.com/story/2019/01/11/nlrb-trump -appointees-1087115.

129   **(OSHA), was gutted, too** See Jordan Barab, "Trump's OSHA: No Standards, No Enforcement, No Problem," *On the Job Safety,* March 2, 2020. Available at: https://jordanbarab.com/confinedspace/2020/03 /02/trumps-osha-no-standards-no-enforcement-no-problem/.

129   **the number of people who die on the job** See "OSHA at 50: 50 Years of Workplace Safety and Health," Occupational Safety and Health Administration, U.S. Department of Labor, 2020. Available at: https://www.osha.gov /osha50.

130   **it would take 165 years to adequately police worksites** See Maryam Jameel and Joe Yerardi, "OSHA's Problematic Pandemic Performance," *Center for Public Integrity,* July 2, 2020. Available at: https://public integrity.org/health/coronavirus-and-inequality/osha-coronavirus -enforcement-failure/.

130   **the agency issued only one citation** See Rachel Leven, "OSHA Receives 20,000 COVID-19 Complaints but Only Issues One Citation," *Center for Public Integrity,* September 2, 2020. Available at: https://publicintegrity .org/health/coronavirus-and-inequality/osha-coronavirus-enforcement -failure/.

130   **"It's like I'm risking my life for a dollar"** See Annie Palmer, "Amazon Workers Speak Out After Employee Dies of COVID-19," *CNBC,* April 14, 2020. Available at: https://www.cnbc.com/2020/04/14/amazon -workers-speak-out-after-employee-dies-of-covid-19.html.

130   **severe shortages of personal protective equipment** See Christopher M. Bartels and Nicole Lurie, "The PPE Crisis Didn't Have to Happen," *Atlantic,* March 20, 2020. Available at: https://www.theatlantic.com /ideas/archive/2020/03/ppe-shortage-health-workers/608908/.

130   **The Trump White House's neglect** See Dan Diamond, "Inside America's Mask Meltdown," POLITICO, April 5, 2020. Available at: https://www .politico.com/news/2020/04/05/america-coronavirus-masks-shortage -166007.

131   **more than 3,600 health-care workers perished** See "Lost on the Frontline," *Guardian* and *Kaiser Health News,* April 2021. Available at:

https://www.theguardian.com/us-news/ng-interactive/2020/aug/11
/lost-on-the-frontline-covid-19-coronavirus-us-healthcare-workers-deaths
-database.

131 **"The total disregard for our safety"** See Chris Hamby, "Doctors and
Nurses Say Shortage of Protective Gear Is Putting Their Lives at Risk,"
New York Times, July 8, 2020. Available at: https://www.nytimes.com
/2020/07/08/us/hospitals-coronavirus-ppe.html.

132 **passed or introduced legislation** See Nina Lakhani, "US States Relax
Child Labor Laws as Violations Rise," *Guardian,* May 26, 2023. Available
at: https://www.theguardian.com/us-news/2023/may/26/us-child-labor
-laws-rollbacks-violations.

132 **more than a 50 percent increase in cases** See Lauren Kaori Gurley,
"America's Exploding Child Labor Crisis," *Washington Post,* July 25, 2023.
Available at: https://www.washingtonpost.com/business/2023/07/25
/child-labor-violations-exploding/.

132 **a sixteen-year-old boy died on the job** See Laura Strickler and Didi
Martinez, "16-Year-Old Dies in Accident at a Mississippi Poultry Plant,"
NBC News, July 18, 2023. Available at: https://www.nbcnews.com/news
/16-year-old-boy-dies-accident-mississippi-poultry-plant-rcna94963.

132 **"an event of overwhelming terror and pain"** See Caitlin Flanagan, "The
Kids Working in Factories Aren't Alright," *Atlantic,* August 2023. Available at: https://www.theatlantic.com/magazine/archive/2023/08/child
-labor-us-factories/674785/.

133 **the air was filled with the pulverized remains** See Philip J. Landrigan et
al., "The Health Impact of 9/11: A Comprehensive Review," *Mount Sinai
Journal of Medicine,* September 2008. Available at: https://www.ncbi.nlm
.nih.gov/pmc/articles/PMC2553156/.

133 **"Anyone who was caught in that cloud"** See author interview with
Dr. Philip Landrigan via Zoom, February 16, 2023. See also Ed Pilking-
ton, "9/11's Dust Cloud Still a Killer," *Guardian,* September 5, 2011.
Available at: https://www.theguardian.com/world/2011/sep/05/911
-dust-cloud-health-fears.

134 **the highly carcinogenic chemical benzene** See "First Long-Term Study of
World Trade Center Rescue and Recovery Workers Shows Widespread
Health Problems Ten Years After 9-11," Mount Sinai, September 6, 2011.
Available at: https://www.mountsinai.org/about/newsroom/2011/first
-longterm-study-of-world-trade-center-rescue-and-recovery-workers-shows
-widespread-health-problems-ten-years-after-911.

134 **that causes burns in the lining of the throat** See Caroline Bankoff,
"What We Know About How 9/11 Has Affected New Yorkers' Health,
15 Years Later," *Intelligencer,* September 10, 2016. Available at: https://
nymag.com/intelligencer/2016/09/15-years-later-how-has-9-11-affected
-new-yorkers-health.html.

134 **EPA administrator Christine Todd Whitman** See Eric Lipton, "E.P.A.
Misled the Public on 9/11 Pollution," *New York Times,* August 23, 2003.
Available at: https://www.nytimes.com/2003/08/23/nyregion/epa
-misled-public-on-9-11-pollution-report-says.html.

135 **"We would've had fewer illnesses"** See author interview with Dr. Philip
Landrigan.

135   **"Within forty-eight hours, we reached out to all the unions"** Ibid. See also Philip Landrigan, "The Mount Sinai Response to 9/11," *Mount Sinai Health System,* 2021. Available at: https://www.mountsinai.org/about /newsroom/2021/mount-sinais-legacy-9-11-legacy.

135   **By the twentieth anniversary of the attacks** See Benjamin Ryan, "The Long-Term Health Toll of 9/11," *NBC News,* September 9, 2021. Available at: https://www.nbcnews.com/health/health-news/long-term -health-toll-9-11-rcna1921.

135   **112,000 people are members of the program** See "Health Effects of 9/11 Still Plague Responders and Survivors," *Scientific American,* September 10, 2021. Available at: https://www.scientificamerican.com/article /health-effects-of-9-11-still-plague-responders-and-survivors/.

136   **(23,000) have at least one type of cancer** See World Trade Center Health Program, "Program Statistics," Centers for Disease Control and Prevention (CDC), updated September 4, 2025. Available at: https:// www.cdc.gov/wtc/ataglance.html.

136   **the James Zadroga 9/11 Health and Compensation Act** See Larry Abramson, "Obama Signs 9/11 Health Bill into Law," NPR, January 2, 2011. Available at: https://www.npr.org/2011/01/02/132585578 /obama-signs-9-11-health-bill-into-law.

136   **"Three nights in a row, Jon Stewart"** See Jordan Freiman, "How Jon Stewart Helped Pass the 9/11 First Responders Bill," *CBS News,* July 29, 2019. Available at: https://www.cbsnews.com/news/jon-stewart-9-11 -victims-compensation-fund-how-he-helped-pass-bill/.

CHAPTER SIX: THE CDC: A CHECKERED HISTORY

137   **he was taking the reins of a "demoralized"** See Marlene Cimons, "To Heal a Nation," *Los Angeles Times,* March 1, 1994. Available at: https:// www.latimes.com/archives/la-xpm-1994-03-01-vw-28674-story.html.

137   **The CDC had been sharply politicized** Ibid.

138   **David Satcher was committed** Ibid.

138   **The bearded and bespectacled physician** See Vincent Coppola, "A Plague of Politics," *Atlanta,* May 1, 1994. Available at: https://www.atlanta magazine.com/great-reads/a-plague-of-politics/.

138   **when he arrived in Atlanta at CDC headquarters** See Cimons, "To Heal a Nation."

138   **Black kids with illnesses like mine** See David Satcher, *My Quest for Health Equity* (Baltimore: Johns Hopkins University Press, 2020), 4–5.

138   **had been arrested and jailed** Ibid., 22.

138   **chaired the family medicine department** See Anne Johnson, "Satcher, David 1941—," Encyclopedia.com, updated June 11, 2018. Available at: https://www.encyclopedia.com/people/history/us-history-biographies /david-satcher.

138   **he was called upon to take over Meharry Medical College** See Peter Applebome, "Conversations/David Satcher; C.D.C.'s New Chief Worries as Much About Bullets as About Bacteria," *New York Times,* September 26, 1993. Available at: https://www.nytimes.com/1993/09/26/weekinreview /conversations-david-satcher-cdc-s-new-chief-worries-much-about-bullets -about.html. See also Satcher, *My Quest for Health Equity,* 29–31.

139 **This was especially the case during the Reagan years** See Coppola, "A Plague of Politics."

139 **President Reagan never even mentioned** See Karen Tumulty, "Nancy Reagan's Real Role in the AIDS Crisis," *Atlantic,* April 12, 2021. Available at: https://www.theatlantic.com/politics/archive/2021/04/full-story -nancy-reagan-and-aids-crisis/618552/.

139 **any research that had a whiff of sexuality** See Coppola, "A Plague of Politics." See also Tumulty, "Nancy Reagan's Real Role in the AIDS Crisis."

139 **We're talking about preventing AIDS** See Coppola, "A Plague of Politics."

139 **the casualties of these cumulative failures** See U.S. Centers for Disease Control and Prevention (CDC), "HIV and AIDS—United States, 1981–2000," *Morbidity and Mortality Weekly Report* 50, no. 21 (June 1, 2001): 430–34. Available at: https://www.cdc.gov/mmwr/preview /mmwrhtml/mm5021a2.htm. See also Rachel Nall and Ashley Williams, "The History of HIV and AIDS in the United States," updated July 7, 2025. Available at: https://www.healthline.com/health/hiv-aids/history.

140 **By 1984, AIDS had claimed more than two thousand lives** See U.S. Centers for Disease Control and Prevention (CDC), "Update: Acquired Immunodeficiency Syndrome (AIDS)—United States," *Morbidity and Mortality Weekly Report* 33, no. 24 (June 22, 1984): 337–39. Available at: https://www.cdc.gov/mmwr/preview/mmwrhtml/00000356.htm.

140 **The gay community was under siege** See United Press International, "Vigils Held for AIDS Victims," *New York Times,* October 9, 1983. Available at: https://www.nytimes.com/1983/10/09/us/vigils-held-for -aids-victims.html.

140 **three times the rate among white Americans** See National Center for HIV, STD, and TB Prevention, "On the Front Lines: Fighting HIV/AIDS in African-American Communities," CDC Stacks, August 1999, 3, 10. Available at: https://stacks.cdc.gov/view/cdc/42659.

140 **"an astonishing 35 percent believed AIDS was a form of genocide"** See "The AIDS 'Plot' Against Blacks," *New York Times,* May 12, 1992. Available at: https://www.nytimes.com/1992/05/12/opinion/the-aids -plot-against-blacks.html.

141 **the CDC's historic role in combating infectious diseases** See U.S. Centers for Disease Control and Prevention, "CDC's 60th Anniversary: Director's Perspective—David Satcher, M.D., Ph.D., 1993–1998," *Morbidity and Mortality Weekly Report* 56, no. 23 (June 15, 2007): 579–82. Available at: https://www.cdc.gov/mmwr/preview/mmwrhtml /mm5623a3.htm.

141 **aggressive plans that would go back to public health's roots** Ibid.

141 **"today most of the incentives"** See Applebome, "Conversations/David Satcher."

141 **Satcher was also keenly aware** See Coppola, "A Plague of Politics."

141 **spearheaded the adoption of broad community-based initiatives** See National Center for HIV, STD, and TB Prevention, "On the Front Lines: Fighting HIV/AIDS in African-American Communities," 4, 6.

141 **especially Black churches** See Applebome, "Conversations/David Satcher."

142   **immunizations, and the self-destructive consequences** See "CDC's 60th Anniversary."

142   **"As early as you can get to people in terms of diet"** See Associated Press, "U.S. Seeks New Partners to Help Prevent Disease," *New York Times*, September 12, 1993. Available at: https://www.nytimes.com/1993/09/12/us/us-seeks-new-partners-to-help-prevent-disease.html.

142   **HIV when there were relatively few infections** See "On the Front Lines: Fighting HIV/AIDS in African-American Communities," 5.

143   **The CDC partnered with local groups** Ibid., 12–18.

143   **"Increasingly, it is becoming an epidemic of color"** Ibid., 1.

143   **Satcher failed to make progress on . . . gun violence** See Coppola, "A Plague of Politics."

143   **"If it's not a public health problem"** See Applebome, "Conversations /David Satcher."

143   **Boots on the ground and data collection** See Maryn McKenna, *Beating Back the Devil* (New York: Free Press, 2004), 20.

144   **Langmuir institutionalized for the nation** See Donna F. Stroup and Jack C. Smith, "Statistical Methods in Public Health: The Influence of Alexander D. Langmuir," *American Journal of Epidemiology* 144, supplement no. 8 (October 15, 1996): S29–33. Available at: https://doi.org/10.1093/aje/144.Supplement_8.S29.

144   **hundreds of military bases and industrial installations** See McKenna, *Beating Back the Devil*, 10–11.

144   **the Office of Malaria Control in War Areas** See Elizabeth W. Etheridge, *Sentinel for Health: A History of the Centers for Disease Control* (University of California Press, 1992), 4.

144   **the newly formed agency would handle all bug-borne illnesses** See McKenna, *Beating Back the Devil*, 10–12. See also Etheridge, *Sentinel for Health*, 14–17.

144   **A tall man with a deep voice and a razor-sharp intellect** See Myron G. Schultz and William Schaffner, "Alexander Duncan Langmuir," *Emerging Infectious Diseases* 21, no. 9 (September 2015): 1635–37. Available at: https://wwwnc.cdc.gov/eid/article/21/9/14-1445_article.

144   **the CDC had plenty of engineers** See Lawrence K. Altman, "Alexander Langmuir Dies at 83; Helped Start U.S. Disease Centers," *New York Times*, November 24, 1993. Available at: https://www.nytimes.com/1993/11/24/obituaries/alexander-langmuir-dies-at-83-helped-start-us-disease-centers.html.

145   **There was a dearth of epidemiologists** See McKenna, *Beating Back the Devil*, 12–13.

145   **a medical CIA comprised of highly trained disease detectives** Ibid., 15–17.

145   **Langmuir advocated what he called "shoe leather epidemiology"** See Altman, "Alexander Langmuir Dies at 83."

145   **He set up a network that connected the CDC** See Stroup and Smith, "Statistical Methods in Public Health."

145   **The data were then analyzed** See McKenna, *Beating Back the Devil*, 17–19.

145   **"When we saw a blip, our mission was to jump on an airplane"** See author interview with Dr. Philip Landrigan.

146   **On April 12, 1955, the tenth anniversary** See Michael E. Ruane, "The Tainted Polio Vaccine that Sickened and Fatally Paralyzed Children in 1955," *Washington Post*, April 14, 2020. Available at: https://www .washingtonpost.com/history/2020/04/14/cutter-polio-vaccine -paralyzed-children-coronavirus/.

146   **in 1952, the nation had experienced the worst polio outbreak** See Etheridge, *Sentinel for Health*, 72.

146   **21,000 were paralyzed, and 3,145 died** See Ruane, "The Tainted Polio Vaccine."

146   **polio vaccine, which had been tested** See Etheridge, *Sentinel for Health*, 71.

146   **Jonas Salk, the polio vaccine inventor** See Ruane, "The Tainted Polio Vaccine."

146   **But in less than two weeks** See Etheridge, *Sentinel for Health*, 72.

146   **On April 25, the CDC received a report** See Neal Nathanson and E. Russell Alexander, "Infectious Disease Epidemiology," *American Journal of Epidemiology* 144, supplement no. 8 (October 15, 1996): S34–38. Available at: https://doi.org/10.1093/aje/144.Supplement_8.S34.

146   **An EIS officer in Napa, California, reported another** See Etheridge, *Sentinel for Health*, 73.

146   **Before that day's end, a total of six cases were identified** Ibid., 74.

146   **EIS officers had interviewed dozens of people** See Ruane, "The Tainted Polio Vaccine."

146   **the vaccines had all come from the Cutter Laboratories** See Etheridge, *Sentinel for Health*, 74.

147   **Dr. Malcolm Merrill . . . canceled the Los Angeles vaccination program** Ibid., 74–75.

147   **Langmuir proposed creating a nationwide polio surveillance network** Ibid., 75–76.

147   **As daily case reports came in over the next five weeks** Ibid., 76.

147   **a bad batch of Cutter vaccines was to blame** See Nathanson and Alexander, "Infectious Disease Epidemiology."

147   **Cutter Laboratories vaccines contained polio viruses** See Etheridge, *Sentinel for Health*, 78.

147   **which ultimately caused ten deaths** See Michael Fitzpatrick, "The Cutter Incident: How America's First Polio Vaccine Led to a Growing Vaccine Crisis," *Journal of the Royal Society of Medicine* 99, no. 3 (March 2006): 156. Available at: https://pmc.ncbi.nlm.nih.gov/articles/PMC1383764/.

147   **The Cutter incident was an inflection point** See Etheridge, *Sentinel for Health*, 79.

148   **there was no telling how many people were already infected** See Frederic E. Shaw et al., "A History of MMWR," *Morbidity and Mortality Weekly Report* 60, no. 4 (October 7, 2011): 7–14. Available at: https:// www.cdc.gov/mmwr/preview/mmwrhtml/su6004a3.htm.

148   **The public health implications were staggering** See David Thorsén, "The First Report—June 5, 1981," *Face of AIDS Film Archive*, Karolinska Institutet University Library, May 18, 2021. Available at: https:// faceofaids.ki.se/theme/MMWR%E2%80%93June-5-1981.

149   **Like so many EIS investigations** See "Global Team Profile: Dr. Phil Landrigan a Champion for Children," Pure Earth, January 7, 2010.

Available at: https://www.pureearth.org/global-team-profile-2/. See also author interview with Dr. Philip Landrigan.

149   **the company had belched out more than 1,000 tons of lead** See Robert A. Wright, "Polluted Town Doesn't Want to Move," *New York Times,* May 17, 1972. Available at: https://www.nytimes.com/1972/05 /17/archives/polluted-town-doesnt-want-to-move.html. See also Lauren Villagran, "Before Flint, Before East Chicago, There Was Smeltertown," NRDC, November 29, 2016. Available at: https://www.nrdc.org/stories /flint-east-chicago-there-was-smeltertown. See also Thomas Matte and Henry Falk, "Human Lead Absorption—Texas," *Morbidity and Mortality Weekly Report* 22 (December 8, 1973): 405–7. Available at: https://www .cdc.gov/mmwr/preview/mmwrhtml/lmrk095.htm.

149   **"Rosenblum wanted the EIS to determine"** See author interview with Dr. Philip Landrigan.

150   **"there was a common source of the lead poisoning outbreak"** See Villagran, "Before Flint."

150   **Landrigan did a large study in 1972** See Philip J. Landrigan et al., "Epidemic Lead Absorption Near an Ore Smelter: The Role of Particulate Lead," *New England Journal of Medicine* 292, no. 3 (January 16, 1975): 123–29. Available at: https://www.nejm.org/doi/full/10.1056 /NEJM197501162920302.

150   **even small levels of lead had a dramatic impact** See Herbert L. Needleman et al., "Deficits in Psychologic and Classroom Performance of Children with Elevated Dentine Lead Levels," *New England Journal of Medicine* 300, no. 13 (March 29, 1979): 689–95. Available at: https:// www.nejm.org/doi/full/10.1056/NEJM197903293001301.

150   **a discovery that helped propel the phaseout** See "Global Team Profile: Dr. Phil Landrigan a Champion for Children."

152   **"I shared their excitement around doing the work"** See author interview with Dr. Diane Rowley via Zoom, March 1, 2023.

152   **with 9.7 deaths per thousand births** See Korbin Liu et al., "International Infant Mortality Rankings: A Look Behind the Numbers," *Health Care Finance Review* 13, no. 4 (Summer 1992): 105–18. Available at: https:// pmc.ncbi.nlm.nih.gov/articles/PMC4193257/.

152   **But in a revolutionary 1992 study** See Kenneth C. Schoendorf et al., "Mortality Among Infants of Black as Compared with White College-Educated Parents," *New England Journal of Medicine* 326, no. 23 (June 4, 1992): 1522–26. Available at: https://doi.org/10.1056/NEJM1992 06043262303.

153   **Black babies were twice as likely to die** See Claire Cain Miller, Sarah Kliff, and Larry Buchanan, "Childbirth Is Deadlier for Black Families Even When They're Rich, Expansive Study Finds," *New York Times,* February 12, 2023. Available at: https://www.nytimes.com/interactive/2023 /02/12/upshot/child-maternal-mortality-rich-poor.html.

153   **Agent Orange, the toxic defoliant used** See Paula Yost, "Agent Orange Study Called Botched or Rigged," *Washington Post,* July 11, 1989. Available at: https://www.washingtonpost.com/archive/politics/1989 /07/12/agent-orange-study-called-botched-or-rigged/6e34800b-0901 -4b70-ad89-5468df4332af/.

154 **Even an abortion study from the 1960s** See Victor Cohn, "Never-Delivered U.S. Report Cites Abortion Benefits," *Washington Post,* July 11, 1981. Available at: https://www.washingtonpost.com/archive/politics /1981/07/12/never-delivered-us-report-cites-abortion-benefits /be64e6c5-840b-4aa5-82c8-01369aeaf02a/.

154 **in the interim, 1,470 children died** See "Delay on Aspirin Warning Label Cost Children's Lives, Study Says," *New York Times,* October 23, 1992. Available at: https://www.nytimes.com/1992/10/23/us/delay-on -aspirin-warning-label-cost-children-s-lives-study-says.html.

154 **Many alarms had been raised over four decades** See Harrison Smith, "Bill Jenkins, Epidemiologist Who Tried to End Tuskegee Syphilis Study, Dies at 73," *Washington Post,* February 27, 2019. Available at: https:// www.washingtonpost.com/local/obituaries/bill-jenkins-epidemiologist -who-tried-to-end-tuskegee-syphilis-study-dies-at-73/2019/02/27 /2319e142-3aa2-11e9-a06c-3ec8ed509d15_story.html.

155 **who was arrested after protesting the whites-only policies** Ibid.

155 **He was forced to travel to Washington, D.C.** See author interview with Dr. Diane Rowley.

155 **alerted him about an ongoing experiment** Ibid.

155 **even the sketchy outlines of the research** See Smith, "Bill Jenkins Dies at 73." See also Susan M. Reverby, "Bill Carter Jenkins (1945–2019)," *Nature* 567, no. 462 (March 18, 2019). Available at: https://www.nature .com/articles/d41586-019-00900-9.

155 **Or that they could inadvertently pass it on** See DeNeen L. Brown, " 'You've Got Bad Blood': The Horror of the Tuskegee Syphilis Experi- ment," *Washington Post,* May 16, 2017. Available at: https://www .washingtonpost.com/news/retropolis/wp/2017/05/16/youve-got-bad -blood-the-horror-of-the-tuskegee-syphilis-experiment/.

156 **they stopped authorities from giving them antibiotics** See Brown, " 'You've Got Bad Blood.' "

156 **he later learned that his supervisor's hands weren't clean** See Smith, "Bill Jenkins Dies at 73." See also Adam Marcus, "William Carter Jenkins," *Lancet* 393, no. 10180 (April 13, 2019): 1498. Available at: https://www .thelancet.com/journals/lancet/article/PIIS0140-6736%2819%2930804 -9/fulltext.

156 **Their concerns were ignored until July of 1972** See Jean Heller, "AP Was There: Black Men Untreated in Tuskegee Syphilis Study," Associated Press, May 10, 2017. Available at: https://apnews.com/article/business -science-health-race-and-ethnicity-syphilis-e9dd07eaa4e74052878a68132c d3803a.

157 **All of this was probably preventable** See Brown, " 'You've Got Bad Blood.' " See also Heller, "AP Was There."

157 **The Tuskegee Health Benefit Program** See Brown, " 'You've Got Bad Blood.' "

157 **"I try to give them the care"** See Katharine Q. Seelye, "Bill Jenkins, Who Tried to Halt Tuskegee Syphilis Study, Dies at 73," *New York Times,* February 25, 2019. Available at: https://www.nytimes.com/2019/02/25 /obituaries/bill-jenkins-dead.html.

157 **He devoted much of his career** See Marcus, "William Carter Jenkins."

157   **When the AIDS epidemic began** See Doug Criss and Madeline Hol-
        combe, "Bill Jenkins, Who Helped End the Infamous Tuskegee Syphilis
        Study, Has Died at Age 73," CNN, February 28, 2019. Available at:
        https://www.cnn.com/2019/02/27/health/bill-jenkins-obit-trnd.

157   **he directed the CDC's first community-based funding program** See
        Smith, "Bill Jenkins Dies at 73."

157   **He believed that increasing the numbers of minorities** See Marcus,
        "William Carter Jenkins."

157   **half of all Black epidemiologists could track their careers** See author
        interview with Dr. Bryan Lindsey via Zoom, February 28, 2023. See also
        Tara Haelle, "'Many Tuskegees' Occur Daily in the U.S.," Association of
        Health Care Journalists, August 8, 2022. Available at: https://health
        journalism.org/blog/2022/08/many-tuskegees-occur-daily-in-the-u-s/.

158   **Dr. Cheryl Blackmore Prince, who was a CDC epidemiologist** See author
        interview with Dr. Cheryl Blackmore Prince via Zoom, February 28, 2023.

159   **"I've worked with these men"** Ibid.

159   **"finally say on behalf of the American people"** See Brown, "'You've
        Got Bad Blood.'"

160   **Yet many are unfamiliar with the gruesome specifics** See Melba
        Newsome, "We Learned the Wrong Lessons from the Tuskegee 'Experi-
        ment,'" *Scientific American,* March 31, 2021. Available at: https://www
        .scientificamerican.com/article/we-learned-the-wrong-lessons-from-the
        -tuskegee-experiment/.

160   **"The numbers in the U.S. are in line, not with our peer nations"** See
        Isabel Wilkerson, "From Jan. 6 to Tyre Nichols, American Life Is Still
        Defined by Caste," *Time,* February 2, 2023. Available at: https://time
        .com/6252144/american-life-caste-isabel-wilkerson/.

CHAPTER SEVEN: THE BURNING BED: WOMEN ARE NOT SAFE

161   **pediatric chief resident** See Amanda D'Ambrosio, "Black Doctor Dies
        After Giving Birth, Underscoring Maternal Mortality Crisis," *MedPage
        Today,* November 2, 2020. Available at: https://www.medpagetoday.com
        /obgyn/pregnancy/89462. See also author interview with Anthony
        Wallace via Zoom, April 12, 2023.

161   **Anthony was a special education teacher** See Nikesha Elise Williams,
        "This Father Had to Turn His Pain into Purpose After Losing His Wife in
        Childbirth," SheKnows, February 16, 2023. Available at: https://www
        .sheknows.com/health-and-wellness/articles/2553864/father-black
        -maternal-mortality-advocate/.

161   **"beloved" "warrior"** See Joelle Goldstein, "'Beloved' Pediatrics Doctor
        Dies from Postpartum Complications After Giving Birth to First Child,"
        People, November 5, 2020. Available at: https://people.com/human
        -interest/indiana-doctor-dies-from-postpartum-complications-after-giving
        -birth-first-child/.

163   **Black patients do better on virtually every metric** See Brad N. Green-
        wood et al., "Physician-Patient Racial Concordance and Disparities in
        Birthing Mortality for Newborns," *Proceedings of the National Academy of
        Sciences* 117, no. 35 (September 1, 2020): 21194–200. Available at:
        https://www.pnas.org/doi/pdf/10.1073/pnas.1913405117.

163   **one groundbreaking 2023 study** See Snyder et al., "Black Representation
        in the Primary Care Physician Workforce."

164   **about 1,200 women who die every year** See Donna L. Hoyert, "Maternal
        Mortality Rates in the United States, 2021," National Center for Health
        Statistics, CDC, 2021. Available at: https://www.cdc.gov/nchs/data/hestat
        /maternal-mortality/2021/maternal-mortality-rates-2021.htm.

164   **nearly three times the rate of white women** Ibid.

164   **Maternal mortality rates of the highest-earning Black mothers** See
        Miller, Kliff, and Buchanan, "Childbirth Is Deadlier for Black Families."

164   **over three times the rate of maternal mortality** See Munira Z. Gunja
        et al., "U.S. Health Care from a Global Perspective, 2022," Common-
        wealth Fund, January 31, 2023. Available at: https://www
        .commonwealthfund.org/publications/issue-briefs/2023/jan/us-health
        -care-global-perspective-2022.

165   **"But the deaths are the tip of the iceberg"** Author interview with
        Dr. Jeffrey Gould, April 27, 2023.

165   **severe maternal morbidity** See John A. Ozimek et al., "Opportunities
        for Improvement in Care Among Women with Severe Maternal Morbid-
        ity," *American Journal of Obstetrics and Gynecology* 215, no. 4 (Octo-
        ber 2016): 509.e1–6. Available at: https://pubmed.ncbi.nlm.nih.gov
        /27210068/.

165   **up to four out of five pregnancy-related deaths** See "Four in 5
        Pregnancy-Related Deaths in the U.S. Are Preventable," CDC Archive,
        September 19, 2022. Available at: https://archive.cdc.gov/#
        /details?url=https://www.cdc.gov/media/releases/2022/p0919
        -pregnancy-related-deaths.html.

165   **more dangerous for a woman to give birth** See "Maternal Mortality
        Rate by Country 2025," World Population Review. Available at: https://
        worldpopulationreview.com/country-rankings/maternal-mortality-rate-by
        -country.

166   **"Addressing the women's health gap"** See "Closing the Women's Health
        Gap: A $1 Trillion Opportunity to Improve Lives and Economies," World
        Economic Forum in collaboration with the McKinsey Health Institute,
        January 17, 2024. Available at: https://www.mckinsey.com/~/media
        /mckinsey/mckinsey%20health%20institute/our%20insights/closing
        %20the%20womens%20health%20gap%20a%201%20trillion%20dollar
        %20opportunity%20to%20improve%20lives%20and%20economies/closing
        -the-womens-health-gap-report.pdf.

166   **The Laws of Chastisement allowed men to discipline their wives** See
        Henry Ansgar Kelly, " 'Rule of Thumb' and the Folklaw of the Husband's
        Stick," *Journal of Legal Education* 44, no. 3 (September 1994): 341–65.
        Available at: https://www.jstor.org/stable/42893341.

167   **spend a quarter of their lives in poor health** See "Closing the Women's
        Health Gap."

167   **higher rates of debilitating headaches** Ibid.

169   **children exposed to abuse** See "About Adverse Childhood Experiences,"
        CDC, October 8, 2024. Available at: https://www.cdc.gov/aces/about
        /index.html.

169   **finally, at long last, get our collective attention** See Anna Boots, " 'The

Burning Bed' Recalls the Case that Changed How Law Enforcement Treats Domestic Violence," *New Yorker,* July 9, 2020. Available at: https://www.newyorker.com/culture/video-dept/the-burning-bed-recalls-the-case-that-changed-how-law-enforcement-treats-domestic-violence.

170   **Hughes was acquitted on a plea of temporary insanity** Ibid.

170   **plunged by about 67 percent** See Claire Goudreau, "Looking Back at the Violence Against Women Act After 30 Years of Protection," Hub, Johns Hopkins University, September 27, 2024. Available at: https://hub.jhu.edu/2024/09/27/violence-against-women-act-30th-anniversary/.

170   **fifty women . . . every month** See Alisa Roth, "An Epidemic of Violence We Never Discuss," *New York Times,* June 7, 2019. Available at: https://www.nytimes.com/2019/06/07/books/review/rachel-louise-snyder-no-visible-bruises.html.

170   **About one in three American women** See "Intimate Partner Violence," American College of Obstetricians and Gynecologists. Available at: https://www.acog.org/topics/intimate-partner-violence.

171   **more than 80 percent of women who are homeless with children** See "Domestic Violence and Homelessness: Statistics (2016)," Administration for Children and Families, 2016. Available at: https://acf.gov/ofvps/fact-sheet/domestic-violence-and-homelessness-statistics-2016.

171   **80 percent of hostage situations** See Roth, "An Epidemic of Violence We Never Discuss."

171   **one in ten said they were victims of domestic violence** See A.E. Bonomi et al., "Ascertainment of intimate partner violence using two abuse measurement frameworks," *Injury Prevention* 12, no. 2 (April 2006): 121–24. Available at: https://pubmed.ncbi.nlm.nih.gov/16595428/.

171   **Mark Fuller was a federal judge** See Margaret Talbot, "Matters of Privacy," *New Yorker,* September 29, 2014. Available at: https://www.newyorker.com/podcast/comment/matters-of-privacy.

172   **In America three women are murdered** See "When Men Murder Women," Violence Policy Center, October 2020. Available at: https://vpc.org/when-men-murder-women/.

172   **male partners are responsible for the deaths** Ibid.

172   **Leaving is often not a viable option** See Jana Kasperkevic, "Private Violence: Up to 75% of Abused Women Who Are Murdered Are Killed After They Leave Their Partners," *Guardian,* October 20, 2014. Available at: https://www.theguardian.com/money/us-money-blog/2014/oct/20/domestic-private-violence-women-men-abuse-hbo-ray-rice.

172   **John Snowling . . . went to a bar and restaurant** See Nathan Solis et al., "What We Know About Cook's Corner Mass Shooter John Snowling," *Los Angeles Times,* August 24, 2023. Available at: https://www.latimes.com/california/story/2023-08-24/cooks-corner-shooting-suspect-john-snowling-worked-for-decades-for-ventura-police-department.

172   **Thomia Hunter was sentenced to life in prison** See Boots, " 'The Burning Bed.' "

173   **homicide is a leading cause of death** See Shaina Goodman, "Intimate Partner Violence Endangers Pregnant People and Their Infants," National Partnership for Women & Families, May 2021. Available at: https://nationalpartnership.org/report/intimate-partner-violence/.

173   **She was only twelve years old** See Charlotte Alter, "She Wasn't Able to
           Get an Abortion. Now She's a Mom. Soon She'll Start 7th Grade," *Time*,
           August 14, 2023. Available at: https://time.com/6303701/a-rape-in
           -mississippi/.

174   **nineteen states across the nation** See Allison McCann and Amy Schoen-
           feld Walker, "Tracking Abortion Laws Across the Country," *New York
           Times*, updated September 8, 2025. Available at: https://www.nytimes
           .com/interactive/2024/us/abortion-laws-roe-v-wade.html.

174   **Half the counties in rural Mississippi** See "Where You Live Matters:
           Maternity Care Access in Mississippi," March of Dimes, 2023. Available at:
           https://www.marchofdimes.org/peristats/reports/mississippi/maternity
           -care-deserts.

174   **medical students . . . don't want to practice** See Andrea González-
           Ramírez, "How *Dobbs* Upended Med Students' Futures," *New York*,
           March 17, 2023. Available at: https://www.thecut.com/2023/03/how
           -dobbs-upended-medical-students-futures.html.

174   **States with abortion bans have the weakest social services** See Emily
           Badger et al., "States with Abortion Bans Are Among Least Supportive for
           Mothers and Children," *New York Times*, July 28, 2022. Available at:
           https://www.nytimes.com/2022/07/28/upshot/abortion-bans-states
           -social-services.html.

175   **tolerates Black women dying in childbirth** See Nina Martin and Renee
           Montagne, "Black Mothers Keep Dying After Giving Birth. Shalon Irving's
           Story Explains Why," NPR, December 7, 2017. Available at: https://www
           .npr.org/2017/12/07/568948782/black-mothers-keep-dying-after
           -giving-birth-shalon-irvings-story-explains-why.

175   **cited a seventeenth-century English jurist** See Ken Armstrong, "Draft
           Overturning Roe v. Wade Quotes Infamous Witch Trial Judge with
           Long-Discredited Ideas on Rape," ProPublica, May 6, 2022. Available at:
           https://www.propublica.org/article/abortion-roe-wade-alito-scotus-hale.

175   **thousands of criminal incidents** See "National Abortion Federation
           Releases 2021 Violence & Disruption Report," National Abortion
           Federation, June 24, 2022. Available at: https://prochoice.org/national
           -abortion-federation-releases-2021-violence-disruption-report/.

176   **"worse than watching people die in a war"** See Alex Traub, "Dr. LeRoy
           Carhart, Fierce Defender of Abortion Rights, Dies at 81," *New York Times*,
           April 30, 2023. Available at: https://www.nytimes.com/2023/04/30
           /obituaries/dr-leroy-carhart-fierce-defender-of-abortion-rights-dies-at-81
           .html.

176   **"For me, the struggles for reproductive rights for women"** See
           Kenneth Edelin, *Broken Justice: A True Story of Race, Sex and Revenge in a
           Boston Courtroom* (Pondview Press, 2008), x.

177   **watching his mother die** See Emily Langer, "Kenneth C. Edelin, Physi-
           cian in Noted Abortion Case, Dies at 74," *Washington Post*, January 1,
           2014. Available at: https://www.washingtonpost.com/national/kenneth-c
           -edelin-physician-in-noted-abortion-case-dies-at-74/2014/01/01
           /45adf9d6-723a-11e3-8b3f-b1666705ca3b_story.html. See also Edelin,
           Broken Justice, 1. See also author interview with Barbara Edelin via Zoom,
           September 1, 2023.

177   **his grandmother had had an illegal abortion** See Langer, "Kenneth C. Edelin Dies at 74."

177   **Lysol, the strong, corrosive disinfectant** See Caitlin Flanagan, "The Dishonesty of the Abortion Debate," *Atlantic*, December 2019. Available at: https://www.theatlantic.com/magazine/archive/2019/12/the-things -we-cant-face/600769/.

177   **between 200,000 and 1.2 million illicit abortions** See Rachel Benson Gold, "Lessons from Before Roe: Will Past Be Prologue?" *Guttmacher Policy Review* 6, no. 1 (March 2003). Available at: https://www .guttmacher.org/gpr/2003/03/lessons-roe-will-past-be-prologue.

178   **more than 60 percent of the desperate women** See Flanagan, "The Dishonesty of the Abortion Debate."

178   **In 1965, there were 235 abortion-related deaths nationwide** See Cohn, "Never-Delivered U.S. Report Cites Abortion Benefits."

178   **The young African American girl on the stretcher** See Edelin, *Broken Justice*, xi–xiv.

179   **the first Black person to be the chief resident** See Langer, "Kenneth C. Edelin Dies at 74." See also Robert D. McFadden, "Kenneth C. Edelin, Doctor at Center of Landmark Abortion Case, Dies at 74," *New York Times*, December 30, 2013. Available at: https://www.nytimes.com/2013 /12/31/us/kenneth-c-edelin-physician-at-center-of-landmark-abortion -case-dies-at-74.html.

179   **"Dr. Edelin, do what you have to do"** See Edelin, *Broken Justice*, 82.

179   **they suspended him from his residency** Ibid., 96.

180   **Dr. Vivian Pinn** Author interview with Dr. Vivian Pinn via Zoom, April 20, 2023.

180   **all-white jury was comprised of nine men and three women** See McFadden, "Kenneth C. Edelin Dies at 74."

180   **he delivered a seven-pound, eight-ounce baby girl** See Edelin, *Broken Justice*, 345.

181   **"I refused to participate and walked out of the room"** See Satcher, *My Quest for Health Equity*, 6–28.

182   **Up until 1968, the American Medical Association** Margaret Vigil-Fowler, "The History Behind America's Devastating Shortage of Black Doctors," *Time*, November 29, 2023. Available at: https://time.com /6333653/black-doctors-racism-history/.

182   **Pinn's mother, who lived in Lynchburg, Virginia** See author interview with Dr. Vivian Pinn, April 20, 2023.

182   **leave of absence from Wellesley College** Ibid. See also Vivian Pinn, "Perspectives from a Pathologist: My Journey on the Path to Women's Health Research, Sex and Gender Policy, and Practice Implications," *Annual Review of Pathology: Mechanisms of Disease* 13 (January 2018): 1–25. Available at: https://www.annualreviews.org/content/journals/10 .1146/annurev-pathol-020117-044020.

183   **"Women and Their Bodies"** See Judy Norsigian, "Our Bodies Ourselves and the Women's Health Movement in the United States," *American Journal of Public Health* 109, no. 6 (June 2019): 844–46. Available at: https://doi.org/10.2105/AJPH.2019.305059. See also Heather Wood Rudúlph, "Why We Need 'Our Bodies Ourselves' Now More than Ever,"

Dame Magazine, April 13, 2018. Available at: https://www
.damemagazine.com/2018/04/13/why-we-need-our-bodies-ourselves
-now-more-than-ever/.

184   **Bernadine Healy** See Robert D. McFadden, "Bernadine P. Healy, a Pioneer at National Institutes of Health, Dies at 67," *New York Times,* August 8, 2011. Available at: https://www.nytimes.com/2011/08/09/us /09healy.html.

184   **Women's Health Initiative** See "Women's Health Initiative," National Heart, Lung, and Blood Institute. Available at: https://www.nhlbi.nih.gov /science/womens-health-initiative-whi.

184   **dangers of hormone replacement therapy** See Anne M. Dranginis, "Why the Hormone Study Finally Happened," *New York Times,* July 15, 2002. Available at: https://www.nytimes.com/2002/07/15/opinion/why-the -hormone-study-finally-happened.html.

185   **her team formulated strategic plans** See Gloria Bachmann and Nancy Woods, "Dr. Vivian Pinn: A Woman Pioneer & Leader," *Women's Midlife Health* 7, December 5, 2021. Available at: https://womensmidlifehealth journal.biomedcentral.com/articles/10.1186/s40695-021-00070-7.

186   **Only 4 percent of Big Pharma's research** See Lucy Pérez et al., "Closing the Women's Health Gap: Biopharma's Untapped Opportunity," McKinsey & Company, January 22, 2025. Available at: https://www.mckinsey.com /industries/life-sciences/our-insights/closing-the-womens-health-gap -biopharmas-untapped-opportunity.

186   **the FDA approved thirty-seven prescription drugs** See Shyam Bishen and Kevin Ali, "Women's Health: Rethinking the Cost as an Investment for Societal Gain," World Economic Forum, January 20, 2023. Available at: https://www.weforum.org/stories/2023/01/davos2023-womens-health -rethinking-the-cost-as-an-investment-for-societal-gain/.

186   **underlying cause of more than 30 percent of pregnancy-related deaths** See "Pregnancy-Related Deaths: Data From Maternal Mortality Review Committees," CDC Maternal Mortality Prevention, August 22, 2025. Available at: https://www.cdc.gov/maternal-mortality/php/data-research /mmrc/index.html.

186   **depression during hospital deliveries has skyrocketed** See Sarah C. Haight et al., "Recorded Diagnoses of Depression During Delivery Hospitalizations in the United States, 2000–2015," *Obstetrics and Gynecology* 133, no. 6 (June 2019): 1216–23. Available at: https://doi.org/10 .1097/AOG.0000000000003291.

186   **almost half of pregnancies in the U.S. are unplanned** See "Family Planning," Healthy People 2030. Available at: https://odphp.health.gov /healthypeople/objectives-and-data/browse-objectives/family-planning.

186   **associated with a nearly 6 percent increase in suicide** See Jonathan Zandberg et al., "Association Between State-Level Access to Reproductive Care and Suicide Rates Among Women of Reproductive Age in the United States," *JAMA Psychiatry* 80, no. 2 (2023): 127–34. Available at: https:// jamanetwork.com/journals/jamapsychiatry/fullarticle/2799597#google _vignette.

187   **cut death rates in half** See Renee Montagne, "To Keep Women from Dying in Childbirth, Look to California," NPR, July 29, 2018. Available

at: https://www.npr.org/2018/07/29/632702896/to-keep-women
-from-dying-in-childbirth-look-to-california.

CHAPTER EIGHT: ENDING THE KILLING FIELDS: PUBLIC HEALTH CONFRONTS THE EPIDEMIC OF GUN VIOLENCE

188   **"Violence is the leading cause of lost life"** See Applebome, "Conversations/David Satcher."

188   **Jevon Standback panicked** See author interview with Jevon Standback, May 23, 2023.

188   **he hit one of the police officers** See "CTA Train Operator, a Convicted Felon, Is Charged with Having Gun in Car, Battering Cop, Driving 100+ MPH to Escape," CWB Chicago, October 27, 2019. Available at: https://cwbchicago.com/2019/10/cta-train-conductor-a-convicted-felon-is-charged-with-having-gun-in-car-battering-cop-driving-100-mph-to-escape.html.

188   **posting bail** See "South Side Man Charged with Illegal Gun Sales," *Chicago Tribune,* updated December 24, 2018. Available at: https://www.chicagotribune.com/2013/09/06/south-side-man-charged-with-illegal-gun-sales-3/.

189   **bullet in his back** See Arne Duncan, "We Know How to Prevent Gun Violence. Now We Need to Scale It.," *Stanford Social Innovation Review,* July 14, 2022. Available at: https://doi.org/10.48558/HKA8-RF51.

190   **more than 48,000 Americans lost their lives** See "Fast Facts: Firearm Injury and Death," Centers for Disease Control and Prevention, Firearm Injury and Death Prevention, July 5, 2024. Available at: https://www.cdc.gov/firearm-violence/data-research/facts-stats/.

190   **the carnage in impoverished neighborhoods** See Lois Beckett, "How the Gun Control Debate Ignores Black Lives," ProPublica, November 24, 2015. Available at: https://www.propublica.org/article/how-the-gun-control-debate-ignores-black-lives.

190   **instead of railroading them into prison** See Duncan, "We Know How to Prevent Gun Violence."

191   **perhaps hundreds of thousands of needless deaths** See Mark L. Rosenberg, "What's Missing from the Gun Debate," POLITICO, February 18, 2018. Available at: https://www.politico.com/magazine/story/2018/02/18/whats-missing-from-the-gun-debate-217022/.

191   **banned the use of federal funds to do research** See John C. Lin et al., "Trends in Firearm Injury Prevention Research Funding, Clinical Trials, and Publications in the US, 1985–2022," *JAMA Surgery* 159, no. 4 (2024): 461–63. Available at: https://jamanetwork.com/journals/jamasurgery/fullarticle/2814720#google_vignette.

191   **policy paralysis thwart the work** See Rosenberg, "What's Missing from the Gun Debate."

191   **almost 50,000 Americans die from gun violence** See John Gramlich, "What the Data Says About Gun Deaths in the U.S.," Pew Research Center, March 5, 2025. Available at: https://www.pewresearch.org/short-reads/2025/03/05/what-the-data-says-about-gun-deaths-in-the-us/.

191   **have enabled us to control infectious diseases** See eds. Mark L. Rosen-

berg and Mary Ann Fenley, *Violence in America: A Public Health Approach* (New York: Oxford University Press, 1991), vii.

191　**But violence has defied efforts by the health profession** Ibid., v, 4.

192　**the number of American adults who smoked** See "Overall Smoking Trends," American Lung Association. Available at: https://www.lung.org /research/trends-in-lung-disease/tobacco-trends-brief/overall-tobacco -trends.

192　**of the five leading causes of premature death** See Rosenberg and Fenley, *Violence in America*, viii.

192　**began to view violence through a public health lens** Ibid.

192　**"We thought the gun violence problem was solvable"** See author interview with Dr. Mark Rosenberg, May 2, 2023.

192　**saved more than 600,000 lives** See "How Vehicle Safety Has Improved Over the Decades," National Highway Traffic Safety Administration. Available at: https://www.nhtsa.gov/how-vehicle-safety-has-improved -over-decades.

192　**Swedish engineers at Volvo focused their efforts on safety** See Douglas Bell, "Volvo's Gift to the World, Modern Seat Belts Have Saved Millions of Lives," *Forbes,* August 13, 2019. Available at: https://www.forbes.com /sites/douglasbell/2019/08/13/60-years-of-seatbelts-volvos-great-gift-to -the-world/.

192　**campaigns to reduce drunk driving** See Mark Rosenberg, "This Myth About Guns Is Killing Us," *Knowable Magazine,* June 20, 2022. Available at: https://knowablemagazine.org/content/article/health-disease/2022 /this-myth-about-guns-killing-us.

193　**have saved hundreds of thousands of lives** See "A Half Century of Highway Safety Innovations—1966 to 2016," Bureau of Transportation Statistics, September 9, 2016. Available at: https://www.bts.gov/archive /publications/passenger_travel_2016/tables/half.

193　**"and would in turn build public trust"** See author interview with Dr. Mark Rosenberg.

194　**of per capita lives lost to gun violence** See Gramlich, "What the Data Says About Gun Deaths in the U.S."

194　**homicides grew by 30 percent** See Chris Rees et al., "Trends and Disparities in Firearm Fatalities in the United States, 1990–2021," *JAMA Network Open* 5, no. 11 (November 29, 2022): e2244221. Available at: https:// jamanetwork.com/journals/jamanetworkopen/fullarticle/2799021#google _vignette. See also John Gramlich, "What We Know About the Increase in U.S. Murders in 2020," Pew Research Center, October 27, 2021. Available at: https://www.pewresearch.org/short-reads/2021/10/27/what-we -know-about-the-increase-in-u-s-murders-in-2020/.

195　**if threat-assessment procedures** See Mark Follman, "The Uvalde Massacre Could Have Been Prevented," *Mother Jones,* May 23, 2023. Available at: https://www.motherjones.com/politics/2023/05/uvalde -robb-elementary-mass-shooting-anniversary-police-investigation-threat -assessment/. See also Zach Despart, " 'Systemic Failures' in Uvalde Shooting Went Far Beyond Local Police," *Texas Tribune,* July 17, 2022. Available at: https://www.texastribune.org/2022/07/17/law -enforcement-failure-uvalde-shooting-investigation/.

195   **according to an investigation** See "Investigative Committee on the Robb
        Elementary Shooting," Texas House of Representatives, July 17, 2022,
        29–34. Available at: https://www.house.texas.gov/pdfs/committees
        /reports/interim/87interim/Robb-Elementary-Investigative-Committee
        -Report-update.pdf.

195   **that an online retailer delivered to his home** Ibid., 29–34.

195   **When the rifle arrived at the gun store on May 20** Ibid.

196   **The real carnage is largely invisible** See Beckett, "How the Gun Control
        Debate Ignores Black Lives."

196   **Americans own nearly 400 million guns** See Scott Simon, "Opinion:
        America's Shameful Obsession with Guns," NPR, April 1, 2023. Available
        at: https://www.npr.org/2023/04/01/1167541925/opinion-americas
        -shameful-obsession-with-guns.

196   **which translates to 67 million more firearms than people** See Evan D.
        Gumas et al., "The Health Costs of Gun Violence: How the U.S. Com-
        pares to Other Countries," Commonwealth Fund, April 20, 2023.
        Available at: https://doi.org/10.26099/a2at-gy62.

196   **The U.S. has the highest death rates from firearms** See Evan Dr. Gumas
        et al., "Comparing Deaths from Gun Violence in the U.S. with Other
        Countries," Commonwealth Fund, October 30, 2024. Available at:
        https://www.commonwealthfund.org/publications/2024/oct/comparing
        -deaths-gun-violence-us-other-countries.

196   **with nearly five times the mortality rates of France** See Gramlich,
        "What the Data Says About Gun Deaths in the U.S."

196   **Firearms are the leading cause of death for children** See Matt
        McGough et al., "Child and Teen Firearm Mortality in the U.S. and Peer
        Countries," KFF, July 18, 2023. Available at: https://www.kff.org/global
        -health-policy/issue-brief/child-and-teen-firearm-mortality-in-the-u-s-and
        -peer-countries/.

196   **guns are the weapon of choice in cases of domestic violence** See Marissa
        Edmund, "Guns and Violence Against Women," Center for American
        Progress, January 5, 2022. Available at: https://www.americanprogress
        .org/article/guns-and-violence-against-women/.

196   **American women are twenty-one times more likely to be killed by
        firearms** See Kelly Drane, "The Devastating Toll of Gun Violence on
        American Women and Girls," Giffords Law Center, February 27, 2025.
        Available at: https://giffords.org/lawcenter/report/the-devastating-toll
        -of-gun-violence-on-american-women-and-girls/.

196   **cost of $1 billion annually** See Gumas, "Health Costs of Gun
        Violence."

196   **accounts for nearly half of inpatient hospital stays** Ibid.

197   **more than $557 billion annually** See "The Economic Cost of Gun
        Violence," Everytown Research & Policy, July 19, 2022. Available at:
        https://everytownresearch.org/report/the-economic-cost-of-gun
        -violence/.

197   **More than half of the people admitted to hospitals** See Gumas, "Health
        Costs of Gun Violence."

197   **die from firearm homicides at a rate that is 22.5 times higher** See Rees,
        "Trends and Disparities in Firearm Fatalities."

197   **among adults and children feeling unsafe** See Beckett, "How the Gun Control Debate Ignores Black Lives."

198   **"This is a made-in-America problem"** See author interview with Arne Duncan, May 23, 2023.

198   **a basic principle of public health** See Duncan, "We Know How to Prevent Gun Violence." See also Alec MacGillis, "When Law Enforcement Alone Can't Stop the Violence," *New Yorker,* January 30, 2023. Available at: https://www.newyorker.com/magazine/2023/02/06/when-law-enforcement-alone-cant-stop-the-violence.

199   **programs have been adopted across the country** See Beckett, "How the Gun Control Debate Ignores Black Lives." See also MacGillis, "When Law Enforcement Alone Can't Stop the Violence."

199   **"We were stitching people up"** See author interview with Dr. Deborah Prothrow-Stith, September 6, 2023.

199   **Prothrow-Stith's *Violence Prevention: Curriculum for Adolescents*** See Deborah Prothrow-Stith, *Violence Prevention: Curriculum for Adolescents,* U.S. Department of Justice Office of Justice Programs, 1987. Available at: https://www.ojp.gov/ncjrs/virtual-library/abstracts/violence-prevention-curriculum-adolescents.

199   **They developed a comprehensive violence-prevention blueprint** See "Dr. Deborah Prothrow-Stith, Ph.D.," *School of Continuing Education.* Available at: https://www.bu.edu/sph/about/departments/community-health-sciences/faculty-and-staff/faculty/deborah-prothrow-stith/.

199   **dropped by nearly two-thirds** See Sandra Johansson, "Boston's Miracle: How America Stopped Young Men Killing Each Other," *Guardian,* December 6, 2018. Available at: https://www.theguardian.com/cities/2018/dec/06/bostons-miracle-how-free-nappies-and-a-little-mentoring-are-curbing.

200   **some 800 homicides, in 2021 alone** See Matt McNulty, "Chicago's Most Violent Year in a Quarter Century," *Daily Mail,* January 1, 2022. Available at: https://www.dailymail.co.uk/news/article-10361741/Chicago-closes-2021-violent-year-quarter-century.html.

200   **"It qualifies as a contagious disease"** See MacGillis, "When Law Enforcement Alone Can't Stop the Violence."

201   **take place in less than 8 percent of the blocks** See "Chicago CRED Impact Analysis," University of Chicago Crime Lab, August 25, 2021. Available at: https://crimelab.uchicago.edu/sites/crimelab.uchicago.edu/files/uploads/ipr-n3-rapid-research-reports-cred-impact-aug-25-2021.pdf.

201   **Shootings dropped by 68 percent** See Duncan, "We Know How to Prevent Gun Violence." See also "Chicago CRED Impact Analysis," University of Chicago Crime Lab.

201   **as much as 73 percent drops in shootings** See Allison Jordan, "6 Ways Cities and Counties Can Reduce Gun Violence," Center for American Progress, October 21, 2024. Available at: https://www.americanprogress.org/article/6-ways-cities-and-counties-can-reduce-gun-violence/.

201   **"after they had just lost their son or daughter"** See author interview with Arne Duncan.

202   **helped hammer out 47 nonaggression pacts** "Chicago CRED Impact Analysis," University of Chicago Crime Lab.

202   **shootings drop to near zero** See Duncan, "We Know How to Prevent
        Gun Violence." See also "Chicago CRED Impact Analysis," University of
        Chicago Crime Lab.

202   **CRED has concentrated its efforts** See Duncan, "We Know How to
        Prevent Gun Violence."

202   **about one thousand people have gone through CRED's comprehen-
        sive program** Ibid.

202   **it costs $37,000 a year to house someone in prison** Ibid.

202   **for scaling up violence prevention efforts is 19–1** Ibid.

202   **each prevented shooting** Ibid.

202   **Hundreds of their graduates** Ibid.

203   **three outreach workers** See Emily Sullivan, "Baltimore Police Make
        Arrest in Killing of Dante Barksdale," WYPR News, May 20, 2021.
        Available at: https://www.wypr.org/wypr-news/2021-05-20/baltimore
        -police-make-arrest-in-killing-of-dante-barksdale.

204   **The impulse to kill oneself is usually a fleeting one** See Matthew Miller
        and David Hemenway, "Guns and Suicide in the United States," *New
        England Journal of Medicine* 359, no. 10 (September 4, 2008): 989–91.
        Available at: https://www.nejm.org/doi/full/10.1056/nejmp0805923.

204   **A 2009 study by a team of Austrian psychiatrists** See Georg Kemmler
        et al., "The Duration of the Suicidal Process: How Much Time Is Left for
        Intervention Between Consideration and Accomplishment of a Suicide
        Attempt?" *Journal of Clinical Psychiatry* 70, no. 1 (January 2009): 19–24.
        Available at: https://pubmed.ncbi.nlm.nih.gov/19026258/.

204   **deliberated for less than five minutes** See "Duration of Suicidal Crises,"
        Means Matter, Harvard T.H. Chan School of Public Health. Available at:
        https://hsph.harvard.edu/research/means-matter/means-matter-basics
        /duration-of-suicidal-crises/.

205   **increases the risks by 300 percent** See Andrew Anglemyer et al., "The
        Accessibility of Firearms and Risk for Suicide and Homicide Victimization
        Among Household Members," *Annals of Internal Medicine* 160, no. 2
        (January 21, 2014). Available at: https://www.acpjournals.org/doi/10
        .7326/m13-1301.

205   **Our children have ten times the gun-suicide rate** See McGough et al.,
        "Child and Teen Firearm Mortality." See also "Firearm Availability and
        Suicide," *Suicide Prevention and Intervention,* NCBI Bookshelf. Available
        at: https://www.ncbi.nlm.nih.gov/books/NBK223849/.

205   **highest rate of firearm suicide** See "Firearm Availability and Suicide." See
        also Heather Saunders, "Do States with Easier Access to Guns Have More
        Suicide Deaths by Firearm?" KFF, July 18, 2022. Available at: https://
        www.kff.org/mental-health/do-states-with-easier-access-to-guns-have
        -more-suicide-deaths-by-firearm/.

205   **Nearly half a million Americans took their own lives** See Saunders, "Do
        States with Easier Access to Guns Have More Suicide Deaths by Firearm?"

205   **As of 2009, suicide has surpassed motor vehicles** See Ian R. H. Rockett
        et al., "Leading Causes of Unintentional and Intentional Injury Mortality:
        United States, 2000–2009," *American Journal of Public Health* 102,
        no. 11 (November 2012): e84–92. Available at: https://pubmed.ncbi.nlm
        .nih.gov/22994256/.

205   **gripped with such anxiety** See David Volk, "Professor Finds Hope After
       Heartache of Husband's Suicide," *University of Washington Magazine*,
       March 2014. Available at: https://magazine.washington.edu/feature
       /professor-finds-hope-after-heartache-of-husbands-suicide/.

206   **"My husband died because no one knew what to do"** See Carol Cruzan
       Morton, "Gun Advocates Take the Lead in Embracing Suicide Prevention
       Message," *Oregonian,* November 28, 2020. Available at: https://www
       .oregonlive.com/pacific-northwest-news/2020/11/gun-advocates-take
       -the-lead-in-embracing-suicide-prevention-message.html.

206   **In states with fewer rules** "Washington: The Latest Washington Annual
       Gun Death Data," Based on CDC data for 2023, Johns Hopkins Center
       for Gun Violence Solutions. Available at: https://publichealth.jhu.edu
       /center-for-gun-violence-solutions/washington.

206   **Even in Washington, nearly two-thirds** Ibid.

206   **85 percent of gun deaths are suicides** See "Utah: The Latest Utah
       Annual Gun Death Data," Based on CDC data for 2023, Johns Hopkins
       Center for Gun Violence Solutions. Available at: https://publichealth.jhu
       .edu/center-for-gun-violence-solutions/gun-violence-data/state-gun
       -violence-data/utah.

206   **58 percent of gun deaths from suicide** Ibid.

206   **"has not been focused on firearm suicide"** See Morton, "Gun Advocates
       Take the Lead."

207   **"So we tested a variety of gun safes"** See author interview with Brett
       Bass, via Zoom, May 2, 2023.

208   **making guns less accessible can lower suicide risks** See Michael Anestis
       et al., "Handgun Legislation and Changes in Statewide Overall Suicide
       Rates," *American Journal of Public Health* 107, no. 4 (April 2017):
       579–81. Available at: https://ajph.aphapublications.org/doi/full/10
       .2105/AJPH.2016.303650.

208   **suicide rates in the IDF dropped by 40 percent** See Gad Lubin et al.,
       "Decrease in Suicide Rates After a Change of Policy Reducing Access to
       Firearms in Adolescents: A Naturalistic Epidemiological Study," *Suicide
       and Life-Threatening Behavior* 40, no. 5 (October 2010): 421–24.
       Available at: https://pubmed.ncbi.nlm.nih.gov/21034205/.

209   **in reducing the rates of illegally trafficked guns** See "Gun Trafficking &
       Straw Purchasing," Brady United. Available at: https://www.bradyunited
       .org/resources/issues/gun-trafficking-straw-purchasing.

209   **guns pose a terrible danger to the families** See Arthur L. Kellermann
       et al., "Gun Ownership as a Risk Factor for Homicide in the Home," *New
       England Journal of Medicine* 329, no. 15 (October 7, 1993): 1084–91.
       Available at: https://doi.org/10.1056/NEJM199310073291506.

209   **"whether having a gun in your home protects you"** See author inter-
       view with Dr. Mark Rosenberg.

211   **writing op-eds and pushing lawmakers** See Rosenberg, "This Myth
       About Guns Is Killing Us."

211   **good science can help us formulate policies** See Jay Dickey and Mark
       Rosenberg, "How to Protect Gun Rights While Reducing the Toll of Gun
       Violence," *Washington Post,* December 25, 2015. Available at: https://
       www.washingtonpost.com/opinions/time-for-collaboration-on-gun

-research/2015/12/25/f989cd1a-a819-11e5-bff5-905b92f5f94b_story
.html.

211   **the administration unveiled a comprehensive strategy** See "FACT
        SHEET: Biden-Harris Administration Announces Comprehensive Strategy
        to Prevent and Respond to Gun Crime and Ensure Public Safety," Ameri-
        can Presidency Project, June 23, 2021. Available at: https://www
        .presidency.ucsb.edu/documents/fact-sheet-biden-harris-administration
        -announces-comprehensive-strategy-prevent-and.

211   **"I think the biggest enemy we have"** See author interview with Dr. Mark
        Rosenberg.

CHAPTER NINE: WASTED LIVES: ENVIRONMENTAL
TOXINS DOOM POOR COMMUNITIES

213   **When Freddie Gray died of a severe spinal injury** See John Woodrow
        Cox, Lynh Bui, and DeNeen Brown, "Who Was Freddie Gray? How Did
        He Die? And What Led to the Mistrial in Baltimore?" *Washington Post*,
        December 16, 2015. Available at: https://www.washingtonpost.com/local
        /who-was-freddie-gray-and-how-did-his-death-lead-to-a-mistrial-in
        -baltimore/2015/12/16/b08df7ce-a433-11e5-9c4e-be37f66848bb
        _story.html.

213   **he had been arrested by police after a foot race** See David Graham,
        "The Mysterious Death of Freddie Gray," *Atlantic*, April 22, 2015.
        Available at: https://www.theatlantic.com/politics/archive/2015/04/the
        -mysterious-death-of-freddie-gray/391119/.

213   **he was dragged into a police van** Ibid.

214   **He remained in a coma and never regained consciousness** See Catherine
        Rentz, "Freddie Gray Remembered as Jokester Who Struggled to Leave
        Drug Trade," *Baltimore Sun*, updated July 1, 2019. Available at: https://
        www.baltimoresun.com/2015/11/22/freddie-gray-remembered-as
        -jokester-who-struggled-to-leave-drug-trade/.

214   **when someone dives headfirst into too-shallow water** See Scott Dance,
        "Freddie Gray's Spinal Injury Suggests 'Forceful Trauma,' Doctors Say,"
        Baltimore Sun, updated June 30, 2019. Available at: https://www
        .baltimoresun.com/2015/04/21/freddie-grays-spinal-injury-suggests
        -forceful-trauma-doctors-say/.

214   **incapable of leading a functional life** See Terrence McCoy, "Freddie Gray's
        Life a Study on the Effects of Lead Paint on Poor Blacks," *Washington Post*,
        April 29, 2015. Available at: https://www.washingtonpost.com/local
        /freddie-grays-life-a-study-in-the-sad-effects-of-lead-paint-on-poor-blacks
        /2015/04/29/0be898e6-eea8-11e4-8abc-d6aa3bad79dd_story.html.

215   **the result of decades of de facto segregation** See Richard Rothstein, *The
        Color of Law: A Forgotten History of How Our Government Segregated
        America* (New York: Liveright, 2017), vii–viii (Preface).

216   **of more than 150 years of laws** Ibid., viii, xii, 54–56.

216   **"inextricably linked and orchestrated"** See author interview with
        DeMarcus Jenkins, assistant professor in the School of Social Policy and
        Practice at the University of Pennsylvania, September 6, 2023.

216   **"not the unintended consequence"** See Rothstein, *The Color of Law*,
        vii–viii (Preface).

217   **three times the rate of white Americans** See Brita Belli, "Racial Disparity in Police Shootings Unchanged Over 5 Years," Yale News, October 27, 2020. Available at: https://news.yale.edu/2020/10/27/racial-disparity-police-shootings-unchanged-over-5-years.

217   **Freddie Gray grew up in Sandtown** See Cox, et al., "Who Was Freddie Gray? How Did He Die?" See also Scott Shane, Nikita Stewart, and Ron Nixon, "Hard But Hopeful Home to 'Lot of Freddies,'" *New York Times*, May 3, 2015. Available at: https://www.nytimes.com/2015/05/03/us/sandtown-winchester-baltimore-home-to-a-lot-of-freddie-grays.html.

217   **A child born in Sandtown isn't expected to live** See "Baltimore City 2011 Neighborhood Health Profile Sandtown-Winchester/Harlem Park," Baltimore City Health Department, December 2011. Available at: https://health.baltimorecity.gov/sites/default/files/47%20Sandtown.pdf.

217   **double the city's rate** Ibid.

217   **four times the city average** Ibid.

217   **Sandtown and the adjacent Harlem Park** See Shane et al., "Hard But Hopeful Home to 'Lot of Freddies.'"

218   **plagued by asthma all of his short life** See McCoy, "Freddie Gray's Life a Study on the Effects of Lead Paint on Poor Blacks."

218   **to do permanent, irreversible neurological damage** See Green & Healthy Homes Initiative, "Lead." Available at: Lead—Green & Healthy Homes Initiative.

218   **two micrograms of lead** See U.S. Food and Drug Administration, "Lead in Food and Foodwares." Available at: https://www.fda.gov/food/environmental-contaminants-food/lead-food-and-foodwares.

218   **more than thirty-seven micrograms per deciliter** See McCoy, "Freddie Gray's Life a Study on the Effects of Lead Paint on Poor Blacks."

219   **yet nothing was done to remove him** See Rentz, "Freddie Gray Remembered as Jokester Who Struggled to Leave Drug Trade."

219   **rarely enforced anything below 45 micrograms** Ibid.

219   **"but there was no redress"** See author interview with Ruth Ann Norton, head of the Green & Healthy Homes Initiative and founding member of the Maryland Lead Poisoning Prevention Commission, June 23, 2023.

219   **This was the result of research** See David Rosner and Gerald Markowitz, "Standing Up to the Lead Industry: An Interview with Herbert Needleman," *Public Health Reports* 120, no. 3 (May–June 2005): 331. Available at: https://pmc.ncbi.nlm.nih.gov/articles/instance/1497712/pdf/16134577.pdf. See also Benedict Carey, "Dr. Herbert Needleman, Who Saw Lead's Wider Harm to Children, Dies at 89," *New York Times*, July 27, 2017. Available at: https://www.nytimes.com/2017/07/27/science/herbert-needleman-dead-lead-poisoning-in-children.html.

220   **"if she has a second episode"** See Rosner and Markowitz, "Standing Up to the Lead Industry."

220   **"a missed case of lead poisoning"** Ibid.

220   **an undetected epidemic in poor urban neighborhoods** See Herbert Needleman et al., "Lead Levels in Deciduous Teeth of Urban and Suburban American Children," *Nature* 235 (January 1972): 111–12. Available at: https://doi.org/10.1038/235111a0.

220   **than their suburban counterparts** Ibid.

220   **a dramatic impact on intellectual development** See Herbert Needleman
        et al., "Deficits in Psychologic and Classroom Performance of Children
        with Elevated Dentine Lead Levels," *New England Journal of Medicine*
        300, no. 13 (March 29, 1979): 689–95. Available at: https://doi.org/10
        .1056/NEJM197903293001301.

221   **In another groundbreaking study** See Herbert Needleman et al., "Bone
        Lead Levels and Delinquent Behavior," *JAMA* 275, no. 5 (February 7,
        1996): 363–69. Available at: https://doi.org/10.1001/jama.1996
        .03530290033034.

221   **Gray's family joined with 480 others in a lawsuit** See Cox et al., "Who
        Was Freddie Gray? How Did He Die?"

221   **the dubious distinction of coming out on top** See Derek Thompson,
        "The Curse of Segregation," *Atlantic,* May 5, 2015. Available at: https://
        www.theatlantic.com/business/archive/2015/05/the-curse-of
        -segregation/392321/.

222   **Freddie Gray had hopes and dreams, too** See Rentz, "Freddie Gray
        Remembered as Jokester Who Struggled to Leave Drug Trade."

222   **city officials switched the city's drinking water** See Mona Hanna-Attisha
        et al., "Elevated Blood Lead Levels in Children Associated with the Flint
        Drinking Water Crisis: A Spatial Analysis of Risk and Public Health
        Response," *American Journal of Public Health* 106, no. 2 (Febru-
        ary 2016): 283–90. Available at: https://doi.org/10.2105/AJPH.2015
        .303003.

223   **About 21 percent of New Yorkers** See "No Excuses, NYC: Replace Lead
        Drinking Water Pipes Now," New York City Coalition to End Lead
        Poisoning, July 18, 2023. Available at: https://nylcv.org/wp-content
        /uploads/NoExcusesNYCReplaceLead.pdf.

223   **downwind from industrial facilities** See "Environmental Racism: How
        Historic Redlining Continues to Affect Communities," RAND, June 27,
        2022. Available at: https://www.rand.org/pubs/articles/2022
        /environmental-racism-how-historic-redlining-continues.html.

223   **intensified in segregated urban neighborhoods** See Stephanie Dutchen,
        "Noise and Health," *Harvard Medicine,* Spring 2022. Available at:
        https://magazine.hms.harvard.edu/articles/noise-and-health.

223   **exposure to the constant drumbeat of loud noises** See S.A. Stansfeld
        et al., "Aircraft and Road Traffic Noise and Children's Cognition and Health:
        A Cross-National Study," *Lancet* 365, no. 9475 (June 2005): 1942–9.
        Available at: https://doi.org/10.1016/S0140-6736(05)66660-3.

223   **have more exposure to ambient light at night** See Shawna M. Nadybal
        et al., "Light Pollution Inequities in the Continental United States: A
        Distributive Environmental Justice Analysis," *Environmental Research* 189
        (October 2020). Available at: https://www.sciencedirect.com/science
        /article/pii/S0013935120308549.

223   **increases the incidence of sleep disorders** See "Blue Light Has a Dark
        Side," Harvard Health, July 24, 2024. Available at: https://www.health
        .harvard.edu/staying-healthy/blue-light-has-a-dark-side.

223   **badly weatherized housing** See "Weatherization and Its Impact on

Occupant Health Outcomes," Green & Healthy Homes Initiative, May 23, 2017. Available at: https://www.greenandhealthyhomes.org/wp-content /uploads/Weatherization-and-its-Impact-on-Occupant-Health_Final_5_23 _2017_online.pdf.

223	**These poor housing conditions** See Khansa Ahmad et al., "Association of poor housing conditions with COVID-19 incidence and mortality across US counties," *PLOS One* 15, no. 11 (November 2, 2020): 1–2. Available at: https://doi.org/10.1371/journal.pone.0241327.

224	**there are places in the rural South** See Katherine Bagley, "Filthy Water: A Basic Sanitation Problem Persists in Rural America," *Yale Environment 360*, December 10, 2020. Available at: https://e360.yale.edu/features /filthy-water-a-basic-sanitation-problem-persists-in-rural-america.

224	**even in the suburbs of St. Louis** See Mike Colombo, "'Just Feces Everywhere': Residents Seek Answers After Sewer Backup Destroys Basements," Fox2now, March 10, 2025. Available at: https://fox2now .com/news/contact-2/just-feces-everywhere-residents-seek-answers-after -sewer-backup-destroys-basements/.

224	**New York City that have sewage backing up** See Samantha Maldonado, "Spike in Sewer Backups Leaves New Yorkers in a Soggy Mess, with Long-Term Fixes Years Away," *The City*, February 8, 2024. Available at: https:// www.thecity.nyc/2024/02/08/sewer-backups-elmhurst-solutions/.

224	**as many as 90 percent of households** See Bagley, "Filthy Water."

224	**were infected with intestinal parasites** See Megan L. McKenna et al., "Human Intestinal Parasite Burden and Poor Sanitation in Rural Alabama," *American Journal of Tropical Medicine and Hygiene* 97, no. 5 (2017): 1623–28. Available at: https://doi.org/10.4269/ajtmh.17-0396.

225	**for the toxic runoff of our industrial society** See "Environmental Racism in Louisiana's 'Cancer Alley' Must End, Say UN Human Rights Experts," UN News, March 2, 2021. Available at: https://news.un.org/en /story/2021/03/1086172.

225	**a state that ranks dead last in most measures** See Alexander C. Kaufman, "UN Says Environmental Racism in Louisiana's Cancer Alley Must End," *Grist*, March 5, 2021. Available at: https://grist.org/justice /united-nations-environmental-racism-cancer-alley-louisiana/.

225	**cancer risks are 95 percent higher** See Naveena Sadasivam, "Real-Time Data Show the Air in Louisiana's 'Cancer Alley' Is Even Worse Than Expected," *Grist*, June 11, 2024. Available at: https://grist.org/science /louisiana-cancer-alley-ethylene-oxide-study/.

225	**during the pandemic, death rates skyrocketed** See Ashley Killough and Ed Lavandera, "This Small Louisiana Parish Has the Highest Death Rate Per Capita for Coronavirus in the Country," CNN, April 16, 2020. Available at: https://www.cnn.com/2020/04/15/us/louisiana-st-john -the-baptist-coronavirus.

225	**levels that were eleven times what is considered acceptable** See Lisa Song and Lylla Younes, "EPA Calls Out Environmental Racism in Louisiana's Cancer Alley," ProPublica, October 19, 2022. Available at: https://www.propublica.org/article/cancer-alley-louisiana-epa -environmental-racism.

225   **parts of Cancer Alley had up to forty-seven times the lifetime cancer risks** Ibid.

226   **"he left us a death sentence"** See Maite Amorebieta et al., "Toxic School: How the Government Failed Black Residents in Louisiana's 'Cancer Alley,'" NBC News, March 16, 2023. Available at: https://www.nbcnews .com/news/us-news/toxic-school-government-failed-black-residents -louisianas-cancer-alley-rcna72504.

226   **wiped off the map by decades of environmental racism** See "'We're Dying Here': The Fight for Life in a Louisiana Fossil Fuel Sacrifice Zone," Human Rights Watch, January 25, 2024. Available at: https://www.hrw .org/report/2024/01/25/were-dying-here/fight-life-louisiana-fossil-fuel -sacrifice-zone. See also Lylla Younes et al., "Poison in the Air," Pro-Publica, November 2, 2021. Available at: https://www.propublica.org /article/toxmap-poison-in-the-air.

227   **These are the communities that were redlined** See "Environmental Racism: How Historic Redlining Continues to Affect Communities."

227   **up to 13 degrees hotter than other communities** See Meg Anderson, "Racist Housing Practices from the 1930s Linked to Hotter Neighborhoods Today," NPR, January 14, 2020. Available at: https://www.npr.org /2020/01/14/795961381/racist-housing-practices-from-the-1930s -linked-to-hotter-neighborhoods-today. See also Jeremy Hoffman et al., "The Effects of Historical Housing Policies on Resident Exposure to Intra-Urban Heat: A Study of 108 US Urban Areas," *Climate* 8, no. 1 (January 13, 2020). Available at: https://doi.org/10.3390/cli8010012.

227   **can add up to 8 degrees in major cities** See Hoffman et al., "The Effects of Historical Housing Policies."

227   **exposed to extreme heat** See "Carbon Pollution Boosted Heat for Billions During Earth's Hottest Summer," Climate Central, September 7, 2023. Available at: https://www.climatecentral.org/climate-matters/global -review-June-August-2023.

227   **more than 250,000 people will die annually** See "Climate change," World Health Organization, October 12, 2023. Available at: https://www .who.int/news-room/fact-sheets/detail/climate-change-and-health.

227   **dying of end-stage kidney failure** See Priyamvada Paudyal et al., "Health and Wellbeing of Nepalese Migrant Workers in Gulf Cooperation Council (GCC) Countries: A Mixed-Methods Study," *Journal of Migration and Health* 7 (2023): 100178. Available at: https://doi.org/10.1016/j.jmh .2023.100178.

227   **leading cause of death in El Salvador** See Carlos Orantes-Navarro et al., "The Chronic Kidney Disease Epidemic in El Salvador: A Cross-Sectional Study," *MEDICC Review* 21, no. 2–3 (April–July 2019): 29–37. Available at: https://doi.org/10.37757/MR2019.V21.N2-3.7.

227   **claim about 800 lives** See Jeffrey T. Howard et al., "Trends of Heat-Related Deaths in the US, 1999–2023," *JAMA* 332, no. 14 (August 26, 2024): 1203–4. Available at: https://pmc.ncbi.nlm.nih.gov/articles /PMC11348089/.

228   **Europe's 2003 heat wave, when more than 70,000 people died** See Jean-Marie Robine et al., "Death Toll Exceeded 70,000 in Europe

During the Summer of 2003," *Comptes Rendus Biologies* 331, no. 2 (2008): 171–78. Available at: https://doi.org/10.1016/j.crvi.2007 .12.001.

228   **Efraín López García, a twenty-nine-year-old farmworker** See Nicole Acevedo, "South Florida Mourns Death of Another Farmworker as Advocates Fight for Heat Protections," NBC News, July 20, 2023. Available at: https://www.nbcnews.com/news/latino/south-florida -mourns-death-another-farmworker-advocates-fight-heat-pro-rcna95378.

228   **Agricultural workers are thirty-five times more likely** See Moussa El Khayat et al., "Impacts of Climate Change and Heat Stress on Farmworkers' Health: A Scoping Review," *Frontiers in Public Health* 10 (February 7, 2022): 782811. Available at: https://doi.org/10.3389/fpubh.2022 .782811.

228   **it was the Lower Ninth Ward** See Tim Padgett, "New Orleans' Lower Ninth: Katrina's Forgotten Victim?" *Time,* August 27, 2010. Available at: https://content.time.com/time/specials/packages/article/0,28804,20 12217_2012252_2012673,00.html.

228   **home to roaming packs of abandoned dogs** See Nathaniel Rich, "Jungleland," *New York Times,* March 21, 2012. Available at: https://www .nytimes.com/2012/03/25/magazine/the-lower-ninth-ward-new-orleans .html.

228   **the nation's first wave of climate refugees** See Laura Bliss, "10 Years Later, There's So Much We Don't Know About Where Katrina Survivors Ended Up," *Bloomberg,* August 25, 2015. Available at: https://www .bloomberg.com/news/articles/2015-08-25/8-maps-of-displacement-and -return-in-new-orleans-after-katrina.

228   **one of the very first suburbs to enact racial covenants** See Elizabeth Evitts Dickinson, "Roland Park: One of America's First Garden Suburbs, and Built for Whites Only," *Johns Hopkins Magazine,* Fall 2014. Available at: https://hub.jhu.edu/magazine/2014/fall/roland-park-papers -archives/.

228   **"a fundamental cause of health disparities"** See author interview with Martine Hackett, professor and director of public health programs at Hofstra University in Hempstead, New York, June 22, 2023.

229   **The HOLC generated color-coded maps** See Rothstein, *The Color of Law,* 63–65, 70–71.

230   **Municipal zoning ordinances** See M. Nolan Gray, "Apartheid by Another Name: How Zoning Regulations Perpetuate Segregation," Next City, July 4, 2022. Available at: https://nextcity.org/urbanist-news/apartheid -by-another-name-how-zoning-regulations-perpetuate-segregation.

230   **The most desirable areas were reserved for the elite** See Rothstein, *The Color of Law,* 48–54.

230   **70 percent of housing developments** Ibid., 79–80.

230   **the swank suburb known as the Black Beverly Hills** See Hadley Meares, "Baldwin Hills, 'The Black Beverly Hills': The Life and Times of the Community," LAist, March 17, 2022. Available at: https://laist.com/news /la-history/baldwin-hills-the-black-beverly-hills-the-life-and-times-of-the -community.

230   **A 2015 Brookings Institution study** See Elizabeth Kneebone, "The

Changing Geography of US Poverty," Brookings Institution, February 15, 2017. Available at: https://www.brookings.edu/articles/the-changing -geography-of-us-poverty/.

231   **about half of the public school students** See Gaby Galvin, "The Suburban Myth of Health and Wealth," U.S. News & World Report, March 26, 2019. Available at: https://www.usnews.com/news/healthiest -communities/articles/2019-03-26/long-island-and-the-suburban-myth -of-health-and-wealth.

231   **"blockbusted" the community** See Alex Boyd, "Despite Prejudice, Roosevelt Perseveres," *LI Herald,* November 21, 2016. Available at: https://www.liherald.com/stories/despite-prejudice-roosevelt -perseveres,85799.

231   **a practice called "welfare dumping"** Ibid.

231   **it's no surprise that infant mortality rates** See Andrew Malekoff, "Birth Justice Warriors Fight for Healthy Moms and Babies," *LI Herald,* April 19, 2019. Available at: https://www.liherald.com/stories/birth-justice -warriors-fight-for-healthy-moms-and-babies,113907.

232   **residents of Roosevelt experience higher rates** See Galvin, "The Suburban Myth of Health and Wealth." See also author interview with Martine Hackett.

232   **numerous court decisions** See Rothstein, *The Color of Law,* 85.

233   **"racially restrictive covenants" were unenforceable** Ibid.

233   **Congress passed the Fair Housing Act** Ibid., ix–x.

233   **the U.S. Commission on Civil Rights** Ibid., 75.

233   **"for an integrated nation had mostly closed"** Ibid., 182.

233   **"in the 1940s and '50s has become permanent"** Ibid., 183.

233   **where the environmental justice movement started** See Vann R. Newkirk II, "Fighting Environmental Racism in North Carolina," *New Yorker,* January 16, 2016. Available at: https://www.newyorker.com/news /news-desk/fighting-environmental-racism-in-north-carolina.

234   **and launched a potent and enduring grassroots movement** See Renee Skelton, Vernice Miller, and Courtney Lindwall, "The Environmental Justice Movement," NRDC, August 14, 2025. Available at: https://www .nrdc.org/stories/environmental-justice-movement.

234   **More than 60,000 tons of toxic PCBs** See Skelton et al., "The Environ- mental Justice Movement."

234   **three out of four toxic landfills in the southern U.S.** See "Siting of Hazardous Waste Landfills and Their Correlation with Racial and Eco- nomic Status of Surrounding Communities," U.S. Government Account- ablility Office, June 14, 1983. Available at: https://www.gao.gov /products/rced-83-168.

234   **A 1987 analysis by the United Church of Christ's Commission** See United Church of Christ Commission for Racial Justice, "Toxic Wastes and Race in the United States," 1987. Available at: https://www.nrc.gov/docs /ML1310/ML13109A339.pdf.

234   **predicter of the location of toxic waste facilities was race** Ibid.

234   **Four decades and $25 million later** See author interview with Deborah Ferruccio, Warren County movement leader, 2025. See also Division of Waste Management, "Warren County PCB Landfill Fact Sheet," North

Carolina Department of Environment and Natural Resources, 2003. Available at: https://web.archive.org/web/20111004053508/http: /wastenot.enr.state.nc.us/WarrenCo_Fact_Sheet.htm.

235 **landmark report** *Unequal Treatment* See eds. Brian D. Smedley, Adrienne Y. Stith, and Alan R. Nelson, *Unequal Treatment: Confronting Racial and Ethnic Disparities in Health Care* (Washington, D.C.: National Academies Press, 2003). Available at: https://nap.nationalacademies.org /catalog/12875/unequal-treatment-confronting-racial-and-ethnic -disparities-in-health-care.

235 **dropped by an astonishing 97 percent** See "Childhood Lead Poisoning Prevention Program," Baltimore City Health Department. Available at: https://health.baltimorecity.gov/lead/lead-poisoning.

235 **Baltimore banned the use of leaded paints** See Luke Scrivener, "Evaluating the Cost of Lead Hazard Control and Abatement in Baltimore City," *Abell Report* 35, no. 2 (April 2022): 2. Available at: https://abell.org/wp -content/uploads/2022/04/2022_Abell_Lead-Control-report_FINAL -web.pdf.

235 **The real changes began in 1994** Ibid., 2–4.

236 **registering of all children starting at twelve months** See "Childhood Lead Poisoning Prevention Program."

236 **"We kept going back to find the holes"** See author interview with Ruth Ann Norton.

236 **in concert with campaigns to weatherize** See Ruth Ann Norton and Brendan Wade Brown, "Green & Healthy Homes Initiative: Improving Health, Economic, and Social Outcomes Through Integrated Housing Intervention," *Environmental Justice* 7, no. 6 (2014): 2–3. Available at: https://www.greenandhealthyhomes.org/wp-content/uploads/GHHI -Improving-Health-Economic-and-Social-Outcomes-through-Integrated -Housing-Intervention-Environmental-Justice.pdf.

236 **Improving these aging homes was salutary** Ibid., 6, Table 5.

236 **a 62 percent increase in school attendance** Ibid., 5, Table 4.

236 **an estimated 85,087 homes in Baltimore** See Scrivener, "Evaluating the Cost of Lead Hazard Control," 1.

237 **at a cost that could exceed $4 billion** Ibid.

237 **"But we still have half a million children a year being poisoned"** See author interview with Ruth Ann Norton.

CHAPTER TEN: THE FIRE NEXT TIME

238 **When Patrick Sawyer was rushed by ambulance** See Muhammed Raji Modibbo et al., "One Woman, One Nation: The Heroic Story of Dr. Stella Adadevoh," *Cureus* 16, no. 10 (October 16, 2024): e71650. Available at: https://pubmed.ncbi.nlm.nih.gov/39417068/.

238 **eventually claiming more than 11,000 lives** See Mercy Corps, "Chapter 2: Major Ebola Outbreaks in Africa," *Ebola Outbreaks in Africa,* March 6, 2019. Available at: https://europe.mercycorps.org/en-gb/blog /ebola-outbreaks-africa-guide/chapter-2.

239 **Nigeria is the largest country in Africa** See "Population, Total— Nigeria," World Bank. Available at: https://data.worldbank.org/indicator /SP.POP.TOTL?locations=NG.

239   **Lagos itself is incredibly dense** See "Nigeria—Lagos: Les Dynamiques
        Urbaines de la Plus Grande Mégapole d'Afrique," Centre National
        d'Etudes Spatiales. Available at: https://cnes.fr/geoimage/nigeria-lagos
        -dynamiques-urbaines-de-plus-grande-megapole-dafrique.

239   **His Ebola test results came back positive** See "Ebola Virus Disease
        Outbreak—Nigeria, July–September 2014," Morbidity and Mortality
        Weekly Report 63, no. 39 (October 3, 2014): 867–72. Available at:
        https://www.cdc.gov/mmwr/preview/mmwrhtml/mm6339a5.htm. See
        also Niniola Soleye, "The Woman Who Helped to Stop an Ebola Epidemic
        in Nigeria," CEPI, March 28, 2019. Available at: https://cepi.net/woman
        -who-helped-stop-ebola-epidemic-nigeria. See also Modibbo et al., "One
        Woman, One Nation."

240   **built a testing and disease surveillance infrastructure** See author
        interview with Dr. Phyllis Kanki, immunology professor at the Harvard
        T.H. Chan School of Public Health, and founder and director of the AIDS
        Prevention Initiative in Nigeria (APIN), July 29, 2021. See also "Zika
        Virus Is Still in Nigeria and People Exposed to Ebola May Have Immu-
        nity," DRASA Health Trust, July 25, 2018. Available at: https://drasatrust
        .org/zika-ebola-immunity/.

240   **AIDS had been present on the African continent** See Richard Knox,
        "Origin of AIDS Linked to Colonial Practices in Africa," NPR, June 4,
        2006. Available at: https://www.npr.org/2006/06/04/5450391/origin
        -of-aids-linked-to-colonial-practices-in-africa.

240   **earmarked more than $100 million in funding** See "FACT SHEET:
        U.S. Response to the Ebola Epidemic in West Africa," The White House
        Office of the Press Secretary, September 16, 2014. Available at: https://
        obamawhitehouse.archives.gov/the-press-office/2014/09/16/fact-sheet
        -us-response-ebola-epidemic-west-africa.

241   **these Ebola hunters made approximately 18,500 face-to-face visits**
        "Ebola Virus Disease Outbreak—Nigeria, July–September 2014."

241   **Nigeria declared victory—the country was free of Ebola** Ibid., 871.

241   **she remains a revered icon** See Modibbo, "One Woman, One Nation."

242   **creating the Africa Centres for Disease Control** See Mosoka Papa Fallah
        et al., "The Role of Africa Centres for Disease Control and Prevention
        During Response to COVID-19 Pandemic in Africa: Lessons Learnt for
        Future Pandemics Preparedness, Prevention, and Response," *BMJ Global
        Health* 9, no. 2 (February 27, 2024): e014872. Available at: https://pmc
        .ncbi.nlm.nih.gov/articles/PMC10900438/.

242   **distributing 500 million doses** See Tyler Pager and Emily Rauhala,
        "Biden Administration to Buy 500 Million Pfizer Coronavirus Vaccine
        Doses to Donate to the World," *Washington Post,* June 9, 2021. Available
        at: https://www.washingtonpost.com/politics/biden-vaccine-donate
        /2021/06/09/c2744674-c934-11eb-93fa-9053a95eb9f2_story.html.

242   **more than a million people died in the Global South** See Heidi
        Ledford, "COVID Vaccine Hoarding Might Have Cost More Than a
        Million Lives," *Nature,* November 2, 2022. Available at: https://www
        .nature.com/articles/d41586-022-03529-3. See also Sam Moore et al.,
        "Retrospectively Modeling the Effects of increased global vaccine sharing
        on the COVID-19 pandemic," *Nature Medicine* 28 (October 27, 2022):

2417, Table 1; 2421. Available at: https://www.nature.com/articles /s41591-022-02064-y.

242 **variants that prolonged the pandemic in rich nations** See Amy Maxmen, "These 7 Radical Changes Would Fortify the U.S. Against the Next Pandemic," *Washington Post,* May 11, 2023. Available at: https://www .washingtonpost.com/opinions/2023/05/10/prevent-next-pandemic -steps/.

243 **we should both learn from and engage with** See Muhammad Ali Pate and Michelle A. Williams, "Building Scientific Talent in the Global South Can Help Prevent Future Public Health Crises," *STAT,* May 8, 2022. Available at: https://www.statnews.com/2022/05/08/build-scientific -talent-global-south-prevent-future-public-health-crises/.

243 **African scientists to lead their own research studies** See Linda Nordling, "How COVID-19 Changed African R&D," *Harvard Public Health,* May 11, 2022. Available at: https://harvardpublichealth.org/policy -practice/how-covid-19-changed-african-rd/.

243 **this lab that first spotted the Omicron variant** See Sophia C. Scott and Dekyi T. Tsotsong, "Harvard-Affiliated Lab Is First to Discover Omicron Variant," *Harvard Crimson,* December 6, 2021. Available at: https://www .thecrimson.com/article/2021/12/6/harvard-botswana-lab-omicron/.

244 **at least 60 percent of vaccines needed in Africa** See Amy Maxmen, "The Radical Plan for Vaccine Equity," *Nature,* July 13, 2022. Available at: https://www.nature.com/immersive/d41586-022-01898-3/index.html.

244 **Within a month after China reported the first cases** See "Novel Coronavirus (2019-nCoV) Situation Report—11," World Health Organization, January 31, 2020. Available at: https://www.who.int/docs/default -source/coronaviruse/situation-reports/20200131-sitrep-11-ncov.pdf.

244 **more than two million Africans died of AIDS** See Stephanie Nolen, "Yes, a Raging Pandemic Can Be Quelled. Recent History Shows How.," *New York Times,* updated January 12, 2022. Available at: https://www .nytimes.com/2022/01/11/health/southern-africa-hiv-aids.html.

244 **provided about $120 billion in funding** See "The U.S. President's Emergency Plan for AIDS Relief (PEPFAR)," KFF, May 13, 2025. Available at: https://www.kff.org/global-health-policy/the-u-s-presidents -emergency-plan-for-aids-relief-pepfar/.

244 **to more than 20 million people in 54 countries** See Apoorva Mandavilli, "The U.S. Program that Brought H.I.V. Treatment to 20 Million People," *New York Times,* March 14, 2023. Available at: https://www.nytimes.com /2023/03/14/health/pepfar-hiv.html.

245 **called it "the most important humanitarian program"** See Nicholas Kristof, "When George W. Bush Was a Hero," *New York Times,* April 8, 2023. Available at: https://www.nytimes.com/2023/04/08/opinion /aids-pepfar-bush.html.

245 **"a model of what can be done"** See Mandavilli, "The U.S. Program that Brought H.I.V. Treatment to 20 Million People."

245 **antiquated equipment** See Sarah Kliff and Margot Sanger-Katz, "Bottleneck for U.S. Coronavirus Response: The Fax Machine," *New York Times,* July 13, 2020. Available at: https://www.nytimes.com/2020/07/13 /upshot/coronavirus-response-fax-machines.html.

245   **anemic budgets, overworked staffers** See Ed Yong, "How the Pandemic Defeated America," *Atlantic,* September 2020. Available at: https://www .theatlantic.com/magazine/archive/2020/09/coronavirus-american -failure/614191/.

245   **left the entire system unequipped** See "The Impact of Chronic Under-funding on America's Public Health System: Trends, Risks, and Recom-mendations, 2023," Trust for America's Health, June 14, 2023. Available at: https://www.tfah.org/report-details/funding-2023/.

246   **nursing homes, prisons** See Yong, "How the Pandemic Defeated America."

246   **needed far better protections** See Mary Van Beusekom, "US Government Failure to Protect Frontline Workers from COVID Led to Thousands of Deaths, Scientists Say," CIDRAP, January 30, 2024. Available at: https:// www.cidrap.umn.edu/covid-19/us-government-failure-protect-frontline -workers-covid-led-thousands-deaths-scientists-say.

246   **for the nearly two million people** See Susan Ferriss and Joe Yerardi, "Trump Attacks Them. COVID-19 Threatens Them. But Immigrants Keep the U. S. Fed.," *Center for Public Integrity,* September 28, 2020. Available at: https://publicintegrity.org/inequality-poverty-opportunity /immigration/immigration-employment/trump-covid-19-immigrants -food-supply-farmworkers/.

247   **a national disgrace** See Michael Grabell, "The Plot to Keep Meatpacking Plants Open During COVID-19," ProPublica, May 13, 2022. Available at: https://www.propublica.org/article/documents-covid-meatpacking-tyson -smithfield-trump.

247   **ignored even the most basic safety precautions** Ibid.

247   **Up to 8 percent of all Covid-19 cases** See Charles A. Taylor et al., "Livestock Plants and COVID-19 Transmission," *PNAS* 117, no. 50 (November 19, 2020): 31706–15. Available at: https://www.pnas.org /doi/10.1073/pnas.2010115117.

247   **responsible for 334,000 illnesses** See Tina L. Saitone et al., "COVID-19 Morbidity and Mortality in U.S. Meatpacking Counties," *Food Policy* 101 (April 8, 2021): 102072. Available at: https://pmc.ncbi.nlm.nih.gov /articles/PMC8026277/.

247   **unable to handle the avalanche of numbers** See Sharon LaFraniere, "'Very Harmful' Lack of Data Blunts U.S. Response to Outbreaks," *New York Times,* September 20, 2022. Available at: https://www.nytimes.com /2022/09/20/us/politics/covid-data-outbreaks.html.

247   **severe data-sharing bottlenecks** See Kliff and Sanger-Katz, "Bottleneck for U.S. Coronavirus Response."

248   **"The CDC has very little ability to innovate new tools"** See author interview with Dr. Julie Gerberding, April 21, 2023.

248   **data collection system has long been broken** See Tom Frieden et al., "Former CDC Directors: Coordinating Our Nation's Health Data Will Save Lives," *Hill,* March 10, 2022. Available at: https://thehill.com /opinion/healthcare/597494-former-cdc-directors-coordinating-our -nations-health-data-will-save-lives/.

248   **"has an anemic surveillance system"** See author interview with Dr. Karen DeSalvo, March 16, 2023.

248   **"Nearly 40 billion was earmarked to digitize health care"** See Kushal T. Kadakia et al., "Modernizing Public Health Data Systems: Lessons from the Health Information Technology for Economic and Clinical Health (HITECH) Act," *JAMA* 326, no. 5 (August 3, 2021): 385–86. Available at: https://pubmed.ncbi.nlm.nih.gov/34342612/.

249   **nearly three thousand state, local, tribal, and territorial health departments** See "Meeting America's Public Health Challenge," Commonwealth Fund, June 21, 2022. Available at: https://www.commonwealthfund.org/publications/fund-reports/2022/jun/meeting-americas-public-health-challenge.

249   **conflicting public guidelines** See Gerald E. Harmon, "AMA: CDC Quarantine and Isolation Guidance Is Confusing, Counterproductive," American Medical Association, January 5, 2022. Available at: https://www.ama-assn.org/press-center/press-releases/ama-cdc-quarantine-and-isolation-guidance-confusing-counterproductive.

249   **direct interagency conflicts** See Dan Diamond, "CDC Blocked FDA Official from Premises," POLITICO, March 3, 2020. Available at: https://www.politico.com/news/2020/03/03/cdc-blocked-fda-official-premises-119684.

250   **The Goldwater–Nichols Act of 1986** See "H.R.3622—Goldwater-Nichols Department of Defense Reorganization Act of 1986," 99th Congress (1985–1986), Congress.gov. Available at: https://www.congress.gov/bill/99th-congress/house-bill/3622.

250   **when everyone puts aside their differences** See Joe Nocera and Bethany McLean, "Operation Warp Speed: The Untold Story of the COVID-19 Vaccine," *Vanity Fair*, October 12, 2023. Available at: https://www.vanityfair.com/news/2023/10/operation-warp-speed-covid-19-vaccine. See also Stephanie Baker and Cynthia Koons, "Inside Operation Warp Speed's $18 Billion Sprint for a Vaccine," *Bloomberg Businessweek*, October 29, 2020. Available at: https://www.bloomberg.com/news/features/2020-10-29/inside-operation-warp-speed-s-18-billion-sprint-for-a-vaccine.

251   **in six months, half the population got vaccinated** See Ivan Pereira, "Half of All Americans Have Now Received At Least 1 Vaccine Dose," ABC News, May 28, 2021. Available at: https://abcnews.go.com/Health/half-americans-now-received-vaccine-dose/story?id=77929916.

251   **Fewer and fewer severely ill patients** See Spencer, "How to Lose a Century of Progress."

251   **there would have been about 1.1 million more deaths** See Eric C. Schneider et al., "The U.S. COVID-19 Vaccination Program at One Year: How Many Deaths and Hospitalizations Were Averted?" Commonwealth Fund, December 14, 2021. Available at: https://www.commonwealthfund.org/publications/issue-briefs/2021/dec/us-covid-19-vaccination-program-one-year-how-many-deaths-and.

251   **"serves as a blueprint"** See Spencer, "How to Lose a Century of Progress."

251   **"the CDC had to be asked by the state"** See Pien Huang, "Battle Over CDC's Powers Goes Far Beyond Travel Mask Mandate," NPR, April 21,

2022. Available at: https://www.npr.org/sections/health-shots/2022/04
/21/1094123780/battle-over-cdcs-powers-goes-far-beyond-travel-mask
-mandate.

252   **deliberately undermined** See Yong, "How the Pandemic Defeated
America."

252   **acts of heroic political defiance** See Lauren Weber and Anna Maria
Barry-Jester, "Over Half of States Have Rolled Back Public Health Powers
in Pandemic," KFF Health News, September 15, 2021. Available at:
https://kffhealthnews.org/news/article/over-half-of-states-have-rolled
-back-public-health-powers-in-pandemic/.

252   **more than one thousand lawsuits challenging Covid-19 measures** See
Lawrence O. Gostin and Sarah Wetter, "Fix the Backlash Against Public
Health," *Science* 379, no. 6639 (March 30, 2023): 1277. Available at:
https://www.science.org/doi/10.1126/science.adh9594.

252   **retail clerks and security guards were threatened** See Neil MacFarquhar,
"Who's Enforcing Mask Rules? Often Retail Workers, and They're Getting
Hurt," *New York Times,* May 15, 2020. Available at: https://www.nytimes
.com/2020/05/15/us/coronavirus-masks-violence.html.

253   **hundreds of high-profile public health officials** See "Public Health
Official Departures," Associated Press via data.world, September 20, 2021.
Available at: https://data.world/associatedpress/public-health-official
-departures.

253   **alerted the public about asymptomatic transmission** See Apoorva
Mandavilli, " 'We Were Helpless': Despair at the C.D.C. as the Pandemic
Erupted," *New York Times,* March 21, 2023. Available at: https://www
.nytimes.com/2023/03/21/health/covid-cdc.html.

253   **36,000 lives would have been saved** See James Glanz and Campbell
Robertson, "Lockdown Delays Cost At Least 36,000 Lives, Data Show,"
New York Times, May 20, 2020. Available at: https://www.nytimes.com
/2020/05/20/us/coronavirus-distancing-deaths.html.

253   **"as lazy and as traitors engaging in sedition"** See Mandavilli, " 'We Were
Helpless.' "

254   **Nearly half of employees** See Jonathon P. Leider et al., "The Exodus of
State and Local Public Health Employees: Separations Started Before and
Continued Throughout COVID-19," *Health Affairs* 42, no. 3
(March 2023): 338. Available at: https://pubmed.ncbi.nlm.nih.gov
/36877909/.

254   **as much as half of the nation's public health workforce** Ibid.

CHAPTER ELEVEN: MISSING AMERICANS: OUR NATION'S EPIDEMIC OF EARLY DEATH

255   **We feed billions of dollars into a medical system** See Berwick, "*Salve
Lucrum:* The Existential Threat of Greed in US Health Care."

255   **"we spend a fraction of that on public health"** See Gregg Gonsalves,
"America Is All Too Happy to Let People Die," *Time,* July 27, 2022.
Available at: https://time.com/6200588/america-is-all-too-happy-to-let
-people-die/.

257   **Longevity in the United States** See Jacob Bor et al., "Missing Americans:

Early Death in the United States—1933–2021," *PNAS Nexus* 2, no. 6 (June 2023). Available at: https://academic.oup.com/pnasnexus/article /2/6/pgad173/7185600.

257   **behind Cuba, Estonia, and Saudi Arabia** See Steven Ross Johnson, "Countries with the Longest and Shortest Life Expectancies," U.S. News & World Report, December 13, 2024. Available at: https://www.usnews .com/news/best-countries/articles/countries-with-the-longest-and -shortest-life-expectancies.

257   **unprecedented in highly developed countries** See Michael Devitt, "CDC Data Show U.S. Life Expectancy Continues to Decline," American Academy of Family Physicians, December 10, 2018. Available at: https://www.aafp.org/news/health-of-the-public/20181210lifeexpect drop.html. See also Roni Caryn Rabin, "U.S. Life Expectancy Falls Again in 'Historic' Setback," *New York Times,* August 31, 2022. Available at: https://www.nytimes.com/2022/08/31/health/life-expectancy-covid -pandemic.html.

257   **compounded by a spike in alcoholism** See Stephen Bezruchka, "Will the U.S. Follow Russia's Health Decline after the Breakup of the Former Soviet Union?" *Random Lengths News,* January 20, 2023. Available at: https://www.randomlengthsnews.com/archives/2023/01/20/will-u-s -follow/43306.

257   **began long before the pandemic** See Bor et al., "Missing Americans."

258   **"was shocking"** See author interview with Jacob Bor via Zoom, July 18, 2022.

258   **the same mortality rates as other wealthy nations** See Bor et al., "Missing Americans," 1.

258   **died before age sixty-five** Ibid., 4, Table 1, 5.

258   **"is unprecedented in modern times"** Ibid., 1.

258   **26.4 million years of lost life in 2021 alone** Ibid., 1.

258   **there is a ripple effect** See Ed Yong, "America Was in an Early-Death Crisis Long Before COVID," *Atlantic,* July 21, 2022. Available at: https://www.theatlantic.com/health/archive/2022/07/us-life-span -mortality-rates/670591/.

258   **Black and Native Americans bore a disproportionate share** See Bor et al., "Missing Americans."

258   **comprised 70 percent of those missing Americans** Ibid., Table 2, Figure 4B, 7.

259   **"Using the experiences of white Americans"** See author interview with Jacob Bor.

259   **People die because of gun violence, traffic accidents** See Bor et al., "Missing Americans."

260   **Nearly 16 million people were dropped** See Caroline Hanson et al., "Health Insurance for People Younger than Age 65: Expiration of Tempo-rary Policies Projected to Reshuffle Coverage, 2023–33," *Health Affairs* 42, no. 6 (May 24, 2023). Available at: https://www.healthaffairs.org/doi /10.1377/hlthaff.2023.00325.

260   **up to 24 million will eventually lose coverage** See Michael Hiltzik, "Millions of Americans Are About to Lose Their Healthcare Coverage. Many Have No Idea," *Los Angeles Times,* July 27, 2023. Available at:

https://www.latimes.com/business/story/2023-07-27/column-millions
-of-americans-are-about-to-lose-their-healthcare-coverage-many-have-no
-idea.

260   **Texas—which quickly dropped 82 percent** See Neelam Bohra, "Nearly 1.7 Million Texans Lose Medicaid as State Nears End of 'Unwinding,'" *Texas Tribune,* December 14, 2023. Available at: https://www .texastribune.org/2023/12/14/texas-medicaid-unwinding/.

261   **"This is the fastest pace in the nation"** See Sarah Huckabee Sanders, "Arkansas Gets Medicaid Back to Normal," *Wall Street Journal,* May 1, 2023. Available at: https://www.wsj.com/politics/arkansas-gets-medicaid -back-to-normal-insurance-healthcare-arkansas-governor-congress-covid -emergency-bd1823b8.

261   **who lost their coverage were children** See Hiltzik, "Millions of Americans Are About to Lose Their Healthcare Coverage."

261   **continue to reliably vote for these same legislators** See Bor et al., "Missing Americans," 10.

261   **deaths among working-age Americans increased** Ibid., 8, Table 2. See also Yong, "America Was in an Early-Death Crisis Long Before COVID."

261   **young white Americans died at three times the rate** See Bor et al., "Missing Americans," 8.

261   **"life in America has excelled at for decades"** See Yong, "America Was in an Early-Death Crisis Long Before COVID."

262   **poorer Americans had scant resources** See Bor et al., "Missing Americans," 10.

262   **66.5 percent of all bankruptcies** See David U. Himmelstein et al., "Medical Bankruptcy: Still Common Despite the Affordable Care Act," *American Journal of Public Health* 109, no. 3 (March 2019): 432. Available at: https://pmc.ncbi.nlm.nih.gov/articles/PMC6366487/.

262   **wave of deregulation that began in the 1980s** See Bor et al., "Missing Americans," 10. See also Yong, "America Was in an Early-Death Crisis Long Before COVID."

262   **after the dissolution of the Soviet Union** See Bezruchka, "Will the U.S. Follow Russia's Health Decline after the Breakup of the Former Soviet Union?"

262   **were dying at astonishing rates** See David Squires and David Blumenthal, "Mortality Trends Among Working-Age Whites: The Untold Story," *Commonwealth Fund,* January 2016. Available at: https://pubmed.ncbi .nlm.nih.gov/26934757/.

262   **more than 600,000 excess deaths** See Atul Gawande, "Why Americans Are Dying from Despair," *New Yorker,* March 16, 2020, 60. Available at: https://www.newyorker.com/magazine/2020/03/23/why-americans-are -dying-from-despair.

262   **were directly correlated with chronic joblessness** Ibid., 61.

263   **breeding the deterioration in social capital** Ibid., 62.

263   **The jobs that are now available are poorly paid** Ibid.

263   **health-care policy costs around $20,000** Ibid., 62–63.

263   **"The grip of financial self-interest in U.S. health care"** See Berwick, "*Salve Lucrum:* The Existential Threat of Greed in US Health Care."

264   **per capita income that is one-sixth** See Atul Gawande, "Costa Ricans

Live Longer than We Do. What's the Secret?" *New Yorker,* August 23, 2021, 32. Available at: https://www.newyorker.com/magazine/2021/08/30/costa-ricans-live-longer-than-we-do-whats-the-secret.

264   **a life expectancy that now approaches eighty-one years** Ibid.

264   **surpassing even the long-lived Japanese** See Luis Rosero-Bixby, William H. Dow, and David H. Rehkopf, "The Nicoya Region of Costa Rica: A High Longevity Island for Elderly Males," *Vienna Yearbook of Population Research* 11 (2013): 109–36. Available at: https://pmc.ncbi.nlm.nih.gov/articles/PMC4241350/.

264   *pura vida,* **or the pure life** See Hanae Armitage, "Longevity's Secret Sauce," *Stanford Medicine Magazine,* January 23, 2023. Available at: https://stanmed.stanford.edu/longevity-secret-costa-rica-area/.

265   **individual health and public health** See Gawande, "Costa Ricans Live Longer than We Do. What's the Secret?," 37.

265   **remote rural regions in the mountains** Ibid., 35–37.

265   **Life expectancy hovered around fifty-five years** Ibid., 32.

265   **their growth was often stunted** Ibid.

265   **which was still in its nascent stages** Ibid.

266   **when kids did get sick** Ibid., 33.

266   **infant mortality had dropped to 2 percent** Ibid.

266   **who will follow them throughout their lives** Ibid., 35–36.

266   **emphasizes prevention and public health** Ibid., 36.

266   **specialists are in short supply** See "The Paradox of Costa Rica's Healthcare: Long Lives, Long Waits," *Tico Times,* May 1, 2025. Available at: https://ticotimes.net/2025/05/01/the-paradox-of-costa-ricas-healthcare-long-lives-long-waits.

267   **have been erased** See Gawande, "Costa Ricans Live Longer than We Do. What's the Secret?" 40.

267   **"health security is national security"** See author interview with Dr. Julie Gerberding.

268   **"We cannot remain indefinitely in our ivory towers"** See Milton Terris keynote address, "Terris Gives Thoughtful, Provocative Address at SER," July 1992. Available at: https://w.epimonitor.net/Keynote-1992.htm.

269   **"shell-shocked about the murder"** See author interview with Dana Peterson, via Zoom, June 18, 2021.

269   **generated an additional $16 trillion** See Saijel Kishan, "Economist Found $16 Trillion When She Tallied Cost of Racial Bias," *Bloomberg Businessweek,* October 20, 2020. Available at: https://www.bloomberg.com/news/articles/2020-10-20/racism-and-inequity-have-cost-the-u-s-16-trillion-wall-street-economist-says.

269   **These disparities along racial fault lines** See Dana M. Peterson and Catherine L. Mann, "Closing the Racial Inequality Gaps," Citigroup GPS report, September 22, 2020, 4. Available at: https://www.citigroup.com/global/insights/closing-the-racial-inequality-gaps-20200922.

269   **on and on** Ibid.

269   **if Black entrepreneurs had had fair and equitable access** Ibid., 7–8.

270   **"that's been left on the table"** See author interview with Dana Peterson.

270   **less than half cast their ballots in midterms** See Hannah Hartig et al., "Voter Turnout, 2018–2022," Pew Research Center, July 12, 2023.

Available at: https://www.pewresearch.org/politics/2023/07/12/voter
-turnout-2018-2022/.

270   **More Republicans than Democrats died in the pandemic** See Yasmin
Tayag, "How Many Republicans Died Because the GOP Turned Against
Vaccines?" *Atlantic,* December 23, 2022. Available at: https://www
.theatlantic.com/health/archive/2022/12/covid-deaths-anti-vaccine
-republican-voters/672575/. See also Jacob Wallace et al., "Excess Death
Rates for Republican and Democratic Registered Voters in Florida and
Ohio During the COVID-19 Pandemic," *JAMA Internal Medicine* 183,
no. 9 (September 1, 2023): 916–23. Available at: https://jamanetwork
.com/journals/jamainternalmedicine/fullarticle/2807617.

270   **When researchers stripped away** See Daniel Wood and Geoff Brumfiel,
"Pro-Trump Counties Now Have Far Higher COVID Death Rates," NPR,
December 5, 2021. Available at: https://www.npr.org/sections/health
-shots/2021/12/05/1059828993/data-vaccine-misinformation-trump
-counties-covid-death-rate.

270   **like lockdowns, masking, social distancing** See Justin Kaashoek et al.,
"The Evolving Roles of US Political Partisanship and Social Vulnerability
in the COVID-19 Pandemic," *PLOS Global Public Health,* December 5,
2022. Available at: https://journals.plos.org/globalpublichealth
/article?id=10.1371/journal.pgph.0000557. See also Nancy Krieger et al.,
"Relationship of Political Ideology of US Federal and State Elected
Officials and Key COVID Pandemic Outcomes Following Vaccine Rollout
to Adults," *Lancet Regional Health—Americas* 16 (December 2022):
100384. Available at: https://www.thelancet.com/journals/lanam/article
/PIIS2667-193X(22)00201-0/fulltext.

271   **residents of blue states live *far* longer** See Haider Warraich et al.,
"Political Environment and Mortality Rates in the United States, 2001–19:
Population Based Cross Sectional Analysis," *BMJ* 377 (June 7, 2022):
e069308. Available at: https://pubmed.ncbi.nlm.nih.gov/35672032/.

271   **according to a 2023 analysis done by Colin Woodard** See Colin
Woodard, "America's Surprising Partisan Divide on Life Expectancy,"
POLITICO, September 1, 2023. Available at: https://www.politico.com
/news/magazine/2023/09/01/america-life-expectancy-regions
-00113369.

271   **There's a difference of nearly five years** Ibid.
271   **what Woodard calls Greater Appalachia** Ibid.
271   **"the gap separating the U.S."** Ibid.
271   **have higher life expectancies** Ibid.
271   **"who have resisted investing tax dollars"** Ibid.
272   **"Speak up, speak out. Get in the way"** See Devan Cole, "John Lewis
Urges Attendees of Selma's 'Bloody Sunday' Commemorative March to
'Redeem the Soul of America' by Voting," CNN Politics, March 1, 2020.
Available at: https://www.cnn.com/2020/03/01/politics/john-lewis
-bloody-sunday-march-selma/.

INDEX

ABOUT THE AUTHORS

MICHELLE A. WILLIAMS is a professor of epidemiology and population health at Stanford University School of Medicine and former Dean of the Faculty at Harvard T.H. Chan School of Public Health, where she also served as the Angelopoulos Professor in Public Health and International Development and currently holds an adjunct professorship. An internationally renowned epidemiologist and award-winning educator, Dr. Williams is a member of the National Academy of Medicine and the American Epidemiological Society. She has authored more than 550 peer-reviewed research articles and is recognized as a leading voice in public health science and global health.

LINDA MARSA is an award-winning investigative journalist and a former *Los Angeles Times* reporter. Her work has been anthologized in *The Best American Science Writing,* and she has authored two previous books, *Prescription for Profits,* about the pharmaceutical industry, and *Fevered: Why a Hotter Planet Will Harm Our Health—and How We Can Save Ourselves,* which *The New York Times* called "gripping to read."

ABOUT THE TYPE

This book was set in Galliard, a typeface designed in 1978 by Matthew Carter (b. 1937) for the Mergenthaler Linotype Company. Galliard is based on the sixteenth-century typefaces of Robert Granjon (1513–89).